Primer of Noninvasive Vascular Technology

Primer of Noninvasive Vascular Technology

Terrence D. Case, M.Ed., R.V.T.
Clinical Instructor in Surgery,
University of Vermont College of Medicine;
Vascular Ultrasound Program Director,
University Health Center,
Burlington, Vermont

Little, Brown and Company
Boston New York Toronto London

First Edition

Library of Congress Cataloging-in-Publication Data

Case, Terrence D.
A primer of noninvasive vascular technology / Terrence D. Case.
p. cm.
Includes bibliographical references and index.
ISBN 0-316-13035-4
1. Blood-vessels—Diseases—Diagnosis. 2. Diagnosis, Noninvasive.
3. Blood-vessels—Imaging. 4. Blood-vessels—Ultrasonic imaging.
5. Doppler ultrasonography. I. Title.
[DNLM: 1. Blood Vessels—ultrasonography. 2. Diagnostic Imaging—methods. 3. Vascular Diseases—diagnosis. WG 141 C337p 1995]
RC691.6.N65C37 1995
616.1'307544—dc20
DNLM/DLC 94-21978
for Library of Congress CIP

Printed in the United States of America

SEM

Editorial: Nancy Megley, Rebecca Marnhout
Copyeditor: Kris Smead
Indexer: Alexandra Nickerson
Composition and Production: Pageworks
Designer: Louis C. Bruno, Jr.
Cover Designer: Linda Dana Willis

To my wife Debra,
and to my children Emily and Tyler

Contents

Preface

Noninvasive vascular technology is one of the most exciting allied medical professions in the health field today. It is a relatively new profession that requires the vascular specialist operating the equipment to function with a certain degree of independence and to be knowledgeable about a variety of medical and vascular conditions. In addition, the vascular specialist must have a particularly strong understanding of not only anatomy, physiology, and clinical medicine, but also the electrical principles and physics associated with the technology.

The field of noninvasive vascular technology has been established for more than 15 years. Formal training, however, is still limited to a handful of independent programs. As a result, many vascular specialists are former nurses, ultrasonographers, medical technologists, physician's assistants, or x-ray technologists, because until only recently there has not been a dedicated program. This diverse background brings to the profession a rich mix of talent and experience, but there remains a void in the consistency of training and experience necessary for a common and general understanding of the physics and technology that underlie the field.

Primer of Noninvasive Vascular Technology is written for the vast majority of individuals who, despite a strong academic and clinical background, require a comprehensive overview of the principles of vascular physics and technology. It is also for those who may not have taken college physics or who don't know the difference between direct current and alternating current, as well as for those who simply need to review the clinical and technological concepts in one comprehensive text. The goal is to help you succeed in the profession of vascular technology.

This book is written in simple language. I have tried to make the text as effective as possible by explaining terminology in detail using illustrations and analogies. If we can take the mystery out of vascular technology and physics and relate those concepts to familiar situations, we can make learning enjoyable and improve examination scores. More important, by understanding these principles we can perform the studies with greater knowledge and confidence and increase the respect vascular specialists have gained over the years.

The challenge has been to develop this approach into a complete text, to make learning interesting, and to take each aspect of noninvasive technology one step at a time, from the circle of Willis to the dorsalis pedis. Enjoy your learning!

T.D.C.

Acknowledgments

I am grateful to a number of people who have contributed to this book in so many different ways: to Michael A. Ricci, M.D., R.V.T., David B. Pilcher, M.D., R.V.T., and Steven R. Shackford, M.D., at the University of Vermont School of Medicine, who have provided to me and this profession the leadership, inspiration, and integrity essential to pursue excellence in the care of patients with vascular disease; to J. Dennis Baker, M.D., Phillip J. Bendick, Ph.D., Peter N. Burns, Ph.D., Ann Marie Kupinski, M.S., R.V.T., and Marcia M. Neumyer, B.S., R.V.T., for their wisdom and contributions in reviewing the material for medical fact; to Professor JunRu Wu, also at the University of Vermont, who worked tirelessly to lead me through the sometimes perilous road of physics; to Frank Gregory, the book's illustrator; and to my countless friends and colleagues, particularly Rob Daigle, who first taught me vascular technology, Jean Primozitch, who continues to do so, and to Sandy Katanick and John Peters, who somehow help to keep it all in perspective.

Primer of Noninvasive Vascular Technology

1 Anatomy

The vascular specialist must know more anatomy than merely that of the arteries and veins. Because blood vessels supply virtually all living tissue, it is essential to understand the general anatomy of all body structures. Knowing the general location and function of the individual organs and parts of organs will assist the specialist in better understanding the physiology of both normal and abnormal blood flow.

TERMS OF ORIENTATION

The following terms are used frequently in discussions of anatomy to describe the orientation of body parts to each other. It is important to know these terms in order to be able to clearly and accurately describe anatomical structures and pathological changes that may appear on a vascular study.

Anterior* or *ventral Lying toward the front ("belly") of the patient

Anterolateral Lying to the front and also to one or the other side

Anteromedial Lying to the front and toward the median plane

Caudad Lying away from the head

Distal Lying away from the origin of something

Lateral Lying away from the midline

Medial: Lying toward the midline

Posterior* or *dorsal Lying toward the back of the patient

Posteromedial Lying toward both the back and the midline

Posterolateral Lying toward both the back and one side

Prone Lying face down (i.e., the position of the body)

Proximal Lying near the origin of something

Quadrant A section of the abdomen. The abdomen is divided into four quadrants (Fig. 1-1): RUQ, right upper quadrant; LUQ, left upper quadrant; RLQ, right lower quadrant; LLQ, left lower quadrant

Superior, cranial, cephalad Lying toward the head (*Cephalad* is the term most commonly accepted for use by vascular specialists.)

Supine Lying on the back with face upward

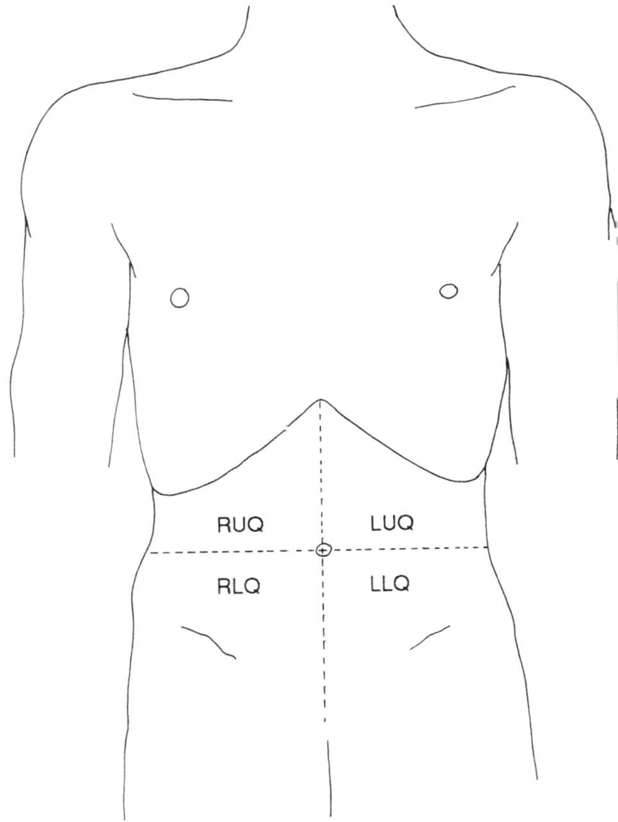

Fig. 1-1. The four quadrants of the abdomen.

Review Exercise

Define the following terms.

1. Anterior or ventral ____________________

2. Distal ____________________

3. Lateral ____________________

4. Medial ____________________

5. Posterior or dorsal ____________________

6. Prone ____________________

7. Proximal ____________________

8. Quadrant ____________________

9. Superior, cranial, cephalad ____________________

10. Supine ____________________

11. Label the quadrants of the abdomen.

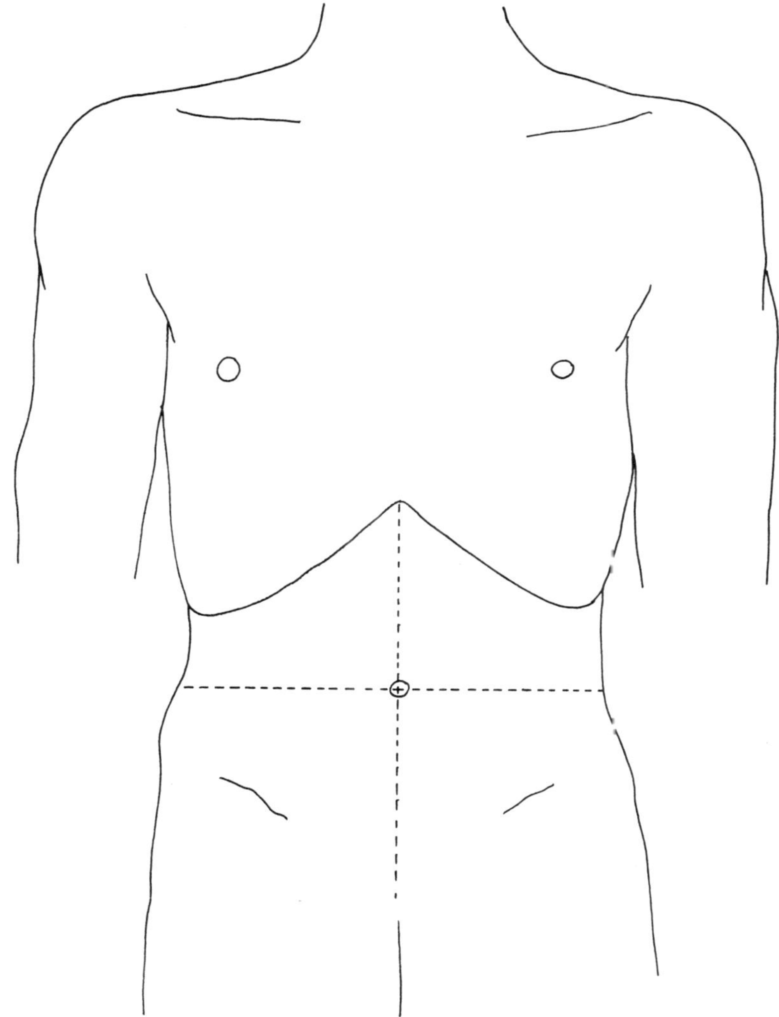

THE NERVOUS SYSTEM

Key Terms

Autonomic nervous system
Brain
Brainstem
Central nervous system
Cerebellum
Cerebrum
Frontal lobe
Left hemisphere
Occipital lobe
Parietal lobe
Peripheral nervous system
Right hemisphere
Spinal cord
Somatic nervous system
Temporal lobe

The nervous system (Fig. 1-2) is responsible for regulating internal body function through response to external stimuli. In humans, as in all vertebrates, the nervous system consists of the *brain*, *spinal cord*, *nerves*, *ganglia*, and parts of the *receptor* and *effector organs*. For vascular specialists, the discussion here is limited to the major components of the system.

The two major divisions of the nervous system are the

- central nervous system
- peripheral nervous system

The Central Nervous System

The *central nervous system* (CNS), the major component of the nervous system, is where information from stimuli is processed and distributed. The brain is one of the primary "vital organs" of the body, on which the body is most dependent. Therefore, blood supply to the brain (and to the kidneys and the heart) is essential for survival. A great deal of our work as vascular specialists is dedicated to the evaluation of blood flow to the brain.

The major components of the central nervous system include the

- brain
- spinal cord

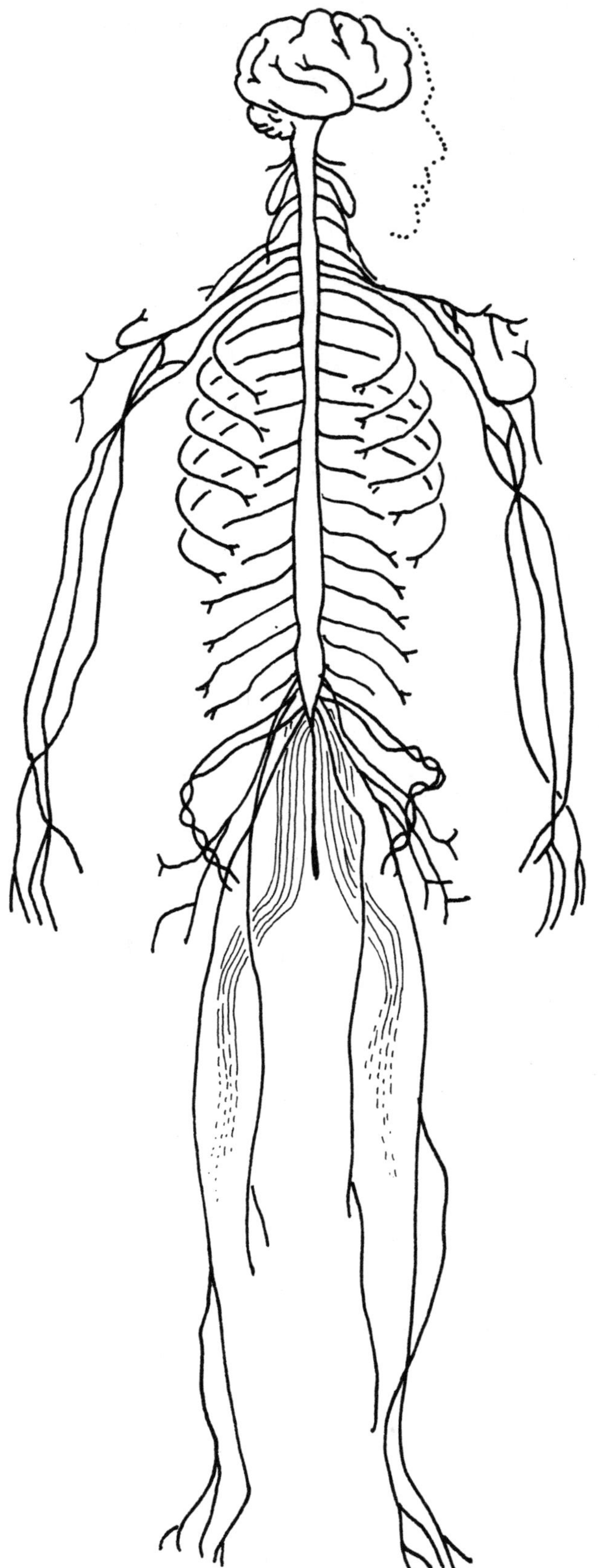

Fig. 1-2. The neural system.

The Brain

As mentioned, the *brain* is one of the major components of the central nervous system and is one of the most essential of all the vital organs. It is the organ that processes information and is contained within the *cranium* (or skull). The brain is divided into several sections, each of which has separate and distinct functions.

The brain consists of two halves, simply named the *left* and the *right hemisphere* (Fig. 1-3). Hemisphere means *half* of a *sphere* (or globe). In this case, the sphere is the brain.

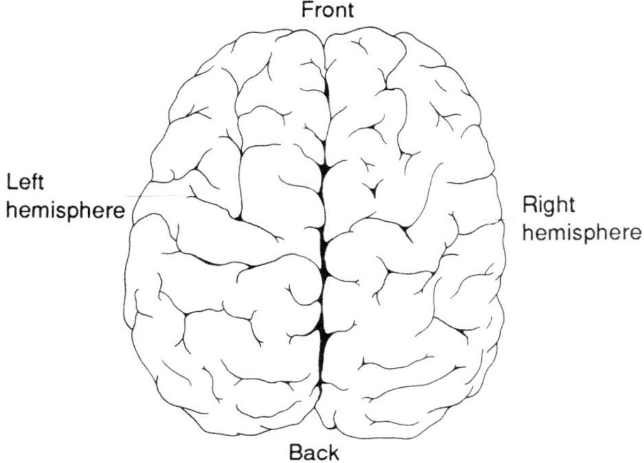

Fig. 1-3. The right and left hemisphere of the brain.

Each *hemisphere* is divided into four lobes named after the bones that cover them (Fig. 1-4):

1. Frontal lobe
2. Temporal lobe
3. Parietal lobe
4. Occipital lobe

The brain also is divided into three principal areas:

- Cerebrum
- Cerebellum
- Brainstem

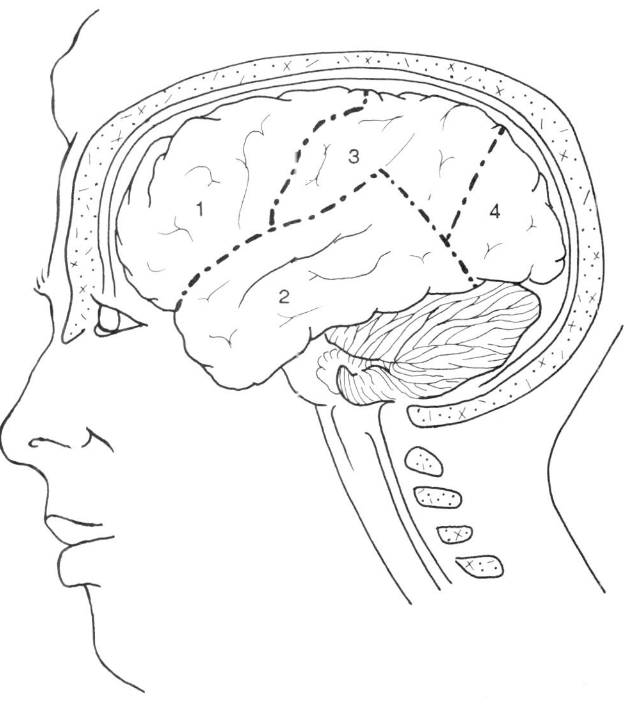

Fig. 1-4. The (1) frontal lobe, (2) temporal lobe, (3) parietal lobe, and (4) occipital lobe.

The Cerebrum

The *cerebrum* is the main portion of the brain, occupying the upper part of the cranial cavity (skull). The two hemispheres are united by the *corpus callosum* and form the largest part of the central nervous system. The functions of the cerebrum are numerous and complex, but in general, it has three primary *functional* areas(Fig. 1-5A):

1. The motor area, which governs muscle movement
2. The sensory area, which is concerned with the interpretation of nerve impulses (e.g., in response to touch)
3. The association area, which is concerned with emotional and intellectual processes

The Cerebellum

The *cerebellum* (Fig. 1-5B) occupies the rear part of the cranium and is connected with the *brainstem*. It is a *motor* area of the brain that controls certain unconscious movements of the body. These movements are required for

1. coordination
2. maintaining posture
3. maintaining balance.

The Brainstem

The brainstem (Fig. 1-5C) is the stem-like portion of the brain connecting the cerebral hemispheres with the spinal cord. It controls the vital functions of the body, including

1. relay of nerve impulses from the body to the brain
2. control of heart and breathing functions
3. interpretation of certain impulses
4. control of muscle movements
5. control of visceral (major organ) functions

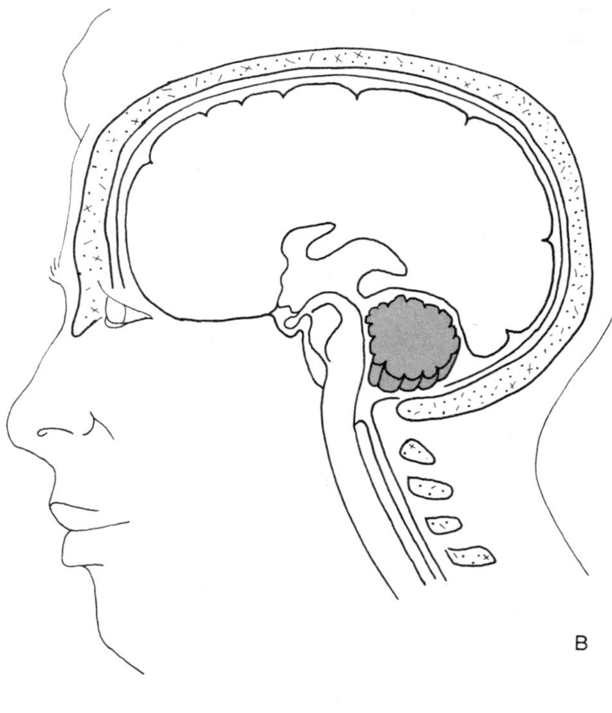

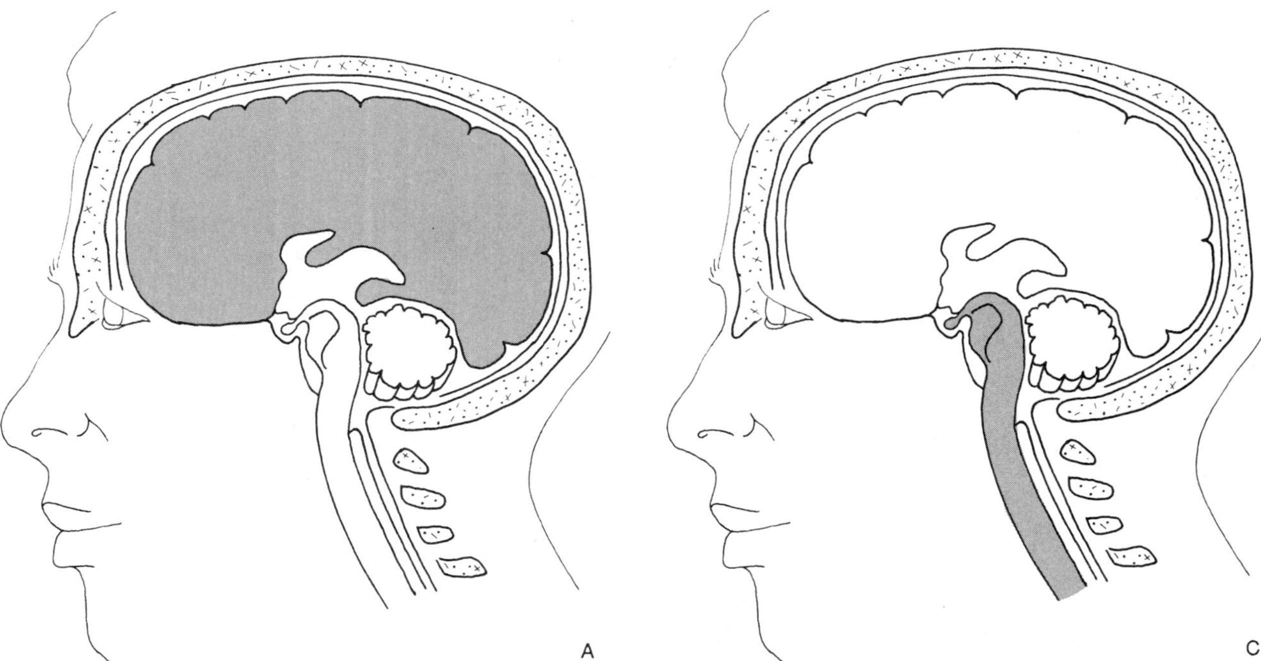

Fig. 1-5. The (A) cerebrum, (B) cerebellum, and (C) brainstem.

The Spinal Cord

The *spinal cord* (Fig. 1-6) is a cylindrical and elongated nerve structure located within the *vertebral canal* (backbone). It serves as a two-way conduction system between the brain and the periphery, and it controls all non-cranial (non-brain) motor reflexes.

The Peripheral Nervous System

The *peripheral nervous system* (PNS) consists of all the nerves that lie outside the brain and spinal cord. This system is essentially responsible for transporting stimuli to the brain where the stimuli are processed and then transmitting the appropriate signal to various parts of the body. Using the analogy of a major power plant, electricity is derived from a hydroelectric dam (the central nervous system) and then distributed to the community through a series of electrical wires (the peripheral nervous system) to homes.

The peripheral nervous system consists of two segments:

- the Autonomic nervous system
- the Somatic nervous system

These two systems are referred to as the *voluntary* and *involuntary* nervous systems, which describes their functions.

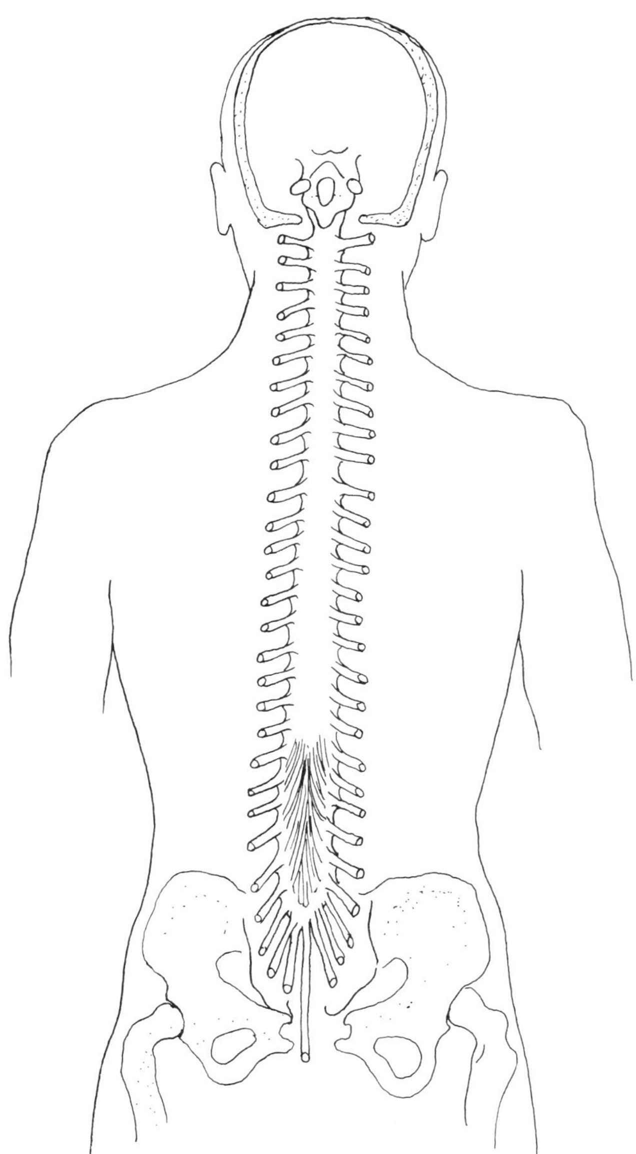

Fig. 1-6. The spinal cord.

The Autonomic Nervous System

The *autonomic*, or involuntary, *nervous system* controls such vital functions as heartbeat and digestive processes, which do not require conscious decisions. For example, when you walk into a dark room, your pupils normally dilate so that you can see better. You don't have to think, "I guess I'll dilate my pupils so I can see better!" Whether you want this to happen or not, it does so automatically.

The Somatic Nervous System

The *somatic*, or voluntary, *nervous system*, is responsible for all movements for which there is some conscious control. For example, if the house is on fire, *you* will tell your body to get moving quickly (Fig. 1-7).

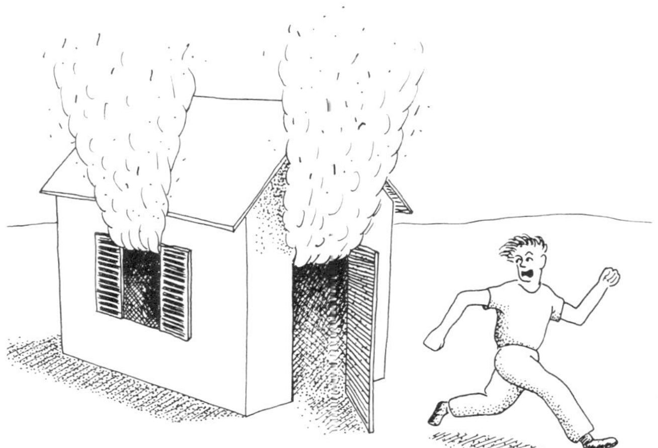

Fig. 1-7. The somatic response to an emergency situation.

Review Exercise

1. The nervous system of the body is divided into which two major systems?

   a. autonomic and somatic **b.** right and left hemisphere
   c. central and peripheral **d.** frontal and temporal

2. The major components of the central nervous system include

   a. ______________________________

   b. ______________________________

3. The brain consists of two halves:

   a. ______________________________

   b. ______________________________

4. The brain is divided into three principle areas:

   a. ______________________________

   b. ______________________________

   c. ______________________________

5. The cerebrum has three primary functional areas:

   a. ______________________________

   b. ______________________________

   c. ______________________________

6. The cerebellum is in the ______________________________ part of the brain and controls ______________________________ movements.

7. Name three basic functions of the cerebellum:

   a. ______________________________

   b. ______________________________

   c. ______________________________

8. Which of the following is *not* a major function of the brainstem?

   a. Control center for muscle movements
   b. Control heart and breathing functions
   c. Control of body temperature, hunger, and thirst
   d. Control of emotional and intellectual processes

9. Each hemisphere of the brain is divided into different lobes and named after the bones that cover them:

   a. ______________________________

   b. ______________________________

   c. ______________________________

   d. ______________________________

10. The spinal cord serves as a two-way conduction system between the ______________ and the ______________________.

11. The spinal cord controls all ______________________ motor reflexes.

12. The peripheral nervous system consists of two segments:

    a. ______________________________

    b. ______________________________

13. The ______________________, or involuntary, nervous system, controls such vital functions as heartbeat and digestive processes.

14. The ______________________, or voluntary, nervous system is responsible for all movements for which there is some conscious control.

THE ABDOMINAL ORGANS

Because we will be discussing vascular anatomy of the *abdominal aorta* and its major branches, it is essential at this point to review the structures and organs that make up the *abdominal cavity* (Fig. 1-8).

Key Terms

Alimentary canal
Bladder
Esophagus
Gallbladder
Kidneys
Large intestines
Liver
Pancreas
Small intestine
Spleen
Stomach
Ureters
Urethra

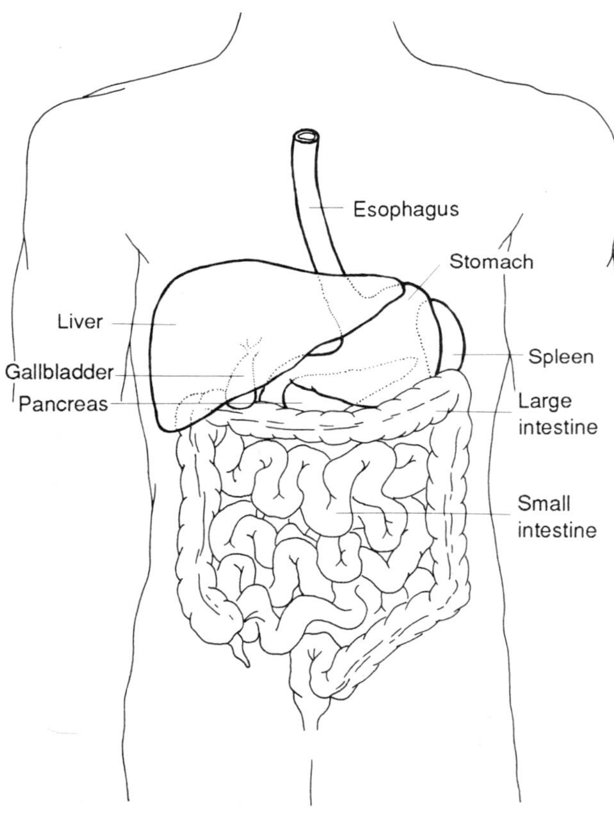

Fig. 1-8. The digestive organs of the abdomen.

The Esophagus and Stomach

The *stomach* is a J-shaped enlargement of the *alimentary* (food) *canal.* The *esophagus* (food pipe) joins the stomach just below the *diaphragm.* A primary function of the stomach is the secretion of digestive juices, such as hydrochloric acid and pepsin, which aid in the digestion of food. Food is "ground" by the muscular motion of the stomach to form a semi-fluid mixture called *chyme,* which makes food suitable for further digestion by the *small intestine.*

The Small Intestine

The *small intestine* performs the major portion of digestion and absorption of nutrients and liquids. It begins at the end of the stomach opening (the pyloric valve) and continues for an average of 20 feet to the beginning of the large intestine. Three additional organs outside the small intestine participate in the digestion of food:

1. The pancreas
2. The liver
3. The gallbladder

The Pancreas

The *pancreas* is a soft carrot-shaped organ that lies close to the stomach. It contains a variety of enzymes that are excreted through the pancreatic duct into the *duodenum,* the first segment of the small intestine. These enzymes further contribute to digestion of food in the small intestine. Some of the cells in the pancreas secrete *insulin,* which helps regulate the breakdown of carbohydrates.

The Liver

The liver is situated in the right upper quadrant of the body, close to the diaphragm. It contains thousands of *lobules,* which are the functional units of the liver. The liver has a double blood supply—from the *hepatic artery* and the *portal vein.* The vital functions of the liver include

1. breaking down poisons to less harmful substances
2. manufacturing anticoagulants
3. transforming and storing glycogen, fat, protein, and glucose
4. storing vitamins A, D, E, and K, as well as some poisons that cannot be broken down
5. manufacturing bile, which is used in the small intestine for the digestion and absorption of fat

The Gallbladder

The *gallbladder* is a sacklike structure attached to the underside of the liver. It stores *bile* until it is required by the small intestine, after which the bile is secreted into the small intestine. Bile also aids in the digestion of food.

The Large Intestine

The *large intestine* is the *distal portion* of the intestine and is about five feet long. It consists of three segments: *cecum*, *colon*, and *rectum* and *anal canal*. The primary functions of the large intestine are the absorption of water and the formation and storage of fecal material (until it is expelled).

The Spleen

The *spleen* is an oval-shaped organ, essentially a large mass of *lymphatic tissue* located in the left upper quadrant of the abdomen just below the diaphragm. Lymphatic tissue plays an important role in the defense against infection. The primary function of the spleen is phagocytosis (eating up) of bacteria and worn-out red blood cells and platelets. The spleen also plays a role in immunity (the body's ability to resist disease). The spleen is not an essential organ and can be removed without important consequences.

The Kidneys, Bladder, and Associated Structures

The *kidneys* are the body's purification units that filter and cleanse the blood of waste products. These organs contain millions of microscopic filtration "loops" called *nephrons*. Nearly 15 gallons of blood are processed through the kidneys each hour.

The main functions of the kidneys include

1. regulation of proper water balance
2. regulation of acid-base concentration
3. excretion of metabolic waste in urine

The kidneys excrete wastes through two tubes known as the *ureters*. These tubes connect with a hollow muscular organ called the *bladder*, which is situated in the pelvic cavity. Once the bladder is full, urine is excreted out of the body through a single tube called the *urethra* (Fig. 1-9).

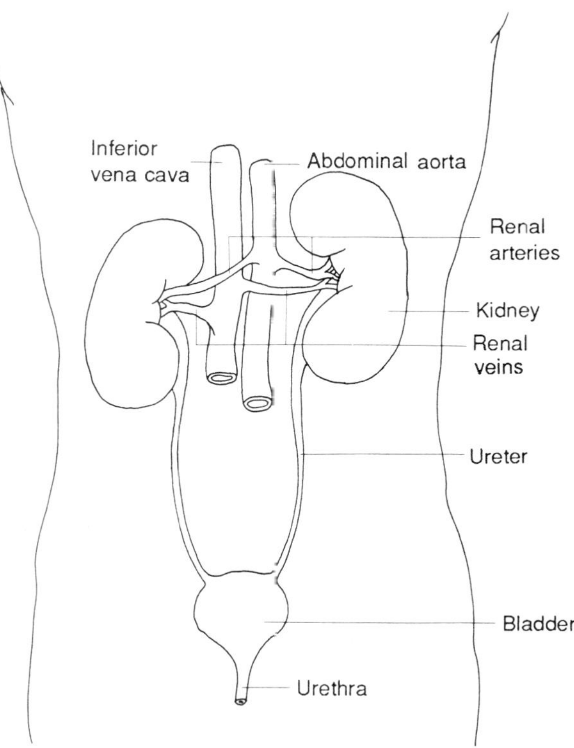

Fig. 1-9. The renal organs and urinary tract system.

Review Exercise

1. The stomach is a J-shaped enlargement of the ______________________ canal.

2. The ______________________, or food pipe, joins the stomach just below the diaphragm.

3. Initially digested food from the stomach is formed into a semi-fluid called ____________.

4. The small intestine performs the major portion of the ______________________ and ______________________ of nutrients and liquids.

5. The pancreas contains a variety of enzymes that are excreted through the pancreatic duct into the ____________________.

6. Some of the cells in the pancreas secrete ______________________, which helps regulate the breakdown of carbohydrates.

7. Which of the following are functions of the liver?

   a. Manufacturing anticoagulants
   b. Storing bile
   c. Secreting insulin
   d. Phagocytosis of worn-out blood cells
   e. Producing lymphocytes
   f. Transforming and storing glycogen, fat, protein, and glucose
   g. Manufacturing bile

8. The ______________________ is a sacklike structure that stores bile.

9. The spleen is an oval-shaped organ, essentially a large mass of

   a. fatty tissue
   b. smooth muscle tissue
   c. monocyte tissue
   d. lymphatic tissue

10. The spleen is situated in the ______________________ quadrant of the abdomen.

11. One of the functions of the spleen is to produce ____________________.

12. The small intestine begins at the end of the ______________________________.

13. The average length of the small intestine is about

a. 20 meters
b. 20 feet
c. 10 meters
d. 15 centimeters

14. The large intestine consists of the following three segments:

a. ______________________________

b. ______________________________

c. ______________________________

15. The main functions of the large intestine include the ______________________ and ______________________ of fecal material.

16. Label the abdominal organs illustrated in Fig. 1-8.

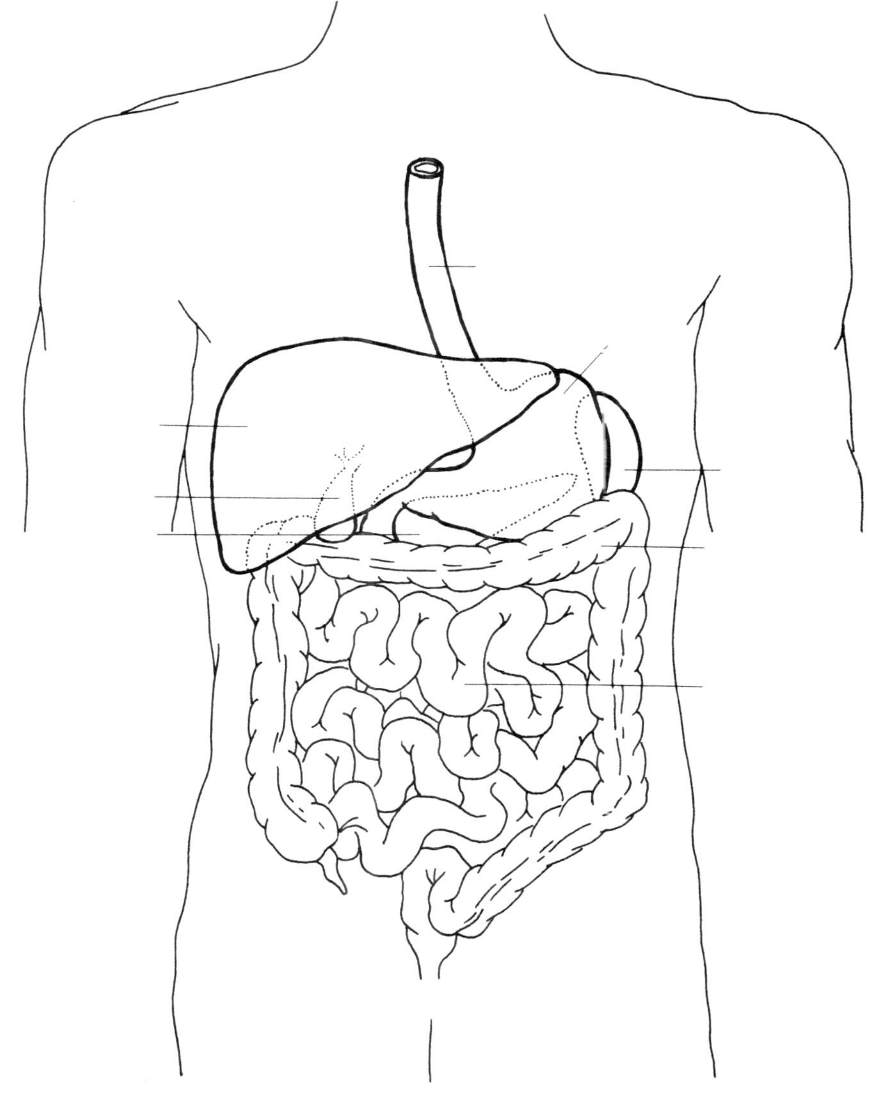

17. The function of the kidneys is to ______________ and ______________ the blood of waste products.

18. Kidneys contain millions of microscopic filter "loops" called

a. ureters
b. urethras
c. renals
d. nephrons

19. Nearly ______________ gallons of blood are processed through the kidneys each hour.

20. Which of the following is *not* one of the main functions of the kidneys?

a. Regulation of proper water balance
b. Regulation of acid-base concentration
c. Excretion of metabolic waste as urine
d. Storage of urine

21. The kidneys excrete wastes through two tubes known as the ______________.

22. The ureters connect with a hollow muscular organ called the ______________, which is situated in the pelvic cavity.

23. Once the bladder organ is full, urine is excreted out of the body through a single tube called the ______________.

24. Label the renal organs illustrated in Fig. 1-9.

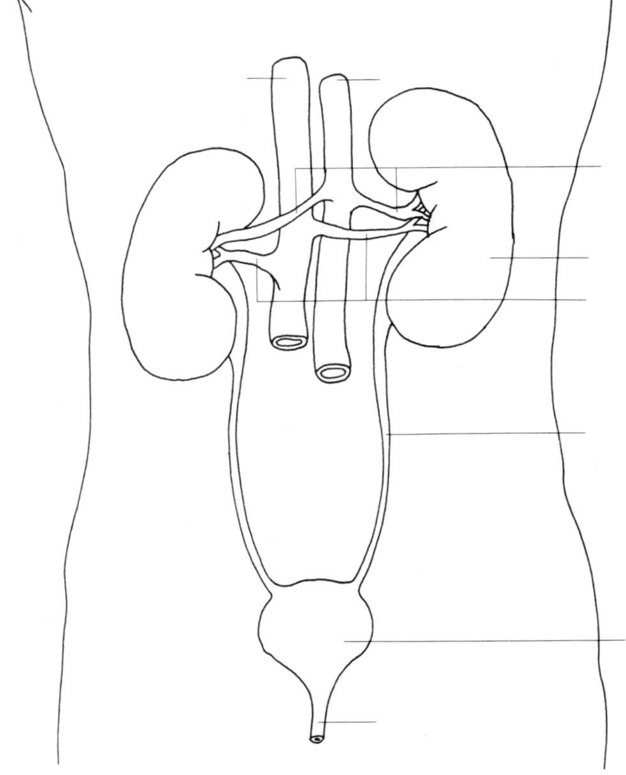

THE HEART

It is essential to understand the *primary pathways* blood takes as it is sent through the body on route to its destination and then back again. The starting point of this journey is the *heart*. The vascular specialist must be able to trace the pathway from the heart, through the *major* and *secondary vessels* to the *capillaries*, and back again through the deep and superficial venous systems. *Collateral circulation* represents alternate routes that blood may take under certain circumstances. (This will be discussed in more detail in Chapter 2.)

Key Terms

Aortic valve
Ascending aorta
Coronary arteries
Capillaries
Left atrium
Left ventricle
Mitral valve
Papillary muscles
Pericardium
Pulmonary artery
Pulmonary valve
Pulse
Right atrium
Right ventricle
Sternum
Tricuspid valve
Veins
Venules

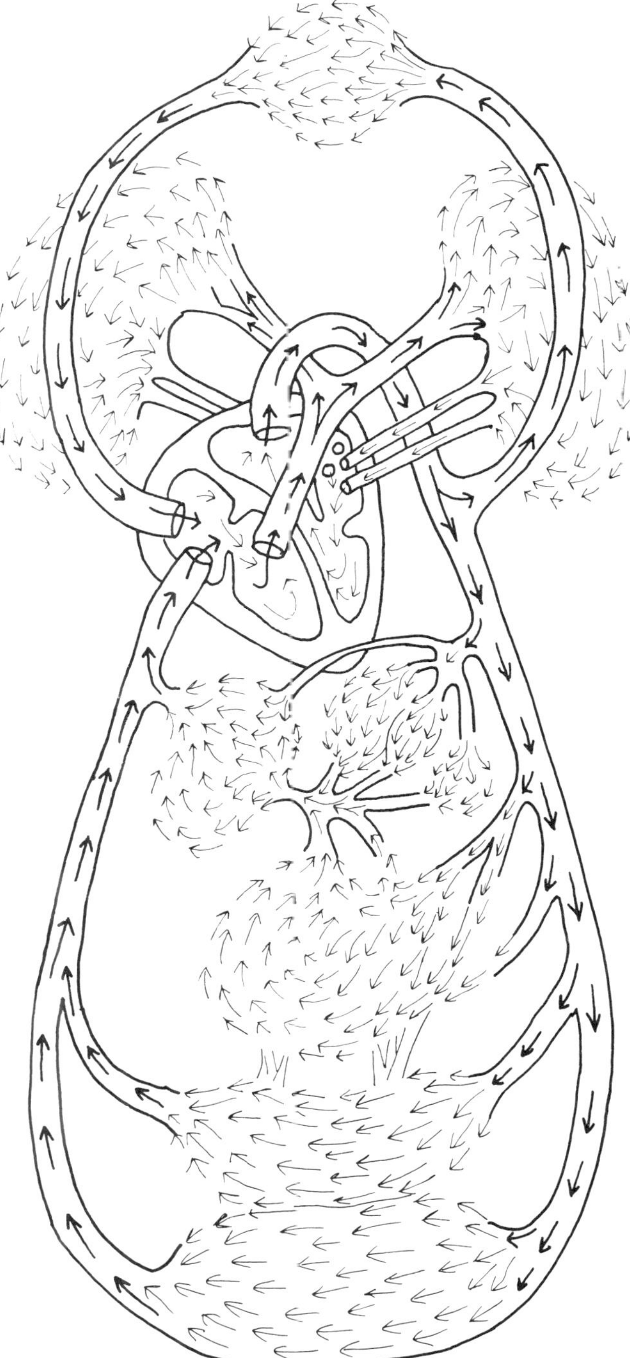

Fig. 1-10. The major circulatory routes of the body.

The Circulatory Pathways

Before we start learning the specific pathways of blood flow, we must have a clear knowledge of the *general* circulatory pathways. These pathways include the

1. cerebrovascular
2. pulmonary
3. abdominal
4. peripheral arterial

In general, the heart pumps oxygenated blood via the *arteries* to all living tissue in the body, and *veins* return deoxygenated blood back to the heart. Figure 1-10 shows the major routes by which blood flows throughout the body.

Cardiac Anatomy

The heart is a cone-shaped organ about the size of your fist. It lies just behind the *sternum* (breastbone) between the lungs (Fig. 1-11) and is slightly slanted to the left. The heart thrusts out from behind the sternum, and it is at this point that it is most easily heard or felt. This positioning gives rise to the mistaken belief that the heart is on the left side of the chest.

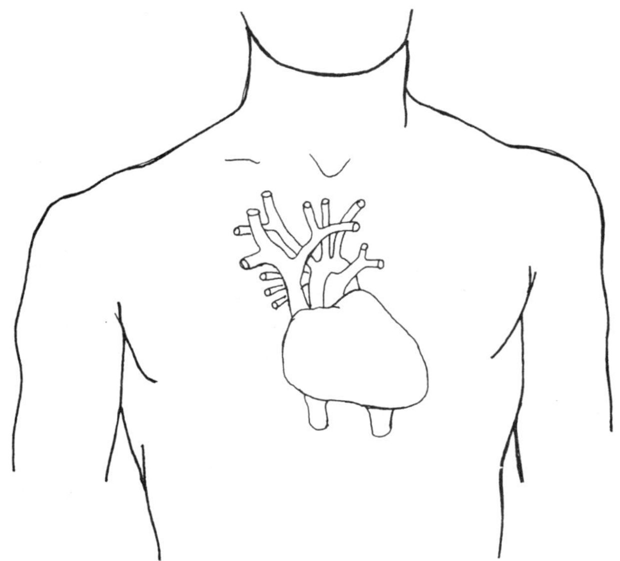

Fig. 1-11. The location of the heart in the chest cavity.

The Pericardium

The *heart muscle* (myocardium) is surrounded by a sacklike structure known as the *pericardium*. Between the pericardium and the *myocardium* is fluid that acts as a lubricant for the heart as it pulsates in the chest cavity.

Movement of Blood Flow through the Heart

Figure 1-12 shows the vessels, chambers, and valves involved with moving blood through the heart.

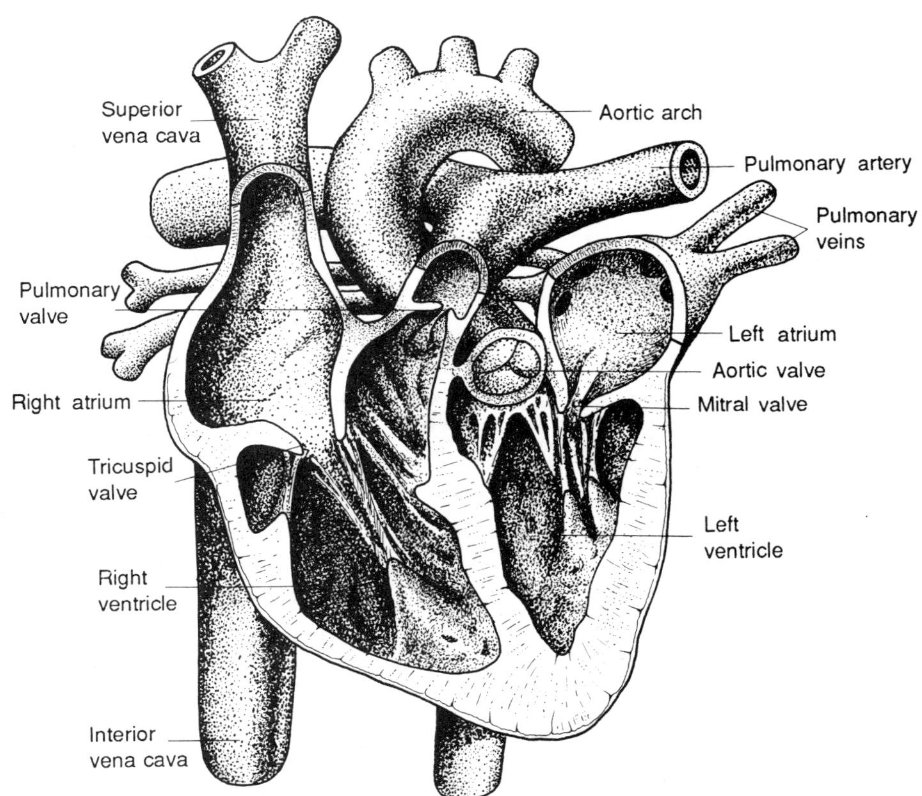

Fig. 1-12. The vessels, chambers, and valves involved in moving blood through the heart.

The Right Atrium and Ventricle

Let's begin with the path a red blood cell takes, beginning in the *right atrium*. Blood passes into the right atrium after it has completed its voyage through the body. At this point, the blood cells are, for the most part, depleted of oxygen. The heart's first task is to correct this condition by rapidly moving blood toward the *lungs*.

Blood flow entering the *right atrium* flows freely past a one-way valve called the *tricuspid valve* and then into the *right ventricle*. By the time the right atrium is full, so is the right ventricle. Now the pumping process begins!

First the right atrium contracts, emptying blood into the right ventricle through the tricuspid valve. When the right ventricle is distended, this portion of the heart almost immediately contracts, sending blood out through the *pulmonary artery* and also back toward the tricuspid valve. This valve slams shut against the pressure and prevents the blood from entering back into the right atrium. The pulmonary artery "gives" a little by expanding to accept the larger volume of blood.

A set of small muscles, attached to the tricuspid valve keeps blood from pushing back through. These muscles (Figure 1-13), known as the *papillary muscles*, reinforce the valve to keep it from collapsing. The papillary muscles tether the edges of the valve to the wall of the right ventricle. This prevents the leaflets from collapsing back into the right atrium when the right *ventricle* contracts.

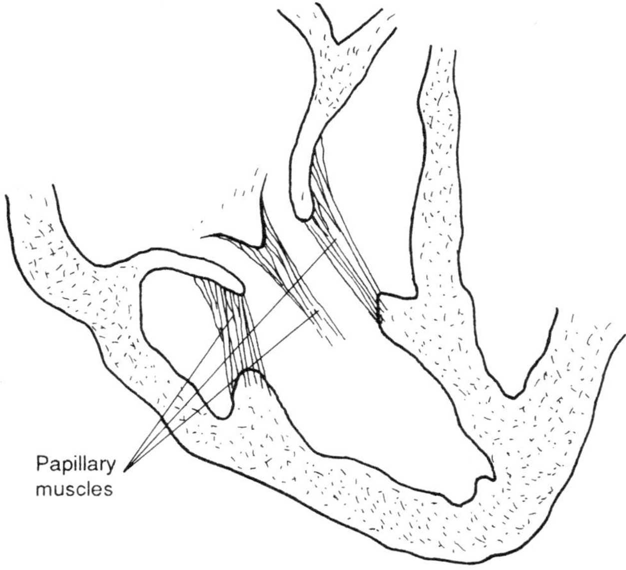

Fig. 1-13. The papillary muscles that provide reinforcement to the heart valves.

The Pulmonary Artery and Vein

At the next stage of the journey, the blood, under a considerable amount of pressure, surges through the only opening available: the pulmonary artery. This is the only *artery* that transports *deoxygenated* blood, an exception to the oxygen-specific role of arteries. (Another exception is that of the pulmonary *vein*, which brings *oxygenated* blood back to the heart.)

Remember that the *right ventricle* has just contracted and sent a surge of blood toward the lungs via the pulmonary artery. Just as the tricuspid valve prevents blood from entering back into the right atrium, the *pulmonary*, or *semilunar, valves* keep blood from entering back into the right ventricle. The pulmonary valve also has papillary muscles attached to its edges to help prevent collapse of the valve into the right atrium.

At this juncture of the blood pathway, the pulmonary artery immediately divides into two branches (one for each lung) and continues dividing and subdividing into *arterioles* and *capillaries*. Here the blood cells are finally oxygenated through the exchange of oxygen from tiny *alveolar sacs* in the lungs. These sacks lie very close to the tiny blood vessels. They are small and thin enough to allow the exchange of oxygen from the lungs to the blood, and carbon dioxide from the blood to the lungs.

The Left Atrium and Ventricle

Freshly oxygenated blood from the pulmonary circulation reenters the heart, passing into the left atrium. From the left atrium the blood flows past another one-way valve, called the *mitral valve*, into the left ventricle. As in the right side of the heart, this valve prevents blood from slipping backward.

The left ventricle has a major task. It must send blood to all parts of the body except the lungs, of course. Although both ventricles contract simultaneously (right or pulmonary circulation to the lungs, left or peripheral circulation to the peripheral body), the left ventricle must do so with six times the force of the right. Consequently, the left ventricle is twice the size of the right ventricle. The contraction of the left ventricle forces the freshly oxygenated blood through the *aortic valve* and into the aorta, the largest single artery in the body.

Keep in mind that the blood flow is still under a lot of pressure. All that blood from the right ventricle has to fit into an artery considerably smaller than the ventricle. Under these circumstances, something has to give! And that is precisely what does happen. The healthy artery will stretch out a bit to accept this increase in blood and then recoil back to normal size as the blood is propelled to the distal circulation. In fact, when a vessel runs close to the skin in the peripheral circulation, you can actually feel the expansion and contraction. This is what is called *pulse*.

On route back to the heart, the blood flows through *venules*, which are very tiny veins leading to the pulmonary vein. By this time, the pulse is completely absorbed by all the divisions and subdivisions, and the blood flows quite smoothly. Because veins do not have to absorb the shock of the powerful thrust of arterial flow, the venous walls are much thinner than the walls of the arteries.

The *ascending aorta* is the major arterial vessel of the heart. The first two branches of the proximal ascending aorta are the *coronary arteries* (Fig. 1-14). These arteries encircle the heart like a crown, from which the name *coronary* is derived. One might think that the heart should be able to get enough nourishment from the blood in the ventricles, but it does not. (*Remember*: only the left side of the heart contains oxygenated blood.) The coronary arteries immediately supply the heart with the nutrients it so richly deserves. Alternately, without the continuous operation of the heart, *no other* organ would be able to receive the nourishment necessary for function.

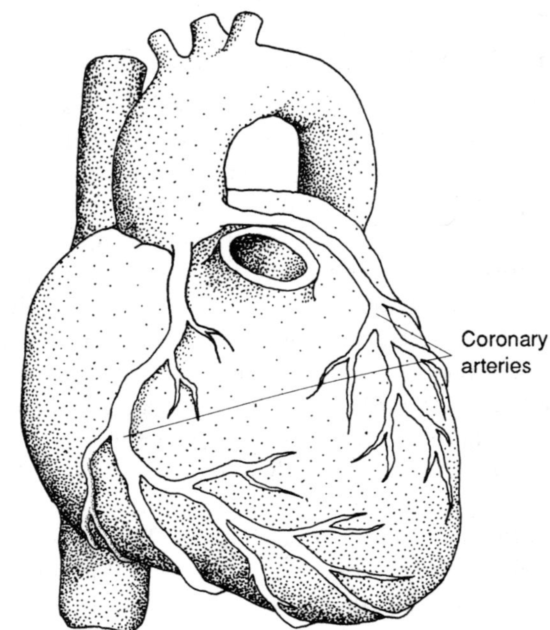

Fig. 1-14. The coronary arteries.

Review Exercise

1. The heart is a cone-shape organ about the size of your ______________.

2. The heart lies to the left of the sternum. True or False?

3. The heart muscle is also called the

   a. endocardium b. myocardium
   c. pericardium d. endometrium

4. The heart is surrounded by a sacklike structure known as the

   a. endocardium b. myocardium
   c. pericardium d. endometrium

5. Between the pericardium and the myocardium is ______________ that acts as a lubricant for the heart as it pulsates in the chest cavity.

6. Which chamber does deoxygenated blood first enter into after it has completed its voyage through the body?

   a. Right ventricle b. Right atrium
   c. Left atrium d. Left ventricle

7. When the blood enters the left atrium from the lungs, the cells are completely ____.

8. Blood flow entering the right atrium, flows freely past a one-way valve called the

   a. aortic valve b. pulmonary valve
   c. mitral valve d. tricuspid valve

9. The right atrium contracts, sending blood into the ______________ ventricle.

10. A set of small muscles attached to the tricuspid valve, called the ____ muscles, prevent blood from flowing back through.

11. Blood is pumped from the right ventricle to the

    a. pulmonary artery b. pulmonary vein
    c. aorta d. right atrium

12. Which valve keeps blood from entering back into the right ventricle?

    a. Pulmonary b. Mitral
    c. Tricuspid d. Aortic

13. The pulmonary artery immediately divides into two branches, essentially one for each ______________.

14. In tissue, the blood flows through ______________, which are very small arteries.

15. On route back to the heart, the blood flows through ____________________________, which are very small veins.

16. The walls of arteries and veins are very similar in size. True or False?

17. Freshly oxygenated blood reenters the heart via the ____________________________.

18. As in the right side of the heart, there is a valve to prevent blood from slipping backward through the pulmonary vein. It is called the:

    a. pulmonary valve
    b. mitral valve
    c. tricuspid valve
    d. aortic valve

19. From the left atrium blood passes another one-way valve called the

    a. pulmonary valve
    b. mitral valve
    c. tricuspid valve
    d. aortic valve

20. Because the ______________ ventricle has to pump blood to the lungs, it is larger than the ______________ ventricle.

21. The contraction of the left ventricle first forces the freshly oxygenated blood into

    a. the carotid arteries
    b. the abdominal aorta
    c. the left atrium
    d. the aortic arch

22. The first two branches of the aorta are the ____ arteries.

THE AORTA

The *aorta* is the first main branch from the heart and is the primary "highway" from which other major vessels depart. This section covers the major branches of the aorta.

Key Terms

Ascending aorta
Brachiocephalic arteries
Clavicle
Common carotid arteries
Innominate artery
Sternum
Subclavian artery

Divisions of the Aorta

The aorta initially courses upward toward the head. It then arches over the *pulmonary artery* and assumes a downward path toward the diaphragm (Fig. 1-15). These three segments of the aorta are called the

- ascending aorta
- aortic arch
- descending aorta

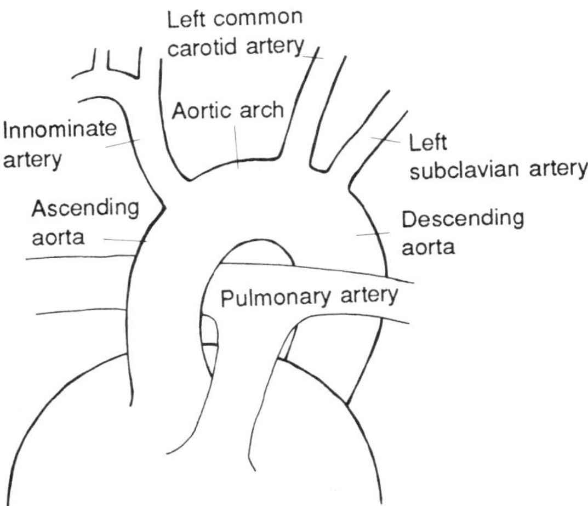

Fig. 1-15. The aortic arch and branches.

Because these three segments of the aorta are essentially in the chest, they are called the *thoracic aorta.* The aorta leaves the chest cavity through a hole (hiatus) in the diaphragm at the level of about the 12th thoracic vertebra. From this point the vessel is termed the abdominal aorta because it is traveling through the *abdominal cavity.*

Major Branches of the Aortic Arch

Three large branches off the aortic arch, which supply the head and arms with blood, are

- the innominate (or brachiocephalic) artery
- the left common carotid artery
- the left subclavian artery

The first branch off the aortic arch on the right is the *innominate artery,* also known as the *brachiocephalic artery.* It is approximately 1½ to 2 inches in length. As it leaves the aortic arch, it reaches the approximate level of the *sternoclavicular junction,* the point at which the *clavicle* (collar bone) connects with the *sternum* (breast bone). The innominate artery then bifurcates into the *right common carotid artery* and the *right subclavian artery.* The term *bifurcate* means to branch into two different arteries.

The *left common carotid artery* originates from the aortic arch just after the innominate artery and ascends toward the head. The *left subclavian artery* originates from the aortic arch just beyond the origin of the left common carotid artery and passes laterally to supply the left arm with blood.

Major Branches of the Descending Aorta

The major branches of the descending aorta, which supply the lungs with blood, are

- the intercostals
- the superior phrenics
- the bronchials
- the esophageals

Review Exercise

1. Name the three large arteries arising from the aortic arch that supply the head and arms with blood:

   a. ______________________________

   b. ______________________________

   c. ______________________________

2. The ______________________ artery is the first branch off the aortic arch (after the coronary arteries).

3. Which two arteries branch off the brachiocephalic?

   a. Right and left common carotid arteries
   b. Right vertebral and right common carotid arteries
   c. Coronary artery
   d. Right subclavian and right common carotid arteries

4. The second branch off the aortic arch after the innominate artery is the

   a. right common carotid artery
   b. left common carotid artery
   c. brachiocephalic
   d. ascending aorta

5. The left common carotid artery, like the right common carotid artery, has

   a. one branch
   b. two branches
   c. three branches
   d. no branches

6. The third branch off the aortic arch is the

   a. left brachiocephalic
   b. left subclavian
   c. left common carotid artery
   d. left vertebral artery

7. The four major branches of the descending aorta are the

   a. ______________________________

   b. ______________________________

   c. ______________________________

   d. ______________________________

7. Label the branches of the aortic arch.

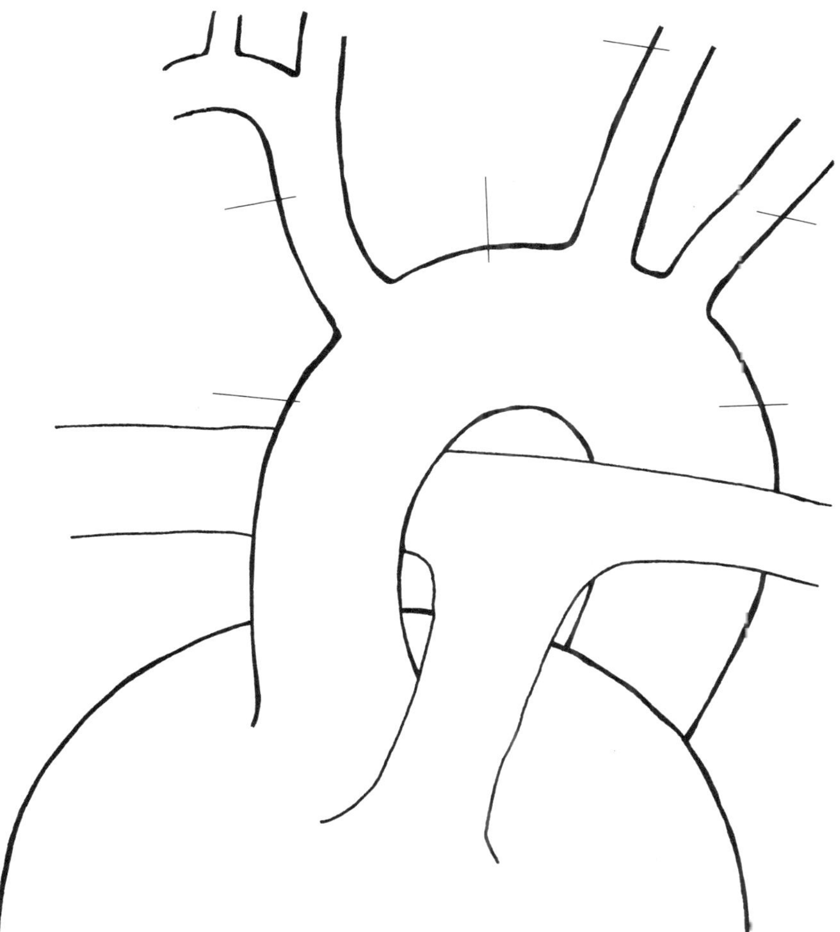

BRANCHES OF THE ABDOMINAL AORTA

In this section, the general anatomy of the abdominal aorta is discussed.

Key Terms

Abdominal aorta
Celiac trunk
Common iliac arteries
External iliac arteries
Gastric artery
Hepatic artery
Internal iliac arteries
Renal arteries
Splenic artery
Superior mesenteric artery

Figure 1-16 shows the arteries that originate from the *abdominal aorta.* The abdominal aorta begins at the level of the 12th thoracic vertebra. It passes through the hiatus (hole) of the diaphragm. There are three major branches off the aorta:

1. Celiac trunk
2. Superior mesenteric artery
3. Renal arteries

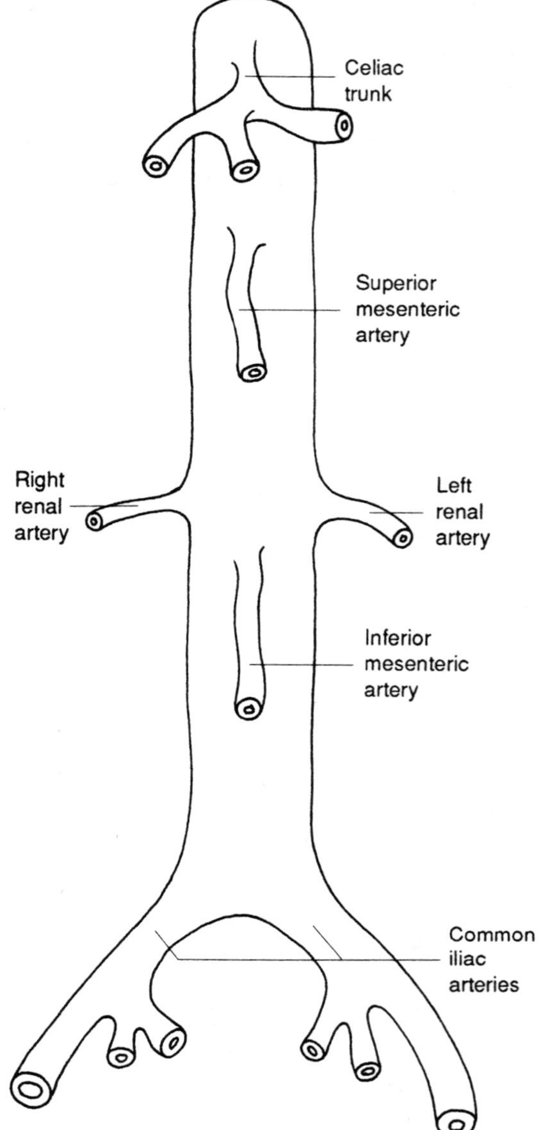

Fig. 1-16. The major vessels of the abdominal aorta.

The Celiac Trunk

The *celiac trunk* is also known as the *celiac axis* or *celiac artery*. It is the first branch off the aorta just below the diaphragm and is fairly short, approximately 1/2 to 3/4 of an inch in length. The celiac trunk has three branches:

1. The hepatic artery, which supplies the liver
2. The left gastric artery, which supplies the stomach
3. The splenic artery, which supplies the spleen, pancreas, and stomach.

The Superior Mesenteric Artery

The *superior mesenteric artery* (SMA) is the next major branch off the abdominal aorta. The SMA exits anterior to the aorta and courses downward, running parallel with the aorta. The SMA distributes blood to the *small intestine* and the first half of the *large intestine*.

The Inferior Mesenteric Artery

The *inferior mesenteric artery* (IMA) primarily supplies blood to part of the *colon* and a greater part of the *rectum*. It arises from the aorta about 2 to 3 inches above the aortic division of the *common iliac arteries*. The IMA is smaller than the superior mesenteric artery and not customarily a vessel that can be investigated in a noninvasive diagnostic laboratory.

The Renal Arteries

The *renal arteries*, which supply the *kidneys* with blood, branch off the lateral aspect of the aorta just below the *superior mesenteric artery*. The *right* renal artery is usually a little higher than the *left* renal artery. The right renal artery courses posteriorly to the *inferior vena cava* and continues to the right kidney. Both renal arteries approach the kidneys slightly posterior to the renal veins.

The Iliacs

At about the level of the 4th lumbar vertebra, near the umbilicus, the abdominal aorta divides into the *right* and *left common iliac arteries*. Each of these arteries passes caudad for only 2 inches and gives rise to two branches: the *internal* and *external iliac arteries*. The internal iliac arteries form two branches that supply the gluteal muscles, medial side of each thigh, urinary bladder, rectum, prostate gland, uterus, and vagina. The internal iliac arteries are sometimes referred to as the *hypogastric arteries*. The external iliac artery continues its path downward to supply the leg with blood.

Review Exercise

1. In the abdominal aorta, the three main vessels branching off the anterior aorta just below the diaphragm are the

   a. ______________________________

   b. ______________________________

   c. ______________________________

2. Which of the following is the first aortic branch below the diaphragm?

   a. Renal artery **b.** Superior mesenteric artery
   c. Hepatic artery **d.** Celiac trunk

3. Match the artery with the organ it supplies.

a. Hepatic artery	____	Spleen
b. Left gastric artery	____	Kidney
c. Splenic artery	____	Stomach
d. Renal artery	____	Liver

4. The celiac trunk is also known as the celiac ______________ or celiac ______________.

5. The celiac trunk is approximately ______________ in length.

6. Distal to the celiac trunk, the next major branch off the abdominal aorta is the ______________________________ artery.

7. The superior mesenteric artery distributes blood to the

   a. small intestine
   b. large intestine and first half of the small intestine
   c. both large and small intestine
   d. small intestine and first half the large intestine

8. The right and left ______________ arteries carry blood to the kidneys.

9. At about the level of the 4th lumbar vertebra, near the level of the umbilicus, the abdominal aorta divides into the right and left

   a. common iliac arteries **b.** common femoral arteries
   c. mesenteric arteries **d.** renal arteries

10. The common iliac arteries bifurcate into

 a. common femoral and external iliac arteries
 b. common femoral and external iliac arteries
 c. superficial femoral and profunda arteries
 d. internal and external iliac arteries

11. The ________________________________ arteries form two branches that supply the gluteal muscles, medial side of each thigh, urinary bladder, rectum, prostate gland, uterus, and vagina.

12. The internal iliac artery supplies the leg with blood. True or False?

13. The inferior mesenteric artery supplies blood to part of the __________ and the __________.

14. Label the major vessels of the abdominal aorta.

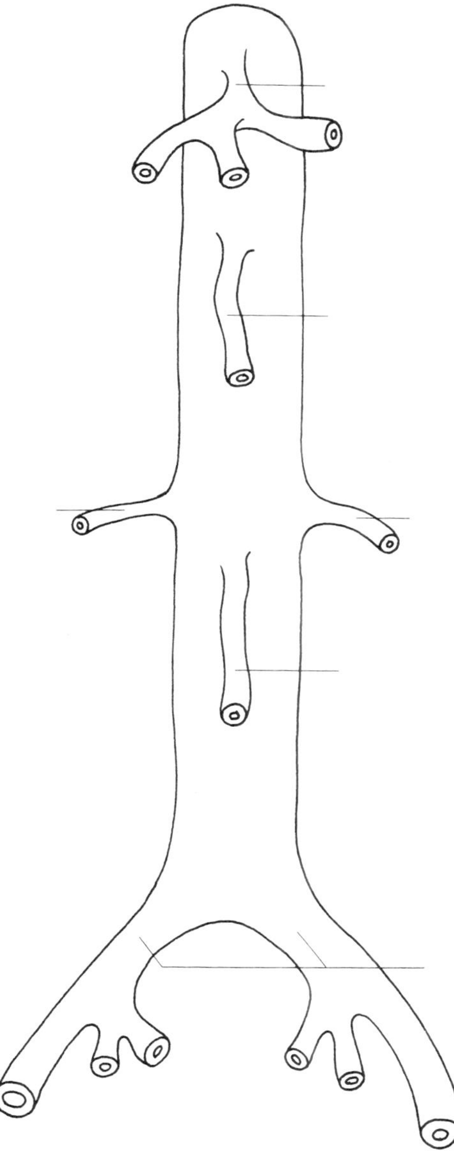

THE CEREBRAL ARTERIAL SYSTEM

This section outlines the general vascular anatomy of the *cerebrovascular circulation* (Fig. 1-17) and the *ophthalmic artery.*

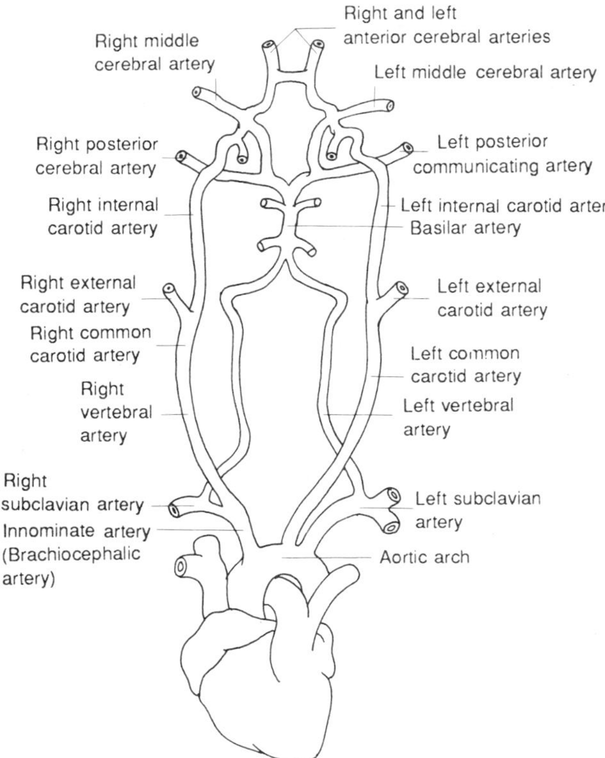

Fig. 1-17. The cerebrovascular circulation.

Key Terms

Anastomose
Anastomosis
Anterior cerebral artery
Anterior cerebrovascular circulation
Anterior communicating arteries
Basilar artery
Bifurcation
Circle of Willis
Common carotid arteries
External carotid artery
Facial artery
Frontal artery
Internal carotid artery
Larynx
Midcerebral arteries
Nasal artery
Ophthalmic artery
Palpate
Periorbital circulation
Posterior cerebral arteries
Posterior cerebrovascular circulation
Siphon
Superficial temporal artery
Supraorbital arteries

Anterior Circulation

The *anterior cerebrovascular circulation* (Fig.1-18), in general, supplies blood to the anterior part of the brain, the eyes, the face, and the scalp. The vessels in this system include the

1. common carotid
2. internal carotid
3. external carotid
4. branches of the external carotid artery

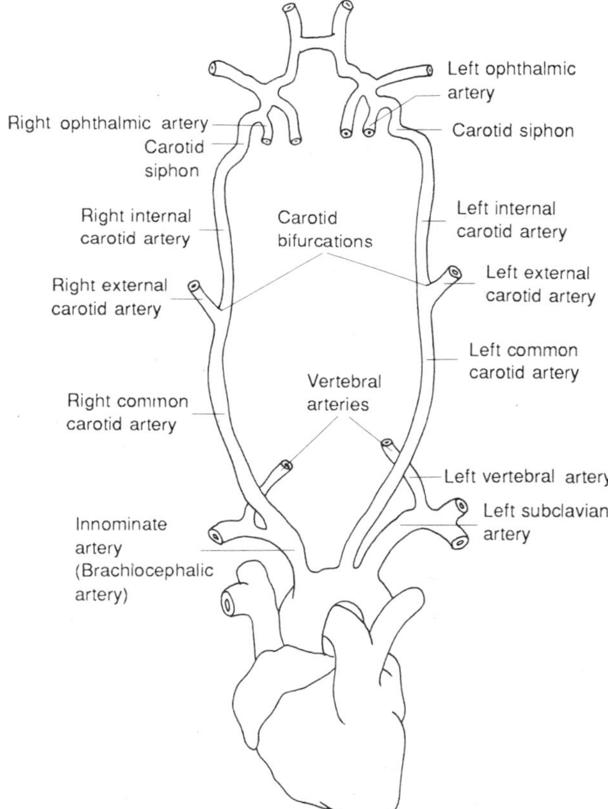

Fig. 1-18. The major arteries of the anterior cerebrovascular circulation.

The Carotid Artery

The *carotid artery* supplies most of the arterial blood, in general, to the anterior part of the brain. Starting on the right side of the chest cavity, the *right common carotid artery* originates off the *bifurcation* of the *innominate artery*. On the left side of the chest cavity, *the left common carotid artery* originates off the *aortic arch*.

At the level of the *larynx* (the voice box), the common carotid artery bifurcates into the *internal carotid artery* and the *external carotid artery*. (This level may be higher or lower in different individuals.) It is the carotid bifurcation that we are most interested in when looking for significant extracranial carotid artery disease. Most disease occurs here because of the flow dynamics typical of a bifurcation.

Internal Carotid Artery

The *internal carotid artery* (ICA) continues straight up the neck into the skull. The primary purpose of the ICA is to supply the brain and eyes with blood. Once inside the skull, the ICA makes a little **S**-shaped bend called the carotid *siphon*. Because it is a bend in an otherwise straight tube, it is a source for stenosis.

The internal carotid artery has *no* branches outside the skull. This is particularly important to remember if the vascular specialist is trying to differentiate between internal and external carotid arteries. The first branch off the ICA is the ophthalmic artery, and, as the name implies, it supplies the eye with blood. (This also is important to remember when discussing indirect methods of assessing cerebral arterial blood flow.) The ICA then terminates at the *anterior cerebral artery*.

External Carotid Artery

The *external carotid artery* (ECA) supplies the face and the scalp with blood. The face, like the brain, is rich in blood supply. A distinction, however, is that vessels supplying blood to the face can terminate in the tissue rather abruptly. The ECA *may* become a source of blood supply to the brain when there is severe disease of the internal carotid artery. It is therefore important to know the major anatomy of the *external artery branches*.

Branches of the External Carotid Artery

The ECA has several branches that start dividing almost immediately after the carotid bifurcation (Fig. 1-19). The first branch is the *superior thyroid artery* (yes, it supplies the thyroid). Other branches off of the ECA include the *lingual*, *facial*, *occipital* and *superficial temporal arteries*. Because only the superficial temporal artery and the branches of the facial artery play a role in possible collateral blood flow, however, we need only concern ourselves with them.

The facial artery branches off the ECA and follows a superficial path over the surface of the angle of the jaw. If you put your fingers lightly on that area, you may *palpate* (feel) a pulse. The facial artery passes through the soft tissue of the face about the area of the cheek, where it connects with (or *anastomoses* with) the nasal branch of the ophthalmic artery.

The superficial temporal artery branches off the external carotid artery just in front of the ear. Here, you should be able to palpate the pulse with your fingers. Some of the branches of the superficial temporal artery traverse across the forehead and form an anastomosis (connection) with branches of the *frontal* and *supraorbital arteries*.

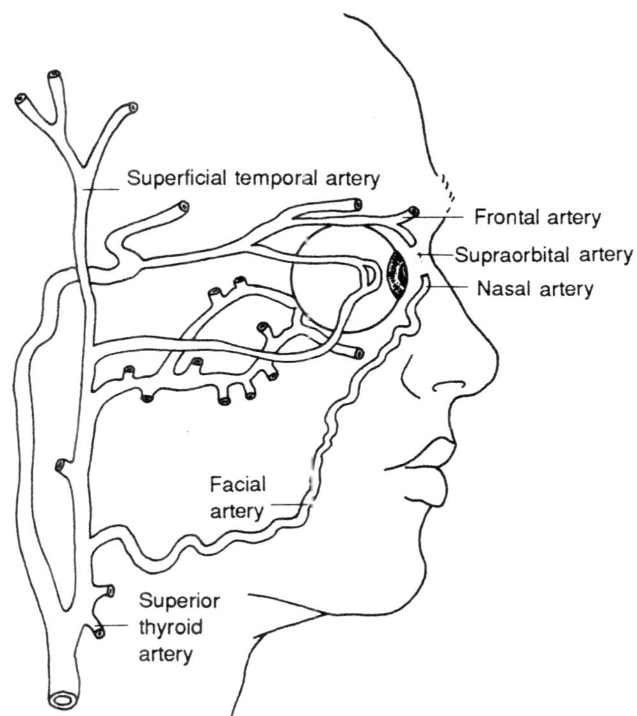

Fig. 1-19. The periorbital circulation.

Review Exercise

1. The anterior cerebrovascular circulation provides circulation primarily to which of the following:

   a. Face and scalp
   b. Frontal lobe
   c. Right hemisphere
   d. Anterior part of the brain and the eyes

2. Both the left and right common carotid arteries originate off the aortic arch. True or False?

3. At the level of the larynx (the voice box), the common carotid artery bifurcates into the ______________________________ and the ______________________________.

4. Because of the flow dynamics typical of a ____________________, most disease occurs at the point indicated in question 3.

5. The primary purpose of the internal carotid artery is to supply the __________ and __________ with blood.

6. Once inside the skull, the internal carotid artery

   a. is perfectly straight
   b. makes a small S-shaped bend
   c. has many branches
   d. terminates at the ophthalmic artery

7. A relatively common anatomic area of the internal carotid artery intracranially (where disease may occur) is called the ____________________.

8. The first branch off the internal carotid artery inside the skull is the:

   a. external carotid artery
   b. anterior cerebral artery
   c. anterior communicating artery
   d. ophthalmic artery

9. The internal carotid artery terminates at the

   a. external carotid artery
   b. anterior cerebral artery
   c. anterior communicating artery
   d. ophthalmic artery

10. The external carotid artery supplies the __________ and the __________ with blood.

11. The __________ carotid artery has several branches that start dividing almost immediately after the carotid bifurcation.

12. The first branch of the internal carotid artery is the

    a. facial artery
    b. superior thyroid artery
    c. superficial temporal artery
    d. ophthalmic artery

13. The superior thyroid artery is an important collateral vessel to the intracranial circulation. True or False?

14. The superficial temporal artery is an important collateral vessel. True or False?

15. The facial artery is an important collateral vessel. True or False?

16. The facial artery branches off the external carotid artery and follows a ______________________________ path over the surface of the angle of the jaw.

17. The term *anastomose* means to

    a. connect with
    b. terminate
    c. bifurcate
    d. make an S-shaped turn

18. The facial artery anastomoses with the nasal branch of the ______________________________ artery.

19. The superficial temporal artery branches off the external carotid artery

    a. just after the ICA/ECA bifurcation
    b. just in front of the ear
    c. just behind the ear
    d. just lateral to the nose

20. The superficial temporal artery is too deep to palpate the pulse with your fingers. True or False?

21. Some of the branches of the superficial temporal artery traverse across the forehead and anastomose with branches of the

    a. facial and frontal arteries
    b. facial and nasal arteries
    c. frontal and supraorbital arteries
    d. frontal and nasal arteries

22. Label the vessels of the anterior circulation.

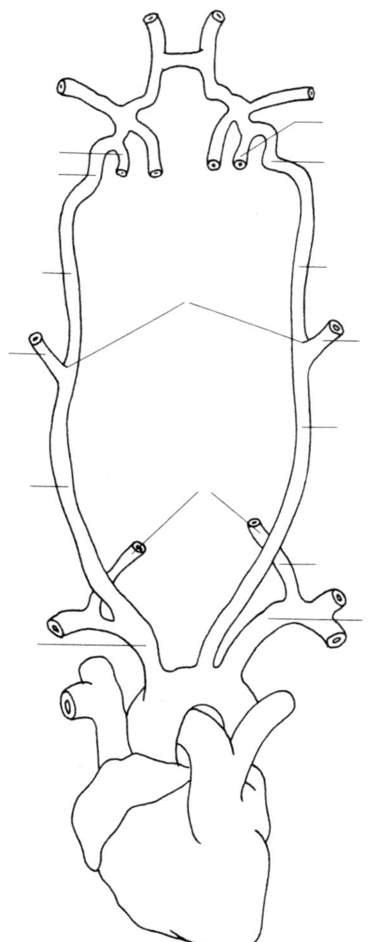

23. Label the vessels of the external carotid circulation.

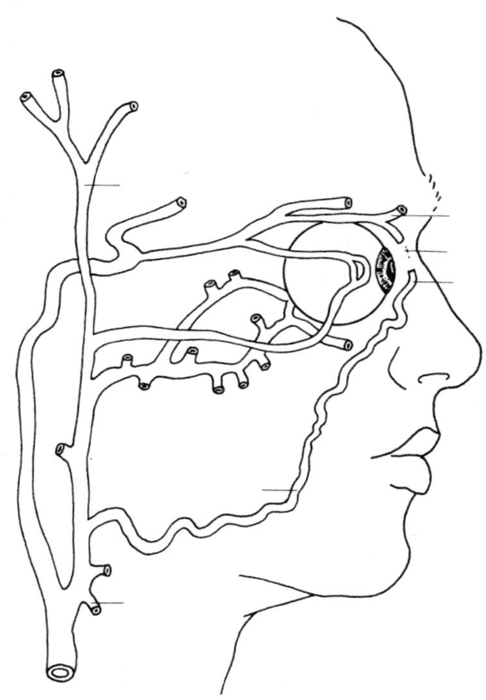

Posterior Circulation

The *posterior cerebrovascular circulation* (Fig. 1-20), in general, supplies the posterior part of the brain with blood. The major vessels in this system include the *basilar* and the *vertebral arteries*. The blood supply from these vessels originates from below the neck.

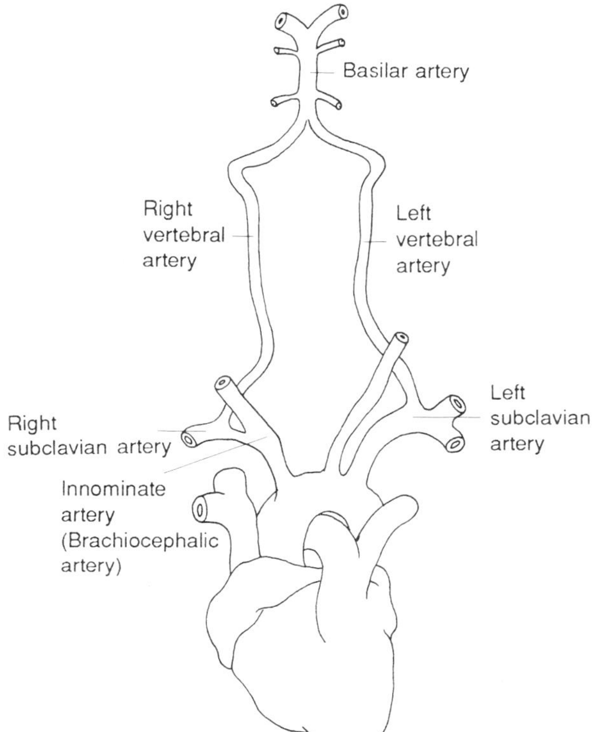

Fig. 1-20. The major arteries of the posterior cerebrovascular circulation.

The Vertebral Artery

The *innominate artery* branches into the *right common carotid artery* and the *right subclavian artery*. The *right vertebral artery* is the first branch off the *right subclavian artery*. It passes cephalad for a short distance and then enters the 6th cervical vertebra in the neck. The right vertebral artery continues through the cervical vertebrae via small holes in the bone (like a string through pearls). At the base of the neck it finally joins with the opposite vertebral artery from the left.

The *left vertebral artery* originates directly off the *left subclavian artery*. It then follows a course through the *left cervical vertebrae* and joins with the *right vertebral artery*. Here the two vessels pass through an opening in the skull via the *foramen magnum*, located at the base of the skull (Fig. 1-21). Shortly after, the two vessels join to form the basilar artery.

The Basilar Artery

The basilar artery, which is intracranial (inside the skull), passes just a short distance and terminates at the two *posterior cerebral arteries*. (More on the intracranial vessels later).

I NEED A "FORAMAN MAGNUM" LIKE I NEED A HOLE IN THE HEAD

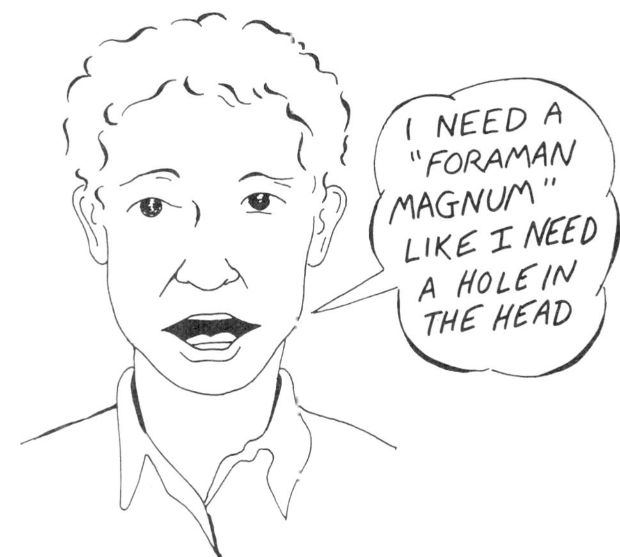

Fig. 1-21.

Review Exercise

1. Which is the first branch off the right subclavian artery?

   a. Right common carotid artery
   b. Right internal carotid artery
   c. Brachiocephalic
   d. Right vertebral artery

2. The right vertebral artery continues through the bones in the neck called the ______________________________ vertebra.

3. The right vertebral artery joins at the base of the neck with the opposite vertebral artery to form the

   a. circle of Willis
   b. posterior communicating artery
   c. posterior cerebral artery
   d. basilar artery

4. The left vertebral artery originates directly off the left ______________________________ artery.

5. The basilar artery passes just a short distance and terminates at the

   a. circle of Willis
   b. posterior communicating artery
   c. posterior cerebral arteries
   d. vertebrobasilar artery

6. Label the vessels of the posterior cerebrovascular circulation.

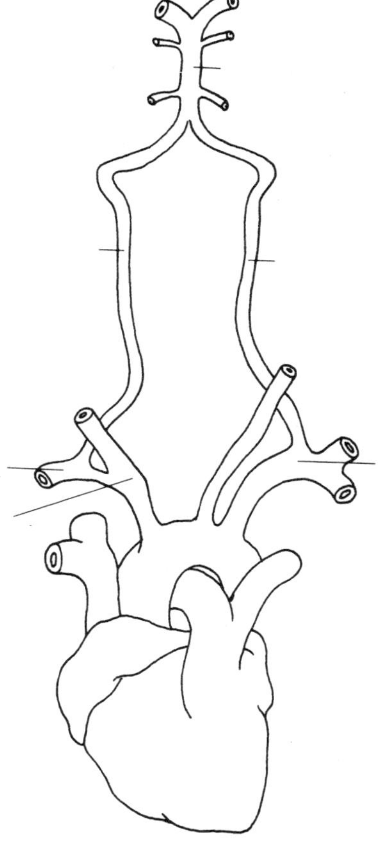

Circle of Willis

The brain is supplied directly by four extracranial vessels. They are the

1. right internal carotid artery
2. left internal carotid artery
3. right vertebral artery
4. left vertebral artery

Inside the cranium, the cerebral branches of the internal carotid arteries and the vertebral arteries are joined at the base of the skull by an arterial loop known as the *circle of Willis* (Fig 1-22), which then distributes blood to the brain via the

1. anterior cerebral arteries
2. midcerebral arteries
3. posterior cerebral arteries

The unique structure and function of the circle of Willis is appreciated when one considers the brain's excessive demand for the body's blood supply. Although the brain accounts for only 2% of the body's weight, it demands nearly 20% of the body's blood supply. Not only does the brain need a lot of blood to function, it cannot last for long without it.

The brain has a high metabolic rate that rapidly consumes oxygen and glucose, leaving little in reserve. It is therefore entirely dependent on the blood supply for its maintenance. That is why when the blood flow to the brain is even temporarily interrupted, brain death may occur in as few as 3 to 8 minutes.

The vital role of the circle of Willis is of particular importance to compensate for a lack of blood supply from one or more of the extracranial arteries. For example, the posterior circulation (vertebral arteries) can support the blood flow needs of the anterior brain in case of a significant reduction of blood flow within the carotid arteries. This hemodynamic assistance also works in reverse; should the vertebral arteries become diseased, the carotid arteries can feed the posterior brain via the circle of Willis.

The vessels forming the circle of Willis can be memorized by using the following analogy. If you use your imagination when studying the branches of the circle of Willis, you will notice that it somewhat resembles a frog (Fig. 1-22), but you will have to remember the stage the frog goes through between tadpole and full grown frog, when it still has a bit of a tail on the rear end, because that will be indicative of the *basilar artery*. You can also think of the two legs as resembling the *posterior cerebral arteries* and the two arms, the *middle cerebral arteries*. The head, with the two protruding eyes, will stand for the anterior communicating arteries.

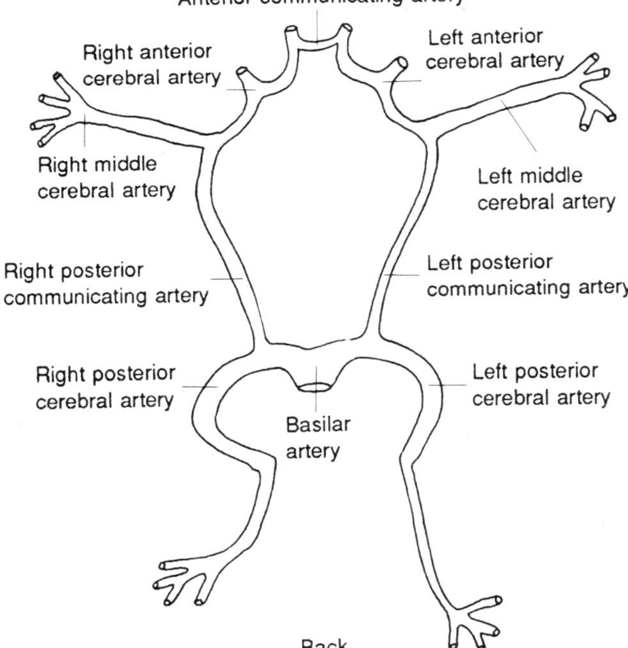

Fig. 1-22. The circle of Willis.

Periorbital Circulation

The *periorbital circulation* is important to the vascular specialist for two reasons. First, when there is a significant stenosis of the ICA, the ECA becomes an important *collateral vessel*. A collateral vessel is a small side-branch of the major vessel that, under certain circumstances, carries blood flow *around* a stenosis. Collateral blood flow will be discussed in detail in the pathophysiology section of this book (chapter 3). Blood flow may be rerouted to the ophthalmic artery and into the circle of Willis through various branches of the ECA.

Second, when testing the cerebrovascular system, the vascular specialist will learn Doppler techniques that will allow detection of flow direction in these vessels, thereby indirectly assessing the severity of ICA disease.

The Ophthalmic Artery and Its Branches

The ICA distributes almost all of its blood supply to *intracranial branches*, with one exception: the *ophthalmic artery*. This artery primarily supplies the eye with blood and then terminates into three branches in the face (see Fig. 1-19). These branches are the

1. nasal artery
2. frontal artery
3. supraorbital artery

The *nasal artery* passes along the lateral portion of the nose and then communicates with a facial branch of the external carotid artery. The *frontal* and *supraorbital arteries* turn upward and pass into the subcutaneous tissues just under the level of the eyebrow. Here they connect with branches of the *superficial temporal artery*. The importance of the connection of the branches will be recognized when we discuss collateral pathways that are used when the ICA is occluded or severely obstructed.

Review Exercise

1. The four main extracranial arteries that supply the brain with blood are the

   a. ______________________________

   b. ______________________________

   c. ______________________________

   d. ______________________________

2. The three main intracranial vessels that supply the brain with blood are the

   a. ______________________________

   b. ______________________________

   c. ______________________________

3. The brain has plenty of oxygen and glycogen reserves. True or False?

4. A main role of the circle of Willis is to ______________________ blood flow from either the anterior to the posterior circulation, or the posterior to the anterior circulation, when a condition of compromised blood flow exists.

5. Label the circle of Willis.

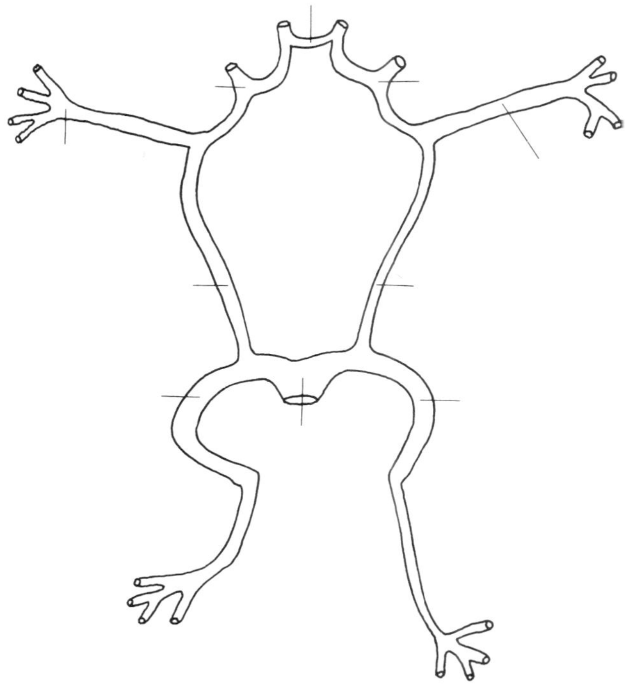

6. The internal carotid artery distributes all of its branches intracranially. True or False?

7. The three primary branches of the ophthalmic artery are

a. ______________________________

b. ______________________________

c. ______________________________

8. The branch that passes along the lateral portion of the nose and then communicates with a facial branch of the external carotid artery is the

a. facial artery
b. frontal artery
c. ophthalmic artery
d. nasal artery

9. The ____________ and ________________________ arteries turn upward and pass into the subcutaneous tissue just under the level of the eyebrow.

10. Label the vessels of the periorbital circulation.

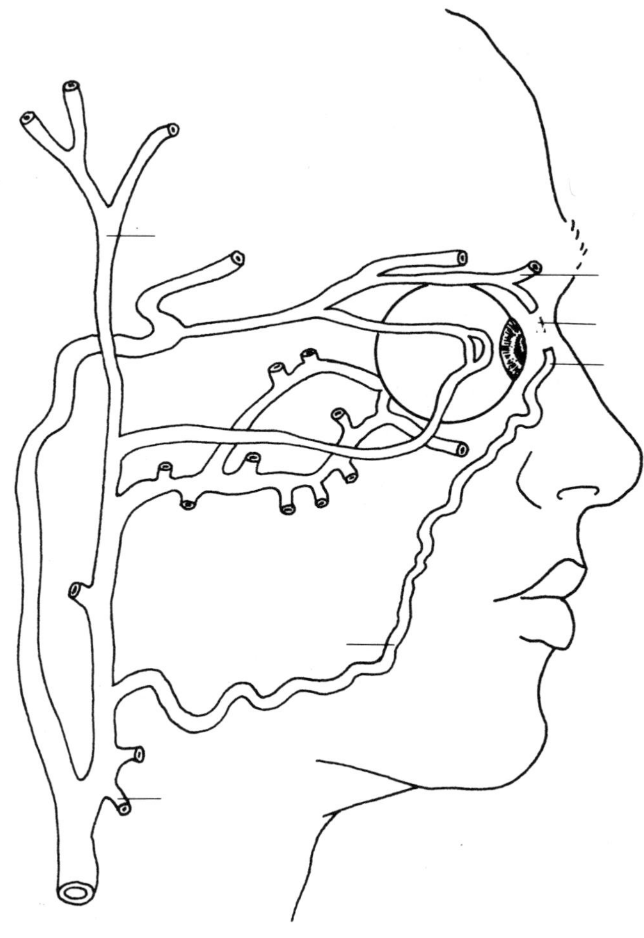

UPPER EXTREMITY ARTERIES

The vessels of the upper extremity are studied noninvasively for a variety of medical and surgical reasons. Although the arms generally have fewer vascular complications than the legs, it is important to be knowledgable about the arterial and venous anatomy.

Key Terms

Axillary artery
Brachial artery
Digital arteries
Innominate artery
Palmar arch
Radial artery
Subclavian artery
Ulnar artery

The Right Subclavian Artery

The *right subclavian artery* (Fig. 1-23) passes from the *innominate artery* just under the first rib. This is important to remember, especially when we study thoracic outlet syndromes. From just beyond the first rib to just beyond the axillary (armpit) region, the vessel takes an anterior course down the upper arm and is called the *axillary artery*.

From the axilla, the axillary artery extends downward and becomes the *brachial artery* in the upper arm. As it passes further down to the bend of the elbow, the brachial artery divides into two arteries: The artery passing along the antecubital fossa near the radius is appropriately named the *radial artery*, and the artery passing along the ulnar bone is named the *ulnar artery*.

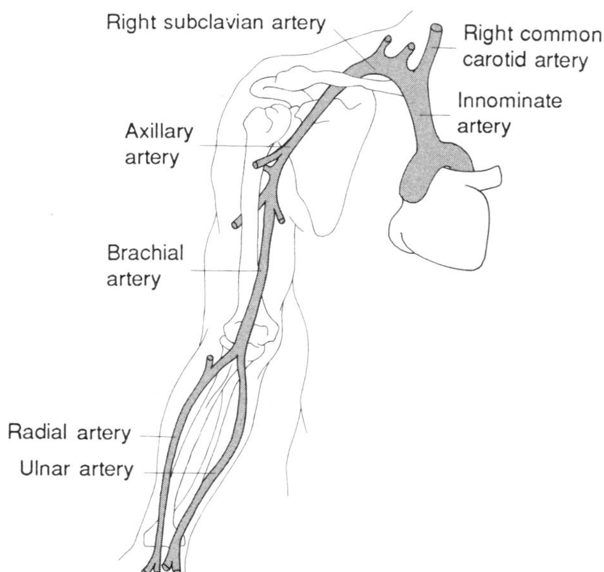

Fig. 1-23. The major arteries of the upper extremity.

Palmar Arch

The radial and ulnar arteries pass down the forearm to the palm, one artery on each side, and anastomose to form two *palmar arches* (Fig. 1-24): the *superficial palmar arch* and the *deep palmar arch*. From these arches arise the *digital arteries*, which supply blood to the fingers and the thumb.

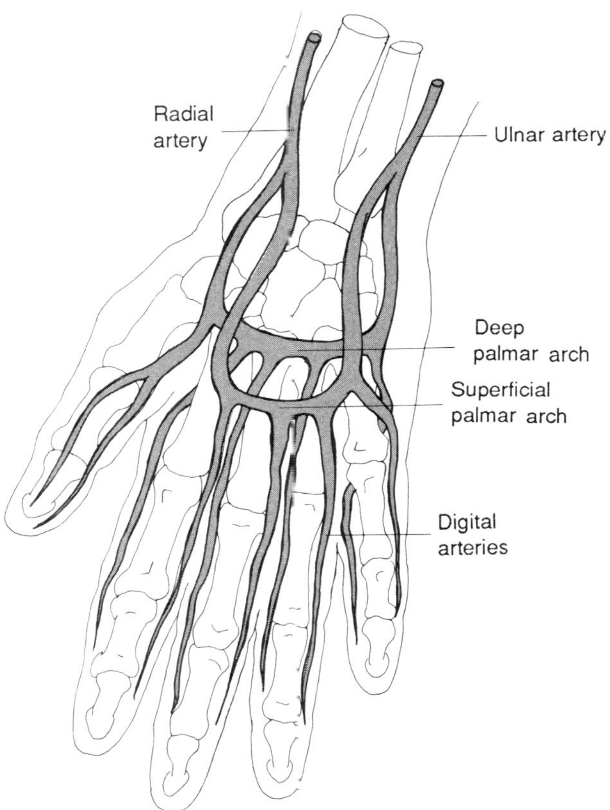

Fig. 1-24. The palmar arches.

Review Exercise

1. The ______________________________ artery passes from the innominate artery just under the first rib to the upper extremity.

2. From the axilla, the axillary artery extends downward and becomes the ______________________ artery in the upper arm.

3. The brachial artery branches into the __________ and the __________ arteries.

4. Label the major arteries of the upper extremities.

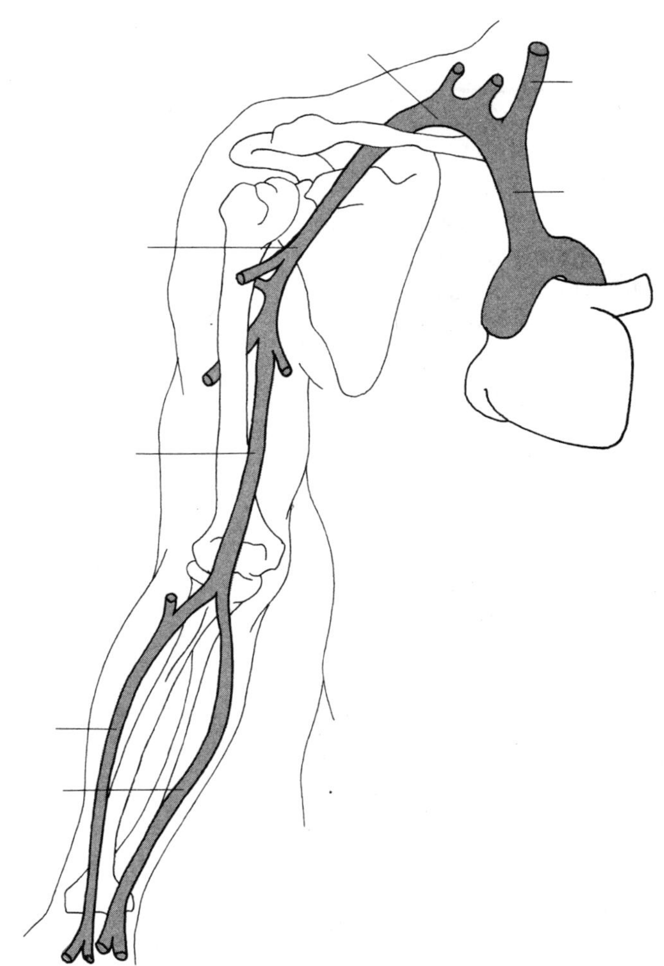

5. The radial and ulnar arteries anastomose to form two palmar arches:

   a. ______________________________

   b. ______________________________

6. From the arches in the palm of the hand arise the ______________, which supply blood to the fingers and the thumb.

7. Label the deep and superficial palmer arch vessels in the hands.

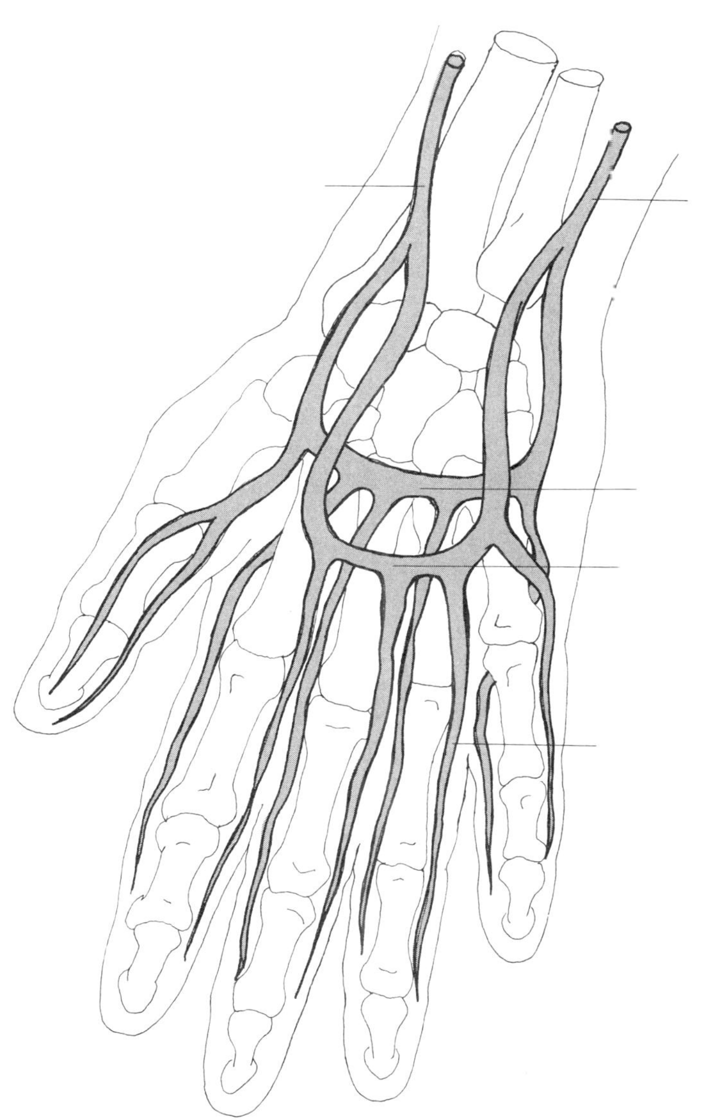

LOWER EXTREMITY ARTERIES

Peripheral arterial disease is a common disorder in the United States, affecting hundreds of thousands of patients each year. The vascular laboratory is the primary source for the initial screening of suspected vascular disease. An understanding of the normal anatomy is essential to perform examinations of the lower extremities. Figure 1-25 shows the routes of the lower extremity arteries.

Key Terms

Adductor canal
Anterior tibial artery
Arcuate artery
Common femoral artery
Digital artery
Dorsalis pedis artery
External iliac artery
Fibula
Hunter's canal
Inguinal ligament
Malleolus
Peroneal artery
Plantar artery
Popliteal artery
Popliteal fossa
Posterior tibial artery
Profunda femoris
Superficial femoral artery
Tibio-peroneal trunk

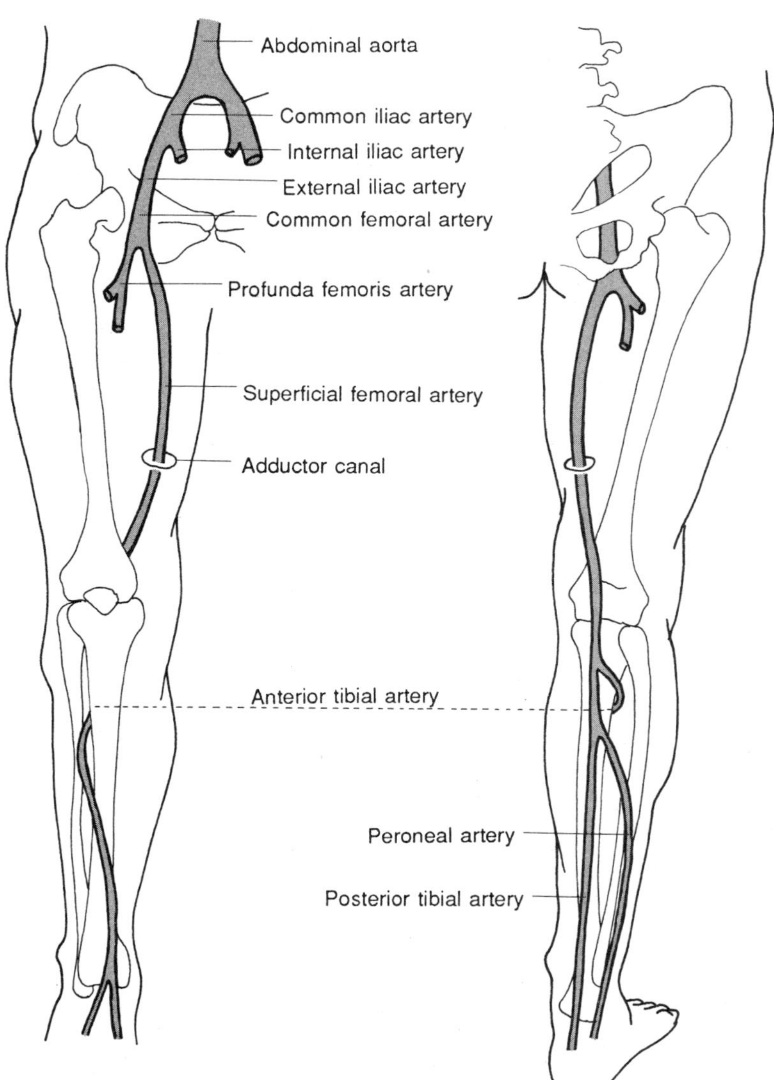

Fig. 1-25. The major arteries of the lower extremities.

Common Femoral Artery

In a previous section, we discussed the anatomy of the aorto-iliac system (aorta and iliac arteries) and some of the major arteries of the abdominal aorta. To continue with that path of blood flow, the *external iliac arteries* supply blood to the lower extremities. At the point where the external iliac artery passes under the *inguinal ligament*, it becomes the *common femoral artery* (CFA).

The inguinal ligament, also known as Poupart's ligament, passes between the iliac crest of the hip and the symphysis pubis. An easy anatomical site to remember is the inguinal crease, that fold of skin in the groin that somewhat divides the lower abdomen from the leg. About an inch beyond the inguinal crease, the common femoral artery bifurcates into the profunda femoris (i.e., the *deep femoral artery*) and the *superficial femoral artery* (SFA).

The Profunda and Superficial Femoral Arteries

The *profunda femoris artery* is posterior and lateral to the *superficial femoral artery*. Branches of the profunda femoris include numerous perforators (branches that penetrate through the muscles). These perforators include the *medial* and *lateral circumflex arteries*.

The superficial femoral artery continues down a medial lateral route until it dives deep through *Hunter's canal* at the middle to lower third of the thigh. The superficial femoral artery must now enter the large quadriceps muscle in order to continue its posterior medial path to the back of the knee. The area in which the vessel enters and exits that muscle is Hunter's canal, also known as the *adductor canal* (Fig. 1-25).

As the superficial femoral artery enters Hunter's canal, it makes a small bend in order to continue its route to the *popliteal fossa* (*fossa* means "space") in the posterior aspect of the leg. *Remember*: Whenever a vessel makes a turn, the area of the bend is susceptible to disease because of the change in flow dynamics that occurs.

Popliteal Artery, Tibials, and Peroneal Artery

The *popliteal artery* is the continuation of the superficial femoral artery and courses behind the knee in the popliteal fossa. Minor branches of the popliteal artery include the *sural* and *genicular arteries*.

The popliteal artery continues downward for a short distance before bifurcating. The first major branch off the popliteal artery is the *anterior tibial artery*. The anterior tibial artery passes laterally and then anteriorly along the tibia and runs deep and anterior to the leg. (To remember which is the bigger of the leg bones, think of *fibula*. *Fib* is a little lie, and fibula is a little bone compared with the tibia.)

After the bifurcation of the anterior tibial artery, the second branch of the *popliteal artery* becomes the *tibio-peroneal trunk* (T-P trunk). The tibio-peroneal trunk passes distally about an inch before dividing into the *peroneal* and the *posterior tibial arteries*. The peroneal artery supplies the medial side of the fibula (small bone). The posterior tibial artery continues a medial and slightly posterior path to the foot.

Dorsalis Pedis Artery (Pedal)

The anterior tibial artery eventually approaches the dorsum (top) of the foot where it becomes the *dorsalis pedis artery* (Fig 1-26). This is often the most distal palpable pulse. The dorsalis pedis then goes on to bifurcate into the *arcuate* and *digital arteries* of the foot.

Posterior Tibial Artery (Pedal)

As the *posterior tibial* reaches the medial side of the ankle, it is situated between the *medial malleolus* (inside ankle bone) and the calcaneal tuberosity (heel bone). The posterior tibial artery then divides into the *medial* and *lateral plantar arteries* of the foot. The arteries of the foot, or *pedal arteries*, are shown in Figure 1-26.

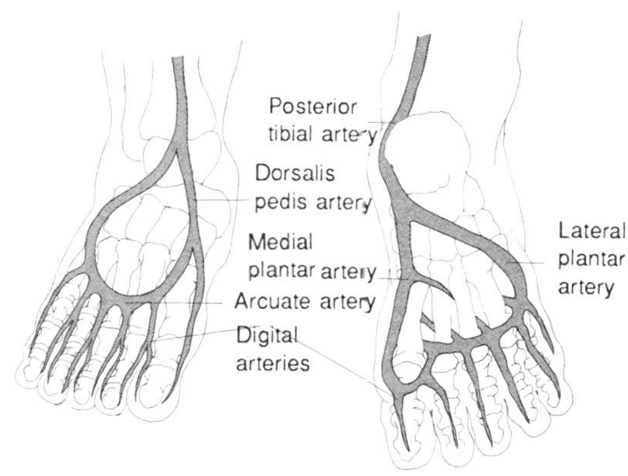

Fig. 1-26. The major arteries of the foot.

Review Exercise

1. At the point where the external iliac artery passes under the inguinal ligament, it becomes the

   a. profunda
   b. common femoral artery
   c. superficial femoral artery
   d. internal iliac artery

2. The common femoral artery divides into the

   a. profunda femoris artery and the deep femoral artery
   b. common femoral artery and the superficial femoral artery
   c. common femoral artery and the profunda femoris artery
   d. profunda femoris artery and the superficial femoral artery

3. The profunda femoris artery is also known as the ______________________________.

4. The superficial femoral artery dives deep through ____________________ canal at about the middle to lower third of the thigh.

5. Behind the knee, the superficial femoral artery becomes the ____________________ artery.

6. The first major branch off the popliteal artery is the

   a. posterior tibial artery
   b. anterior tibial artery
   c. deep posterior artery
   d. peroneal artery

7. The anterior tibial artery gradually approaches the top of the foot where it becomes the

   a. arcuate artery
   b. peroneal artery
   c. malleolus artery
   d. dorsalis pedis artery

8. Once in the foot, the dorsalis pedis artery divides into

   a. ______________________________

   b. ______________________________

9. The tibial peroneal trunk divides into the

   a. anterior tibial and posterior tibial arteries
   b. anterior tibial and peroneal arteries
   c. posterior tibial and peroneal arteries
   d. popliteal and anterior tibial arteries

10. Label the arteries of the leg.

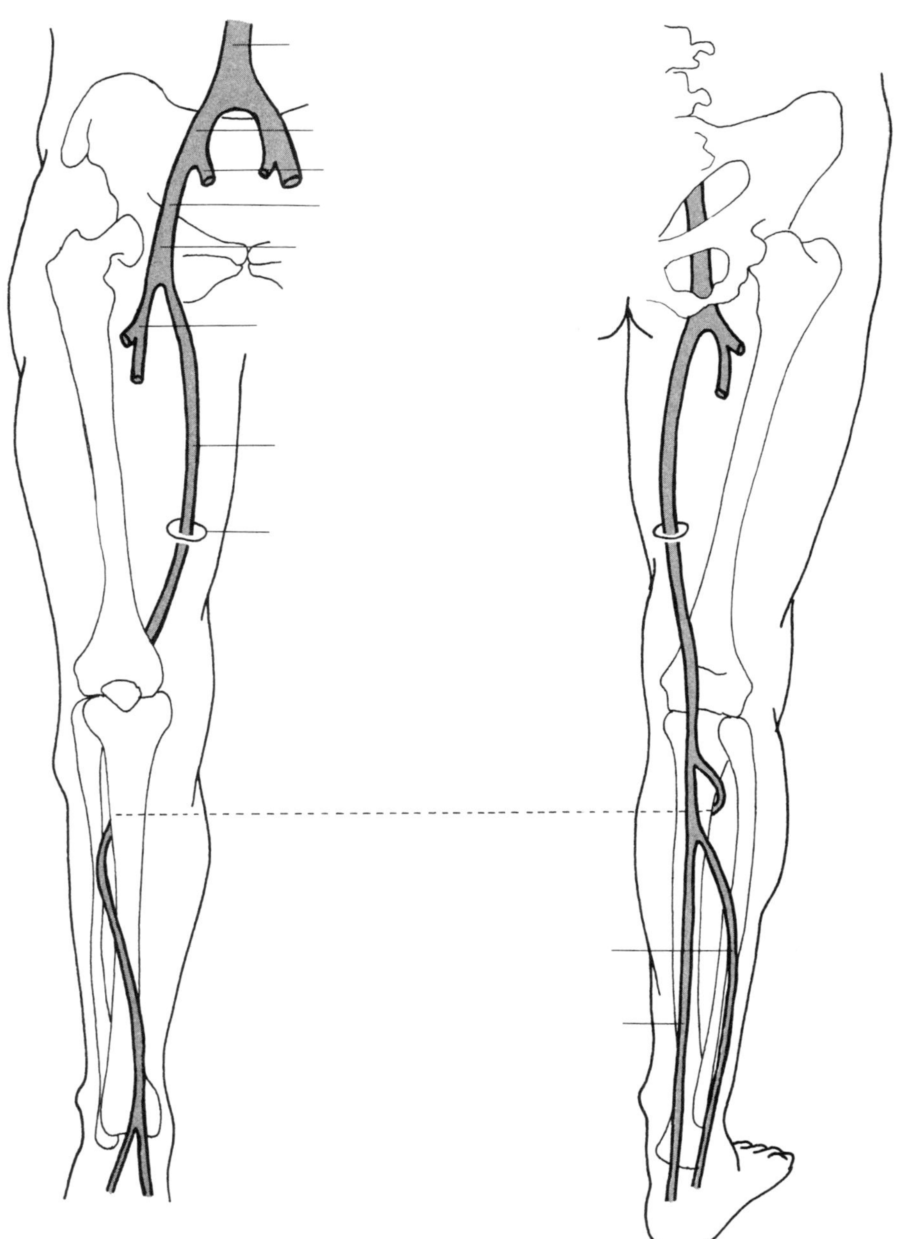

11. Once the posterior tibial reaches the foot, it is situated between the ______________________ and the ______________________ and further divides into the ____________ and ____________ arteries.

12. Label the arteries of the foot.

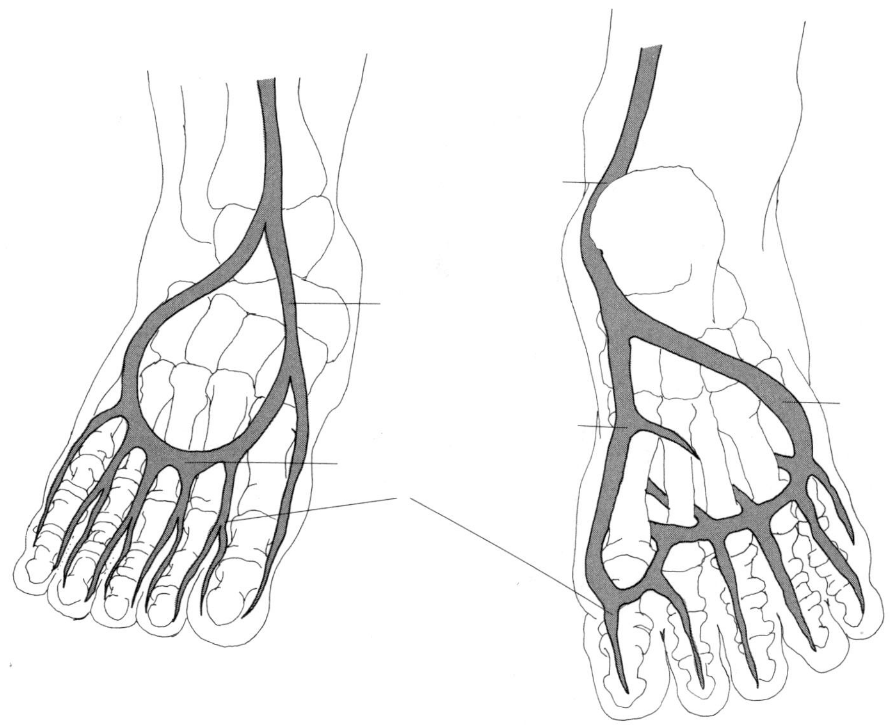

THE VENOUS SYSTEM

Venous anatomy is a little more difficult to grasp than arterial anatomy because there are more variations on what is considered normal. For example, veins usually run in pairs below the knee, but they can sometimes run in threes as well. Because practitioners are becoming more and more dependent on the vascular lab, it is critical that the vascular specialist be particularly knowledgable about the normal venous anatomy.

Key Terms

- Anterior tibial vein
- Axillary vein
- Basilic vein
- Cephalic veins
- Common femoral vein
- Coronary sinus
- Deep femoral vein
- Deep venous system
- Gastrocnemius muscle
- Greater saphenous vein
- Iliac vein
- Inferior vena cava
- Lesser saphenous vein
- Perforator veins
- Peroneal vein
- Popliteal vein
- Portal vein
- Posterior tibial veins
- Saphenofemoral junction
- Soleus muscle
- Subclavian vein
- Superficial femoral veins
- Superficial venous system
- Superior mesenteric vein
- Superior vena cava
- Thrombus
- Venous sinusoids
- Venous valves

Veins of the Lower Extremity

Several characteristics of the venous system account for the complexity of venous anatomy. First of all, there are *deep* and *superficial venous systems*. Veins in the calf tend to run in pairs, coursing along the artery on each side. There are also communicating, or *perforator, veins* that connect the deep and superficial systems. Finally, veins have one-way valves that allow blood to flow in one direction only. Figure 1-27 shows the veins of the lower extremity.

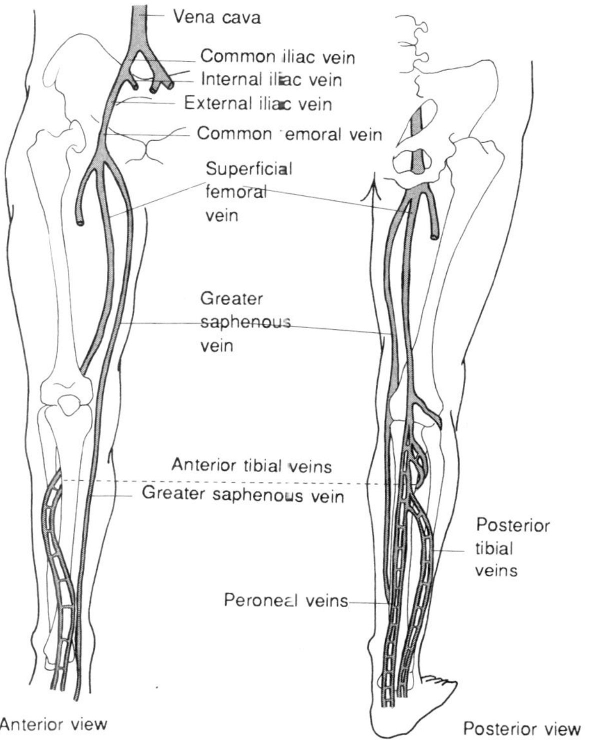

Fig. 1-27. The major veins of the lower extremities.

Deep Veins

Posterior Tibial Veins

The *posterior tibial vein* is formed by the union of the medial and lateral plantar veins just behind the medial malleolus (the ankle bone). Remember: Plantar is to the foot as palm is to the hand. From the medial malleolus, the posterior tibial vein dives deeply into the calf muscle, receives blood from the *peroneal vein*, and unites with the *anterior tibial vein* just below the knee.

Anterior Tibial Vein

The *anterior tibial vein* is an upward continuation of the *dorsalis pedis vein* of the foot. It runs between the tibia and fibula and unites with the posterior tibial vein to form the *popliteal vein*.

Popliteal Vein

The *popliteal vein*, located behind the knee, receives blood from the anterior and posterior tibial veins and the *lesser saphenous vein* in the calf muscle. It is medial to the *popliteal artery* and courses laterally through the *adductor canal*.

The Profunda, Superficial Femoral, and Common Femoral Veins

The *superficial femoral vein* is a continuation of the popliteal vein just above the knee. The superficial femoral vein runs up the medial aspect of the leg alongside the superficial femoral artery and drains deep structures of the thigh. After receiving the blood from the greater saphenous vein in the groin, the superficial femoral vein continues briefly before becoming the common femoral vein. The *profunda vein*, or *deep femoral vein*, courses the thigh along the profunda artery. The *profunda* and *superficial femoral veins* unite in the groin to form the *common femoral vein*.

Iliac Veins

The *iliac vein* is a continuation of the common femoral vein. The *right* and *left internal iliac veins* receive blood from the pelvic wall, viscera, external genitals, buttocks, and medial aspect of the thigh. The right and left internal iliac veins join the left and right external iliac veins to form the *common iliac veins*. The common iliac veins join to form the *inferior vena cava*.

Superficial Veins

Greater Saphenous Vein

Beginning just anteriorly and laterally to the medial malleolus, the *greater saphenous vein* (the longest vein in the body) passes upward medially along the calf and thigh. If you don't have socks on and you're sitting at your desk, you may see branches of the greater saphenous vein in your foot. It contains numerous branches. From the thigh, the greater saphenous vein enters the common femoral vein in the groin.

Saphenofemoral Junction

The junction of the *proximal greater saphenous vein* and the common femoral vein forms an important anatomic location referred to as the *saphenofemoral junction*. It is an important landmark for the vascular specialist when identifying the varied and sometimes confusing venous anatomy in the groin.

Lesser Saphenous Vein

The *lesser saphenous vein* begins just posterior to the lateral malleolus and runs upward along the posterior aspect of the calf where it joins into the popliteal vein.

Review Exercise

1. Which statement is *not* true about veins?

   a. Veins in the calf tend to run in pairs.
   b. Veins usually follow the same course as arteries.
   c. Venous anatomy rarely varies.
   d. Most veins have valves.

2. Veins have ______________ to allow blood flow in one direction only.

3. The vein formed by the union of the medial and lateral plantar veins just behind the medial malleolus is the

   a. peroneal vein
   b. posterior plantar vein
   c. medial plantar vein
   d. posterior tibial vein

4. Which vein dives deeply into the calf muscle, receives blood from the peroneal vein, and unites with the anterior tibial vein just below the knee?

   a. Peroneal vein
   b. Posterior plantar vein
   c. Medial plantar vein
   d. Posterior tibial vein

5. Which vein runs between the tibia and fibula and unites with the posterior tibial vein to form the popliteal vein?

   a. Peroneal vein
   b. Posterior plantar vein
   c. Anterior tibial vein
   d. Posterior tibial vein

6. The popliteal vein, located behind the knee, receives blood from the

   a. ____
   b. ____
   c. ____

7. The ____ is a continuation of the popliteal vein just above the knee.

8. Which veins receive blood from the pelvic wall, viscera, external genitals, buttocks, and medial aspect of the thigh?

   a. Common femoral veins
   b. Internal iliac veins
   c. External iliac veins
   d. Common iliac veins

9. The ____ join the ____ to form the common iliac veins.

10. The common iliac veins join to form the inferior vena cava. True or False?

11. Which is the longest vein in the body?

    a. The inferior vena cava
    b. The superficial femoral vein
    c. The posterior tibial vein
    d. The greater saphenous vein

12. The posterior lateral vein begins just posterior to the lateral malleolus and runs upward along the posterior aspect of the calf. True or False?

14. Label the veins of the lower extremity.

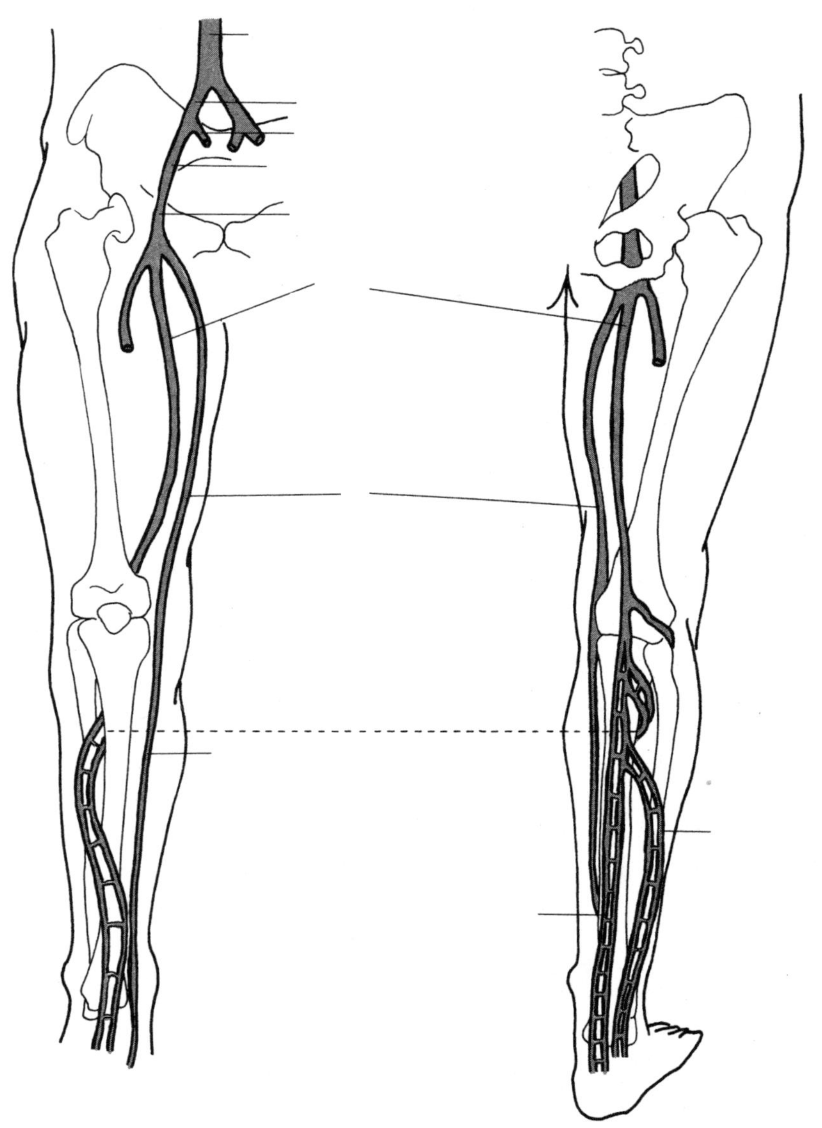

Perforator Veins

Perforator veins connect the deep and superficial venous systems. Of particular interest are approximately six medial calf perforators that join the *posterior tibial vein* and the *greater saphenous vein* through a series of communicating veins known as the *posterior arch vein*. Other perforators connect the *peroneal vein* with superficial tributaries of the *greater saphenous vein*.

These perforators are generally more numerous in the calf but are often found in the thigh as well. The *Hunterian perforator* (named after the Hunter of Hunter's canal) connects the *superficial femoral vein* to the greater saphenous vein.

Venous Sinuses

The term *sinus* means "cavity." In the calf, there are venous sinuses called *sinusoids*. When you add *oids* at the end of a word, it means "similar to"; *sinusoids* therefore means "sinus-like." The *venous sinusoids* are spindle-shaped veins that collect venous drainage from the *soleus* and *gastrocnemius muscles* in the calf. The soleal muscles are the inner calf muscles and the gastrocnemius muscle is the outer calf muscle.

Venous sinusoids are important for two reasons, one beneficial and the other not. They are beneficial because they act as "bellows" of the muscle pump to assist the return of venous blood upward. They may *not* be beneficial because these cavities essentially hold venous blood until the muscle pumps it out. Thus, if the patient has been immobile for a period of time, because of illness, trauma, or long periods of sitting, the sinusoids become an ideal site for venous blood clots, or *thrombi* (plural of *thrombus*). (The development of venous thrombi will be discussed in detail in the chapter 3.)

The soleal sinusoids drain into the posterior tibial and peroneal veins. The gastrocnemius sinusoids empty into the popliteal vein.

Review Exercise

1. Veins that drain venous blood from the superficial system to the deep venous system are called the

   a. saphenous system b. perforator veins
   c. vena cava d. venous sinusoids

2. The ________________________ connects the superficial femoral vein to the greater saphenous vein.

3. The term *sinus* means:

   a. blockage b. congestion
   c. pressure d. cavity

4. In the calf, there are venous sinuses called ________________.

5. Venous sinusoids are spindle-shaped veins that collect venous drainage from the ________ and ________________________.

6. Venous sinusoids are beneficial because these cavities retain blood until the muscle pumps it out. True or False?

7. The soleal sinusoids drain into the ________________________ and ________________ veins.

8. The gastrocnemius sinusoids empty into the popliteal vein. True or False?

Veins of the Upper Extremity

Blood from the upper extremity is returned to the heart by deep and superficial veins. As in the lower extremities, both sets of veins contain valves.

Superficial Veins

The *superficial veins* of the upper extremity anastomose extensively with each other and the deep veins. In this section, we will limit discussion of the superficial venous anatomy to the following:

1. Superficial veins of the hands, fingers, and forearm
2. Superficial radial and ulnar veins
3. Median basilic vein
4. Cephalic and basilic veins.

Superficial Veins of the Hands, Fingers, and Forearm

The superficial veins of the hands drain venous blood to the *superficial ulnar* and *radial veins.* The superficial ulnar veins receive blood from numerous branches and form the *basilic vein* in the upper arm. The superficial radial veins also receive blood from numerous branches in the forearm and ascend to the upper arm to form the *cephalic vein* (Fig. 1-28). The *medium basilic vein* is a superficial vein that lies in front of the brachial artery in the anterior segment of the elbow. This is the vein most commonly used for blood drawing or venipuncture.

Cephalic Veins

The *cephalic vein* originates at the radial side of the back of the hand (dorsal arch) and winds up the arm along the radial bone and artery of the forearm. At this point, just below the bend of the elbow, the cephalic unites with the accessory vein to form the cephalic vein of the upper arm. It continues into the axillary vein, which is just proximal to the first rib.

Basilic Veins

The *basilic vein* of each forearm originates at the ulnar aspect of the arm and, as you may have guessed, winds up along the *ulnar artery* and *vein* (Fig. 1-28). The basilic vein extends along the posterior aspect of the forearm and then courses laterally up the forearm.

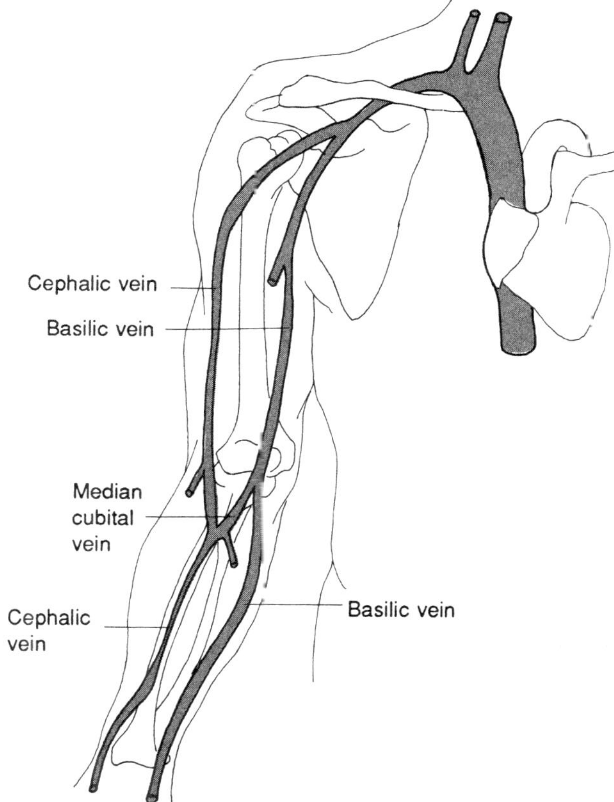

Fig. 1-28. The major superficial veins of the upper extremities.

Deep Veins

The *deep veins* of the upper extremity course along the sides of the arteries and are named according to their proximity to a particular artery. Keep in mind that there are both superficial and deep veins with the same name (i.e., superficial and deep ulnar vein); it is important to be specific in your references to them. Because you have already learned the names of the arteries in the upper extremities, you will recognize the following names:

1. Deep ulnar and radial veins
2. Brachial vein
3. Axillary vein
4. Subclavian vein

Deep Radial and Ulnar Veins

The *deep palmar veins* of the hand drain blood from the digits and hand and communicate with the *deep radial* and *ulnar veins*, which course with their corresponding arteries. These two veins terminate at the *brachial vein* at the *antecubital fossa* (anterior space of the elbow).

Brachial and Axillary Veins

Brachial veins course on either side of the brachial artery, receiving blood from numerous branches in the forearm. The brachial vein joins the *axillary vein*, which is a continuation of the basilic vein. The axillary vein is a large vein that terminates at the first rib to become the *subclavian veins*.

Subclavian Veins

The right and left *subclavian veins* lie just below the clavicle. They unite with the internal jugular vein to form the *brachiocephalic veins*. The subclavian veins usually have a large valve positioned about 3/4 of an inch from the *innominate vein*.

Review Exercise

1. The five deep veins of the upper extremities are

   a. ______________________________

   b. ______________________________

   c. ______________________________

   d. ______________________________

   e. ______________________________

2. The main superficial veins in the upper segment of the arm are

   a. ______________________________

   b. ______________________________

3. The radial and ulnar veins drain blood from the ______________________________.

4. The ______________________________ originates at the radial side of the dorsal arch in the hand and winds up the arm along the radial bone and artery of the forearm.

5. The ______________ vein of the forearm originates at the ulnar aspect of each arm and extends along the posterior aspect of the forearm.

6. Which vein is a continuation of the basilic vein at the upper arm?

   a. Median cubital vein
   b. Axillary vein
   c. Brachial vein
   d. Ulnar vein

7. The right and left subclavian veins unite with the internal jugular vein to form the ______________________________ veins.

8. Label the veins.

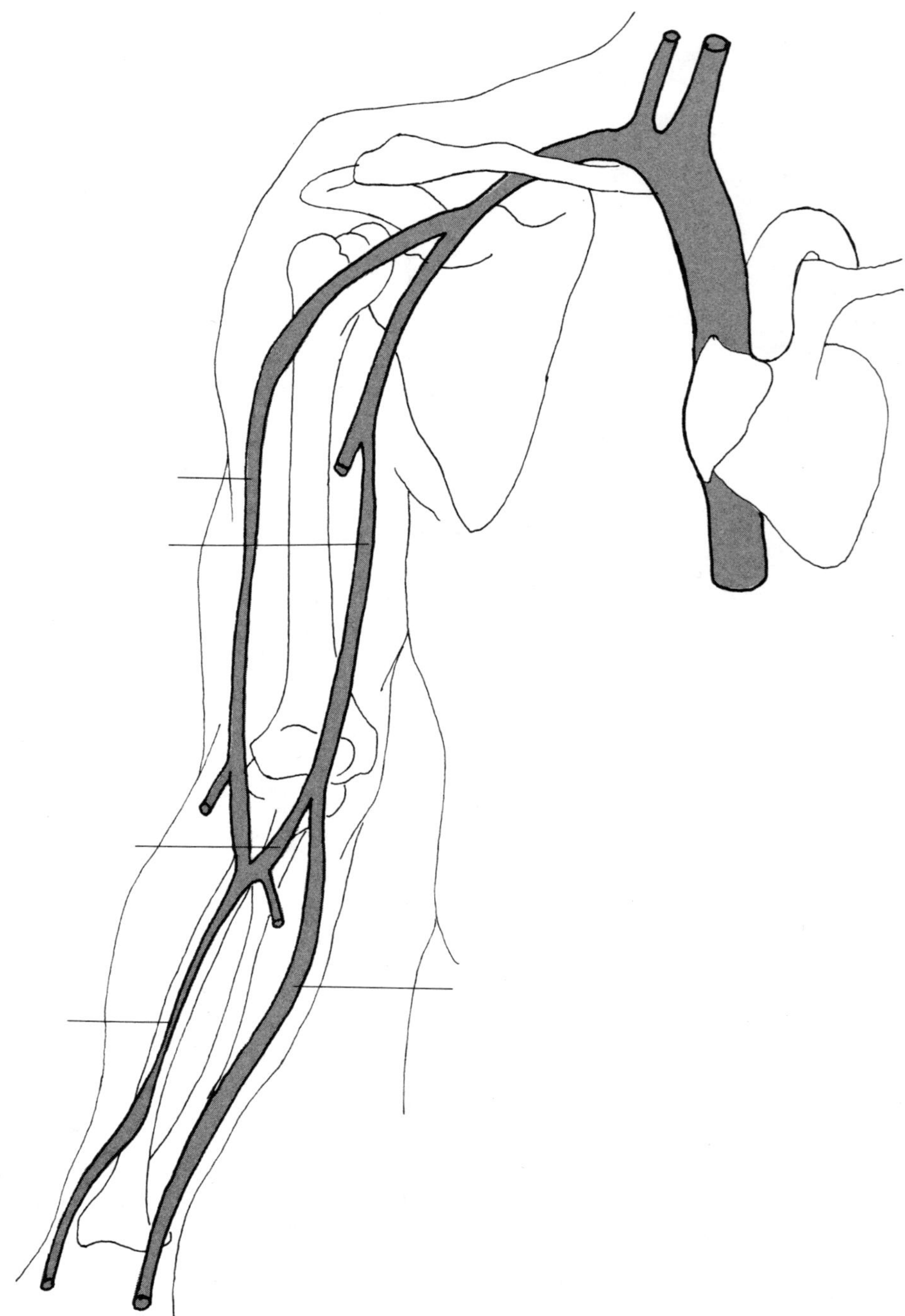

Central Veins

Vena Cavas and Cardiac Veins

All veins return blood to the *right atrium* though one of three large vessels:

1. The coronary sinus
2. The superior vena cava
3. The inferior vena cava

The return flow from the coronary arteries is taken up by the *cardiac veins*, which empty into the large vein of the heart called the *coronary sinus*. From here, the blood empties into the right atrium of the heart.

The veins that empty into the *superior vena cava* (Fig. 1-29) are the veins of the

1. head
2. neck
3. upper extremities
4. thorax
5. azygous vein

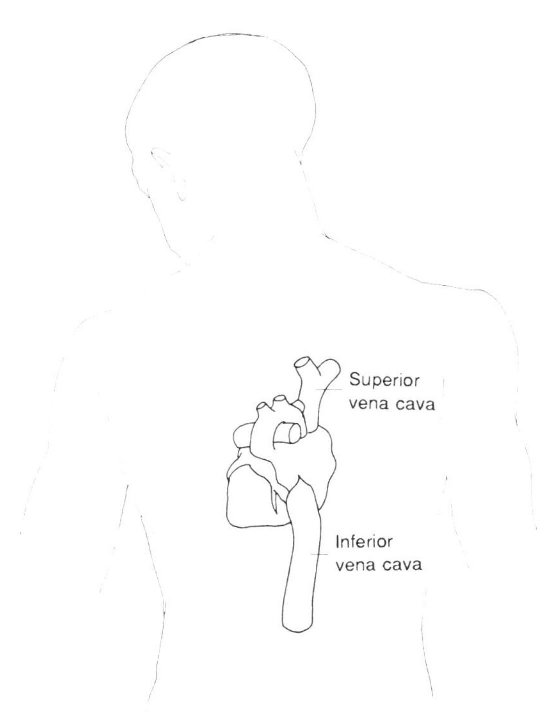

Fig. 1-29. The azygous of the heart.

The veins that empty into the *inferior vena cava* (Fig. 1-29) are the veins of the

1. abdomen
2. pelvis
3. lower extremities
4. azygous vein

Note that the *azygous vein* connects together the inferior and superior vena cavas.

Portal Veins

The *portal system* (Fig. 1-30) includes veins that drain blood from the pancreas, spleen, stomach, intestines, and gallbladder. Drained blood is then transported to the *portal vein* of the liver. The portal vein is formed by the union of the *superior mesenteric vein*, the *inferior mesenteric vein*, and the *splenic vein*.

Portal venous blood, unlike venous blood in general, is rich from nutritive substances that have been absorbed from the digestive tract. Recall that the role of the liver is to monitor and filter these substances before they are passed into general circulation. For example, the liver stores nutrients such as glucose, modifies other digested substances so they may be more easily absorbed by cells, and detoxifies harmful substances.

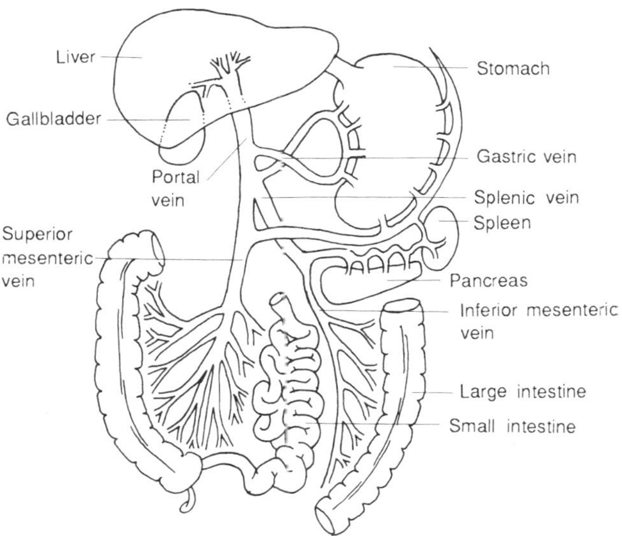

Fig. 1-30. The portal venous circulation.

Review Exercise

1. All systemic veins return blood to the right atrium through one of three large vessels:

   a. ______________________________

   b. ______________________________

   c. ______________________________

2. The return blood flow from the coronary arteries is taken up by the ______________________, which empty into the large vein of the heart called the coronary vein.

3. The veins of the head, neck, upper extremities, and thorax empty into the

   a. subclavian veins b. superior vena cava
   c. innominate veins d. azygous

4. The veins of the abdomen, pelvis, and the lower extremities empty into the

   a. iliac veins b. femoral veins
   c. inferior vena cava d. azygous

5. The azygous vein empties blood from the ______________________ and the ______________________.

6. Label the vessels.

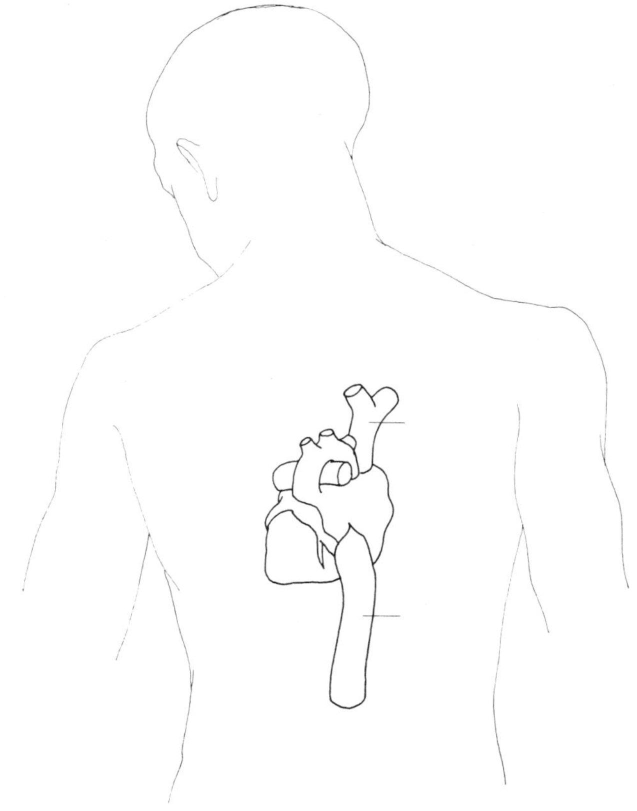

7. The portal system includes veins that drain blood from the

a. ______________________________

b. ______________________________

c. ______________________________

d. ______________________________

e. ______________________________

8. The portal vein of the liver is formed by the union of the ______________________________ and the ____________________ veins.

9. Portal blood is rich from substances that have been absorbed from the ______________________________.

10. Label the veins.

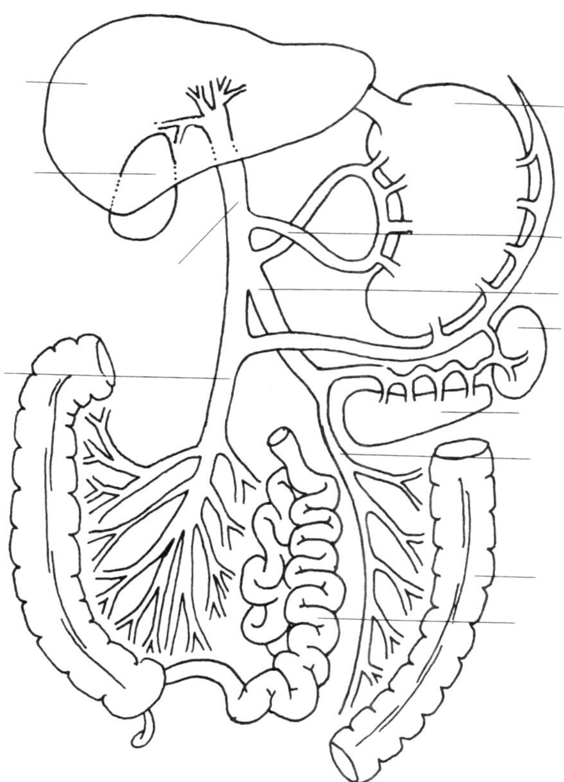

STRUCTURAL ANATOMY OF THE BLOOD VESSELS

Now that we are getting into the specific anatomy of the vascular system, more detail will be provided. The *structural anatomy* is important, not only because it will help the student better understand physiology, but also because as vascular professionals, you will be imaging the structures of the vessels in detail.

Key Terms

Adventitia
Arterioles
Bicuspid valves
Connective tissue
Contractility
Elasticity
Elastic tissue
Endothelial cells
Intima
Lumen
Media
Tunica

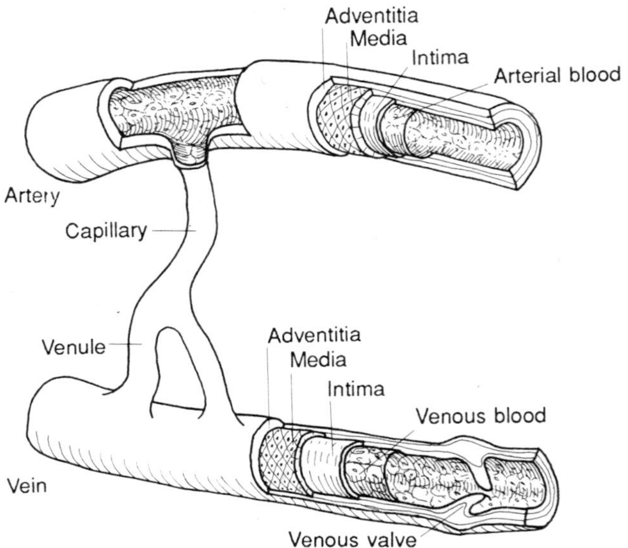

Fig. 1-31. Cross-sectional anatomy of the artery and vein.

Arteries

Arteries have walls constructed of three coats called *tunica* and a hollow middle called a *lumen*. (Think of tunica as tunics [like a toga] worn in ancient times.) The innermost wall (layer) of the artery is called the *intima* (Fig. 1-31). It is composed of *endothelial cells* that are in contact with the blood. The middle layer, or *media*, is usually the thickest layer and contains a layer of *elastic* and *connective tissue* that consists of elastic fibers and smooth muscle. The outer layer of the arterial wall is called the *adventitia*, which is principally composed of *fibrous tissue* that prevents the artery from collapsing when cut.

Elasticity and Contractility

Because of the structure of the media, arteries have two very important properties: *elasticity* and *contractility*. As discussed earlier, the ventricles of the heart contract and send a surge of blood into the arterial system; the artery normally expands a little to contain the extra volume of blood. Then, as the ventricle relaxes, the elastic recoil of the subsequently relaxing vessel propels the blood further down its path toward the *arterioles*.

Veins

Veins are fairly similar in construction to the arteries except for the size of their walls. Both have three layers (Fig. 1-31), but because veins are not subject to the repeated pressure from a pumping ventricle, the walls of a vein are much thinner. Veins also have the ability to collapse when the pressure in the lumen is less than that of the outside tissue.

Venous Valves

A significant feature of veins, not found in arteries, is the presence of *bicuspid valves* (Fig. 1-32). *Bicuspid* refers to the valves as having two cusps. These valves, when working properly, prevent blood flow from moving backward down the leg or arm.

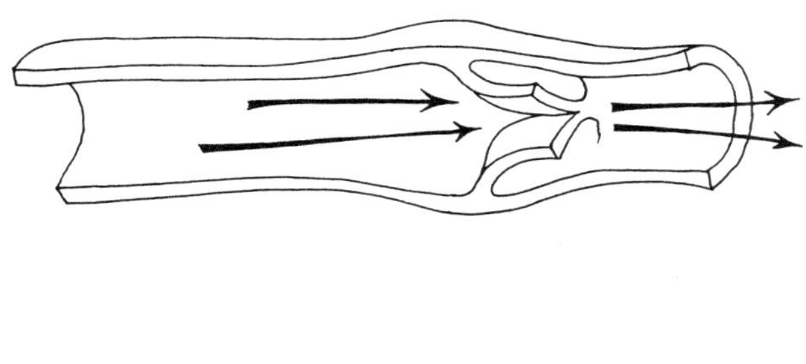

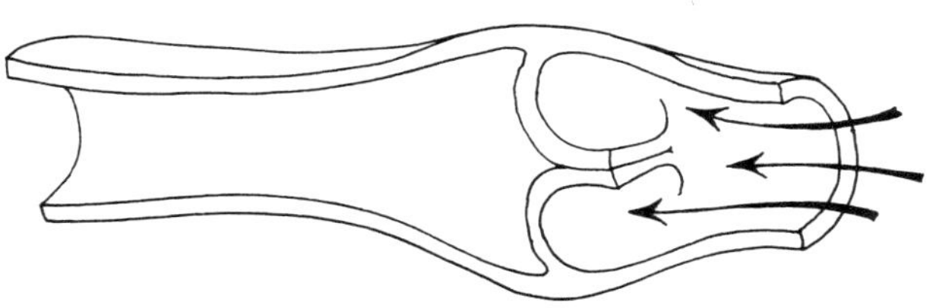

Fig. 1-32. Bicuspid valves of veins.

Valves are more numerous in the calf than in the thigh. The reason for this is that there is greater hydrostatic pressure in veins. *Hydrostatic pressure* refers to the weight of a column of blood. (This will be discussed in greater depth in chapter 2.) In the calf, valves can be found every inch or so. The popliteal vein usually has just one valve, and the superficial femoral vein typically has three.

The perforator veins also have valves, usually two. These valves assist the shunting of blood from the superficial to the deep system. The saphenous veins in the leg usually have seven to nine valves. Only about 25% of iliac veins have valves, but the vena cava has none.

Review Exercise

1. The intima is composed of ______________________________ cells that are in contact with the blood.

2. The media is usually the thickest layer. It consists of ____________ and ______________________ tissue.

3. The adventitia is principally composed of ____________ tissue.

4. Arteries have two very important properties:

   a. Pulsatility and rigidity
   b. Pulsatility and elasticity
   c. Elasticity and contraction
   d. Elasticity and contractility

5. Veins are exactly the same in construction and size as arteries. True or False?

6. A significant feature of veins, not found in arteries, is the presence of tricuspid valves, which prevent blood flow from moving backward. True or False?

7. Valves are more numerous in the calf than in the thigh. True or False?

8. The number of valves in the popliteal vein usually number about

   a. 0
   b. 1
   c. 2-3
   d. 3
   e. 5-7

9. The number of valves in the superficial femoral vein usually number about

   a. 0
   b. 1
   c. 3
   d. 3-5
   e. 5-7

10. The number of valves in the saphenous veins usually number about

    a. 0
    b. 1-2
    c. 2-3
    d. 3-5
    e. 7-9

11. Only about ____________ of iliac veins have valves.

    a. 1%
    b. 25%
    c. 50%
    d. 75%

12. The number of valves in the vena cava usually number about

    a. 0
    b. 1-2
    c. 2-3
    d. 3-5
    e. 5-7

13. The perforator veins have valves that assist the shunting of blood from the ______________________________ to the _______________ system.

14. Label the vessels and the layers of the arterial and venous walls.

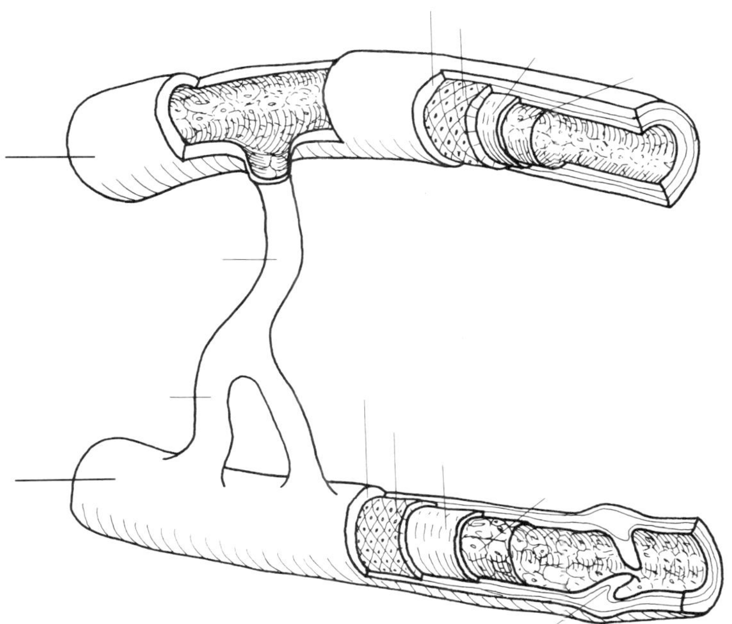

2 Hemodynamics

As recently as the 1500s, most people, including physicians, believed that blood just sort of ebbed and flowed in the body. It was not until the late 1500s that William Harvey, an English physician, explained that blood actually circulated throughout the system. Since that time, a great deal more has been learned about the physiology of blood flow. In this section, we will concentrate primarily on how blood moves throughout the body and what controls the vascular system utilizes to monitor pressure in various resting, exercise, normal, and diseased states.

FUNDAMENTALS OF HEMODYNAMICS

Key Terms

Acceleration
Average blood pressure
Bernoulli effect
Blood pressure
Cardiac cycle
Cardiac output
Deceleration
Elasticity
Energy gradient
Flow
Friction
Inertia
Myocardial infarction
Poiseuille's law
Pressure/flow relationship
Pulsatile flow
Resistance
Steady flow
Velocity
Viscosity
Volume

Bernoulli Principle

Daniel Bernoulli (1700-1782) was a Swiss mathematician, sometimes referred to as the founder of mathematical physics. Bernoulli unified the study of hydrodynamics under what became known as the conservation of energy, which states that energy can be changed but it cannot be destroyed. He is best known in the noninvasive vascular field for the Bernoulli effect, which is the reduction in pressure that accompanies the increase of velocity of fluid flow.

Energy Gradient

What makes blood flow? Blood flows through its system of closed vessels because of an energy gradient. An energy gradient is the difference in pressure at one point within the vessel when compared with another. Blood always flows from regions of higher pressure to lower pressure (Fig. 2-1).

The *average blood pressure* in the aorta is about 100 mmHg. (The abbreviation mmHg refers to millimeters of mercury.) This pressure continually decreases to about 45 mmHg after the blood flows from the aorta through the arteries to the arterioles (Fig. 2-2).

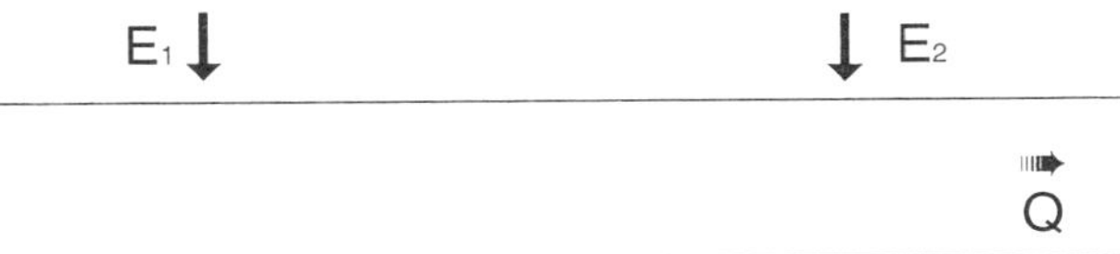

Fig. 2-1. An energy gradient (E_1–E_2) is required to cause flow (Q) between any two points in a vessel. Because there are energy losses due to friction and inertia between E_1 and E_2 flow will occur.

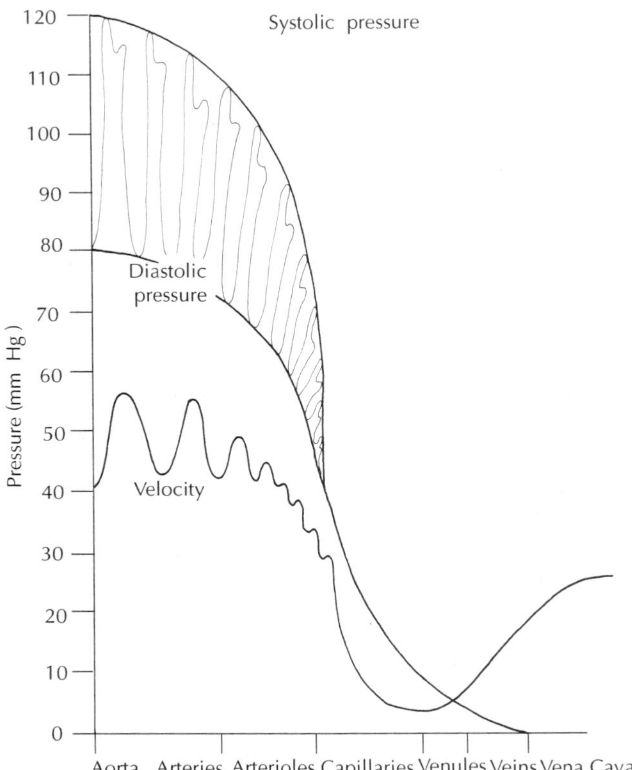

Fig. 2-2. Schematic relationship between blood pressure and flow. Note that while blood pressure continues to drop in the venules and veins, blood flow velocity actually increases slightly.

Capillary blood pressure averages about 10 mmHg, which is less than the pressure in the arterioles but greater than the pressure in the venules. Therefore, an energy gradient exists that drives blood from the aorta through the capillaries and into the venules.

Blood Pressure

Poiseuille's law summarizes the interrelationship between the pressure gradient across an arterial segment. Before we try to decipher the components of that *equation*, however, let's first review how arterial blood pressure occurs.

Arterial blood pressure is determined by two factors:

1. The *volume* of blood (*cardiac output*) delivered to the artery during a given amount of time
2. The amount of *resistance* exerted against the flow.

These two factors and their relationship can be summarized as follows:

Pressure = flow (vol/min) × resistance

If either the flow or the resistance is increased, the pressure will rise. For example, if you want to increase the pressure in a garden hose, you can either turn the faucet on more (increase the volume of water) or increase the resistance to flow by narrowing the opening in the nozzle (Fig. 2-3).

In the circulatory system, turning the faucet on more is equal to increasing the flow pumped out of the heart, that is, increasing cardiac output. Narrowing the nozzle of the hose has the same effect as *reduction of arterial diameter*; they both increase the pressure. The *arterioles* are the last small branches of the arterial system and act as the control valves analogous to the nozzle. The arterioles have strong muscular walls that are capable of opening (dilating) or closing (constricting) the arteriole. This opening and closing of the arteriole will alternate resistance and with it, blood pressure and flow.

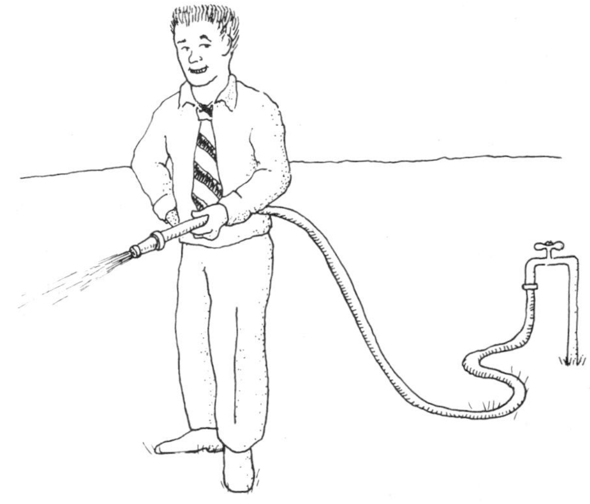

Fig. 2-3. What might happen if the man opens the faucet completely (increasing flow) and tightens down (increasing resistance)?

Cardiac Output

Cardiac output is defined as the amount of blood pumped out of the heart each minute and is an important determinant of arterial blood pressure. Cardiac output is affected by the strength of each contraction of the heart, the heart rate (or number of contractions each minute), and amount of blood pumped out of the heart with each contraction. If the heart muscle is weak due to an injury, such as a *myocardial infarction* (injured heart muscle), the heart will have difficulty keeping pressure up. If the heart rate is slow or irregular due to an arrhythmia (irregular heartbeat), pressure will likely decrease. If a patient has lost a lot of blood due to a hemorrhage, the heart will have too little blood to pump out with each contraction and blood pressure will fall.

Resistance

Resistance in the blood vessels can also increase pressure. This resistance can be modified to adapt to changes and demands of the body. For example, if you get hurt or even think you are close to getting hurt, what happens? Do you notice that your hands get cold and clammy? That change is a result of vasoconstriction (blood vessel constriction) of the arteries in the skin.

Distensibility and Elasticity

During systole, the ventricles contract, forcing blood into the arterial system, which is already filled with blood. Because of the *distensibility* of the blood vessels, the arteries stretch out to accommodate the extra volume of blood. Once the force of the contraction has passed, the elastic nature of the arteries causes them to snap back to their original shape, which helps force the blood toward the capillaries.

If the aorta and arteries were like steel pipes, the pressure created in the aorta each time the heart contracted would be twice (or more) as high as that normally observed. In reality, the pressure in the aorta does not rise to such heights because in the normal vessel, the increased pressure load is canceled out by the expansion of the arterial wall. During diastole, the "resting" phase of the cardiac circle, as the ventricles relax, the *elasticity* of the arterial wall bounces back and propels the blood farther down the vessel toward the capillaries. The distensibility and elasticity of the aorta and arteries prevent blood pressure from fluctuating too much.

The effects of the pumping of the heart in systole and the snap-back of the arteries during diastole help the blood to flow in a more steady state rather than in squirts or "boluses" of blood. By the time blood reaches the capillaries, flow in a normal and healthy body is generally slow, smooth, and steady; this is ideal for the exchange of nutrients and wastes (Fig. 2-4).

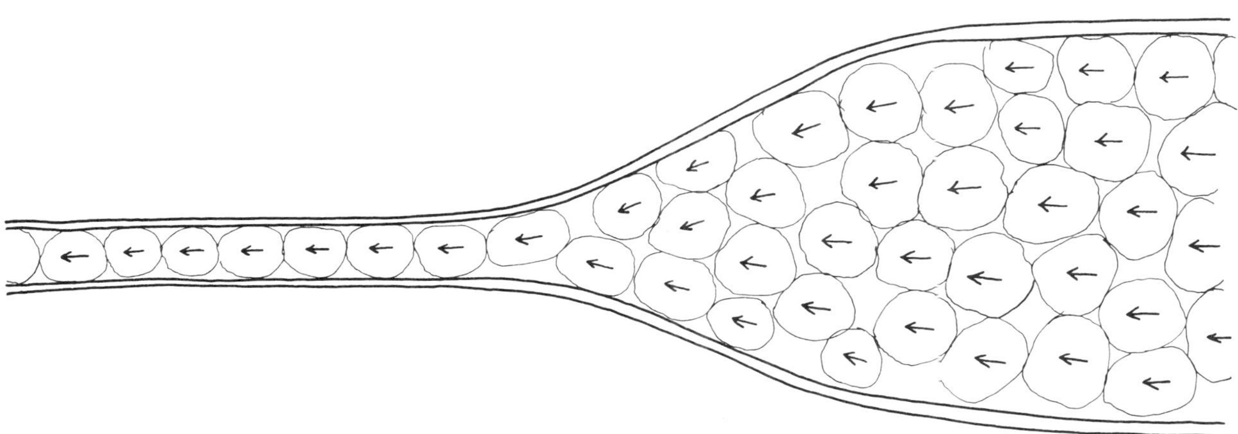

Fig. 2-4. When blood flow is smooth and steady, the red cells can move through the capillaries in an orderly manner and at a speed that is ideal for the exchange of nutrients and wastes.

Review Exercise

1. Blood flows through its system of closed vessels because of

   a. the Bernoulli effect b. vessel elasticity
   c. vessel contractility d. an energy gradient

2. An energy gradient is the difference in ____________ at one segment of the vessel when compared with another.

3. Blood always flows from regions of ____________ pressure to ____________ pressure.

4. The average blood pressure in the aorta is about

   a. 100 mmHg b. 10 mmHg
   c. 50 mmHg d. 150 mmHg

5. The pressure continually decreases once it leaves the aorta and travels through the arteries to the arterioles to a reading of about

   a. 100 mmHg b. 10 mmHg
   c. 45 mmHg d. 150 mmHg

6. Capillary blood pressure averages about

   a. 100 mmHg b. 10 mmHg
   c. 50 mmHg d. 150 mmHg

7. Which law summarizes the relationship of the pressure gradient across an arterial segment?

   a. Bernoulli's Law b. Poiseuille's law
   c. Ohm's law d. Murphy's law

8. Blood pressure is determined by which two factors?

   a. Cardiac output b. Vessel elasticity
   c. Vessel contractility d. Vessel resistance

9. The two factors selected in question 8 and their relationship can be summarized as follows:

   Pressure = ______________________ x ______________________

10. What three factors determine the force in which blood is delivered into the system?

    a. ______________________________

    b. ______________________________

    c. ______________________________

11. Vasoconstriction will ______________ blood pressure.

12. Blood is forced into the arterial system during

a. systole
b. diastole
c. both a and b
d. none of the above

13. Because of the distensibility of the blood vessels, the arteries are able to accommodate the extra volume of blood during

a. systole
b. diastole
c. both a and b
d. none of the above

14. Once the force of the contraction is passed, the elasticity of arteries forces the vessels to snap back to their original shape, which helps

a. increase blood pressure
b. decrease blood pressure
c. increase cardiac output
d. propel blood down the vascular tree

15. The blood pressure does not rise to extreme levels each time the ventricles contract because in normal arteries the increased load is canceled out by which of the following actions?

a. Cardiac output
b. Vessel elasticity
c. Vessel contractility
d. Vessel resistance

16. As the ventricles relax, the arteries snap back and propel the blood farther down the vessel toward the capillaries during

a. systole
b. diastole
c. both a and b
d. none of the above

17. The effects of the pumping of the heart in ______________ and the recoil of the arteries during ______________ help the blood to flow in a more steady state.

18. The Bernoulli effect states that the ______________________________ in pressure accompanies an ______________ in velocity of fluid flow.

Average Blood Pressure

The *average blood pressure* leaving the left ventricle is approximately 100 mmHg. If that pressure were to reach the fragile capillaries, the result would be disastrous. Also, the average *velocity* of blood leaving the left ventricle is quite fast, between 80 and 100 cm/sec. If the velocity were to continue at that rate, there would not be enough time for the exchange of nutrients to take place at the capillary level (Fig. 2-5).

We have covered how cardiac output and the distensibility and elasticity of the vessels help influence the pressure of blood as it moves through the circulatory system. There are other factors that contribute to this essential energy gradient as well. They are *viscosity*, *friction*, and *inertia*. These produce a resistance to flow, which dissipates the pressure energy in the arteries as blood flows through them.

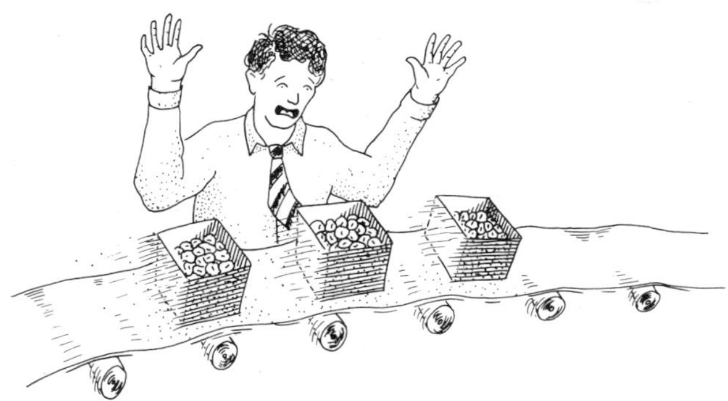

Fig. 2-5. What happens when blood flows through the capillaries too rapidly? The cells cannot obtain the oxygen and nutrients they need. It is like the worker can't take anything from the boxes because they are moving too rapidly along the conveyor belt.

Viscosity

Viscosity refers to the thickness of blood itself. In a thick fluid, molecules tend to be attracted to each other and resist flowing. Take a plastic squeeze bottle of water and another of maple syrup and squeeze them both from the same height and angle. Clearly, the thick, viscous maple syrup comes out more slowly than the water. If you apply more pressure (squeeze the maple syrup container harder), you can produce a more rapid flow of maple syrup from the opening. Thus, the more viscous the material you are attempting to move, the more slowly it moves, unless you apply more pressure.

Friction

An energy gradient is necessary to move blood from one part of the vessel to another; how is this energy lost and where does it go?

The resistance of the blood moving against itself and the arterial walls produces *friction*. Friction causes energy loss in the form of heat. Take the palms of your hands and rub them together hard and fast; notice the heat caused by the friction.

Any time friction occurs, such as against the vessel walls, some of the pressure (or potential energy) is converted into heat and energy escapes. It is like the racecar driver who accidentally brushes against the wall as he is racing around the track. He may not crash, but it sure will slow him down (Fig. 2-6).

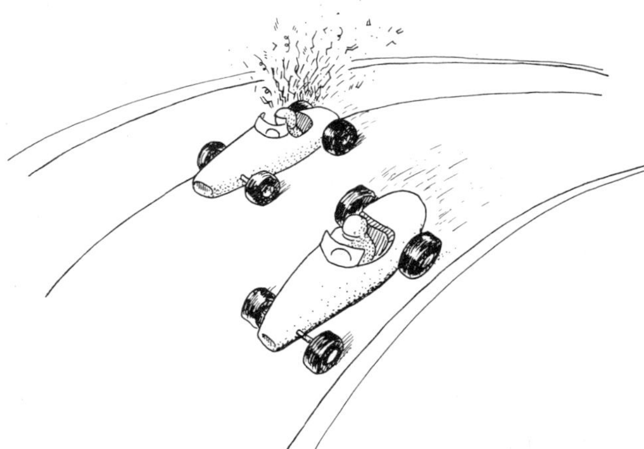

Fig. 2-6. The racecar driver on the outside wall is experiencing some unwanted friction and it's slowing him down!

Therefore, as blood passes through the arteries en route to the capillaries, it continually loses pressure as it rubs against the walls of the vessel. The narrower and longer the vessel, the more friction occurs. The more friction, the more heat loss and subsequent loss of pressure.

Inertia

Inertia is a property of all matter that causes an object at rest to stay in a resting situation and an object in motion to stay in motion, unless some outside force changes these situations. A rolling ball will eventually come to a rest because of the force of friction that opposes the motion of the ball. The same is true for the blood cells. By nature, the moving blood cells will start to slow down unless there is a constant push. Inertial losses contribute to the diminishing energy gradient along the arterial circuit.

Acceleration and Deceleration

Intertial loss of energy occurs in the cardiovascular system due to the *acceleration* and *deceleration* of the blood flow. It's like the gas (energy) consumed in stop-and-go traffic as opposed to the mileage a car gets on an open highway. In addition, more energy is used as the blood flows through branches and around bends. The descending aorta is wide and straight; there is minimal inertia loss, and you would not want there to be. Those cells have a long way to go before they reach the foot. Once down in the lower leg, however, vessels begin dividing and subdividing, causing extensive inertial loss.

Equations

Most people who have been out of school for a few years panic when they see equations, the strange and feared conglomeration of letters where numbers should be, intermixed with strange Greek symbols that everybody seems to understand but you (Fig. 2-7). Some people avoid equations altogether and others only memorize them for examinations. To perform the profession of vascular technology, however, one must truly understand the concepts behind these equations. In this and every section of this book, great care will be taken to demystify what the equations are all about so that you, the vascular specialist, can understand the principles they provide. Let's start with Poiseuille's law.

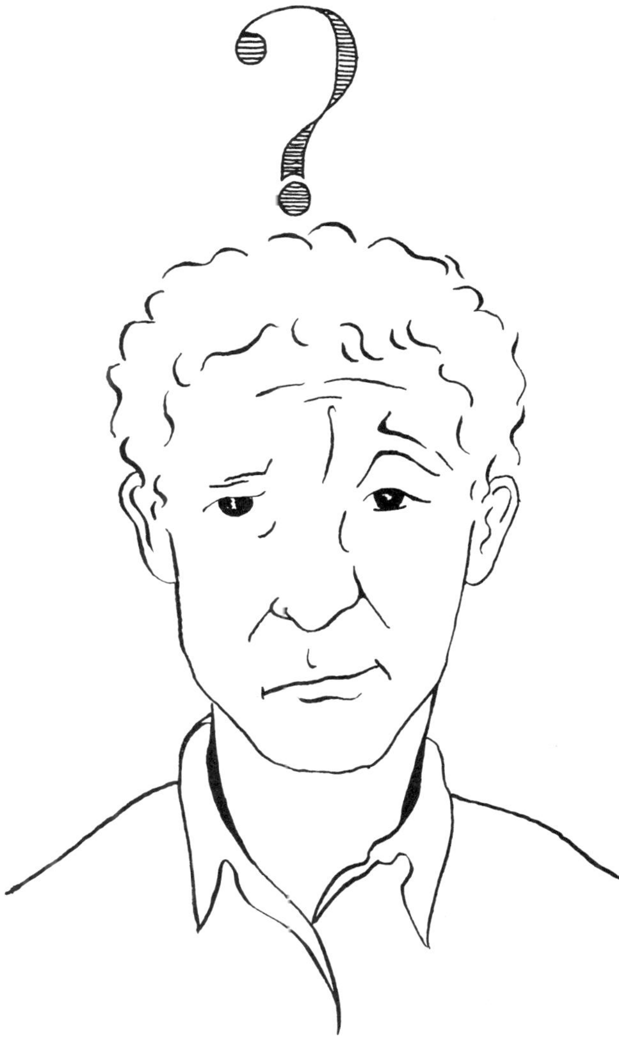

Fig. 2-7. "It's all Greek to me!"

Poiseuille's Law

Poiseuille's law summarizes the relationships among the factors producing a pressure gradient across an arterial segment.

$$P = \frac{Q\ 8Ln}{\pi r^4}$$

where, P = pressure gradient, L = length, r = radius, Q = flow, and n = viscosity of blood.

By understanding this equation, one can discern why average pressure *drops* once it leaves the left ventricle on its way down the arterial tree. The following questions pertain to the factors that affect pressure gradient:

1. How *long* is the vessel?
2. How *wide* is the vessel?
3. How *much* blood flow is going through the vessel?
4. How *thick* is the blood in the vessel?

For a given pressure gradient, if you wanted blood flow to be very low in the blood vessels, what type of situation would you create, given the previous equation? First, you would want the vessel to be long to increase frictional losses, narrow to increase frictional losses, and filled with thick blood to increase viscosity and its related losses.

Conversely, if you want the flow to travel fast, you would construct a vessel that is short to reduce inertial losses and wide to reduce frictional losses, and put in a small amount of thin blood to reduce viscosity and its related losses.

Any change in diameter or length of vessel or the viscosity of the blood affects the pressure gradient or energy loss. However, none is more significant than the reduction in diameter. For example, a 50% reduction in vessel diameter would increase energy losses not by a factor of 2, but of 16 (2 x 2 = 4 x 2= 8 x 2 = 16).

The velocity of blood flow is inversely proportional to the cross-sectional area of a vessel. Inversely proportional means the smaller the vessel, the greater the velocity.

Pressure Gradient in the Veins

Pressure in the venules is higher than it is in the large veins, which helps propel blood back to the heart. The calf-muscle pump and one-way valves assist this process.

Review Exercise

1. What are three factors that contribute to the essential energy gradient?

   a. ____________________

   b. ____________________

   c. ____________________

2. Resistance results in

   a. hypertension
   b. atherosclerosis
   c. increased viscosity
   d. energy loss

3. Viscosity refers to the ____________________ of blood itself.

4. In a thick fluid, molecules tend to

   a. repel each other and resist flow
   b. attract each other and increase flow
   c. attract each other and resist flow

5. An energy ____________________ is necessary to move blood from one part of the vessel to another.

6. The resistance of the blood moving against the arterial walls produces

   a. turbulence
   b. disturbed flow
   c. endothelial damage
   d. friction

7. Friction causes energy loss in the form of

   a. pressure
   b. energy
   c. viscosity
   d. heat

8. Any time __________ occurs, some of the energy is converted into heat.

9. As blood passes through the arteries on route to the capillaries, it continually

   a. maintains pressure
   b. increases pressure
   c. loses pressure
   d. none of the above

10. The narrower and longer the vessel, the __________ friction occurs.

11. The more __________, the more heat loss and subsequent loss of pressure.

12. By nature, a moving object wants to

    a. speed up
    b. stay the same
    c. come to a resting situation
    d. none of the above

13. Moving blood cells tend to slow down unless there is a constant push due to

a. viscous losses
b. kinetic losses
c. frictional losses
d. inertial losses

14. Another factor contributing to inertial loss is the constant ______________ and ______________ of pulsatile flow.

15. More energy is used as the blood flows through ______________ and around ______________.

16. The descending aorta is wide and straight; therefore, there is

a. minimal inertial loss
b. maximum inertial loss
c. no change in inertial loss
d. total inertial loss

17. The loss of energy provides the necessary energy ______________ for blood to flow.

18. Which law summarizes the relationships among the factors producing a pressure gradient across an arterial segment?

a. Ohm's law
b. Bernoulli's law
c. Murphy's law
d. Poiseuille's law

19. In the following equation, define the terms that compose it.

$$P = \frac{Q\ 8Ln}{\pi r^4}$$

P = ______________

Q = ______________

L = ______________

n = ______________

r = ______________

20. The questions pertaining to the factors that affect pressure gradient are

a. How ______________ is the vessel?

b. How ______________ is the vessel?

c. How ______________ is the blood in the vessel?

d. How ______________ blood flow is in the vessel?

21. If you wanted blood flow to be very low in the blood vessels, what type of situation would you create, given the determinants in question 20? (Select three.)

a. Long vessel
b. Short vessel
c. Wide vessel
d. Narrow vessel
e. Thick blood
f. Thin blood

22. A long vessel would increase

a. inertial losses
b. viscous losses
c. frictional losses
d. no losses

23. Thick blood would increase

a. inertial losses
b. viscous losses
c. frictional losses
d. no losses

24. Any decrease in vessel diameter or increase in length or blood volume or viscosity ______________ the pressure gradient and energy loss.

25. No factor is more significant to energy loss than the ____ of a vessel.

26. The velocity of blood flow is ____________________________ proportional to the cross-sectional area of a vessel.

27. A 50% reduction in vessel diameter would increase energy losses by a factor of

a. 2
b. 4
c. 8
d. 16

28. Which of the following are significant factors that assist venous return back to the heart?

a. Calf-muscle pump
b. Energy gradient
c. One-way valves
d. All of the above

29. By increasing the vessel radius by 2, you reduce the energy gradient by a factor of

a. 2
b. 4
c. 8
d. 16

Velocity and Flow

A common mistake made in the vascular profession is using the terms *flow* and *velocity* interchangeably, as if they mean exactly the same thing. They do not. *Flow* refers to the amount of blood over time:

$$\text{flow} = \text{volume} \times \text{time } (F = V \times T)$$

Flow is usually expressed in milliliters per minute (e.g., 45 ml/min).

Velocity refers to distance moved over a period of time:

$$\text{velocity} = \text{distance} \times \text{time } (V = D \times T)$$

How would you feel if you had to pay your water bill by its velocity entering your house as opposed to the volume of water entering your house? *Volume* is a measurement of quantity.

Velocity refers to the speed of blood, usually expressed in distance over time (e.g., 100 cm/min). The average or mean velocity of blood flow, like the average pressure, continually diminishes as it moves to the extremities. The systolic velocity actually increases as flow moves distally.

Pressure/Flow Relationships

If we rewrite the formula for flow, we find that the less resistance blood meets, the greater its flow. To obtain the equation for flow, simply divide both sides by resistance:

If $\quad \text{pressure} = \text{flow (vol/min)} \times \text{resistance}$

Then $\quad \text{flow} = \dfrac{\text{pressure}}{\text{resistance}}$

As mentioned earlier, a larger vessel offers much less peripheral resistance than a smaller vessel. The average blood pressure is thus greater in the aorta and lowest in the capillaries (Fig. 2-8).

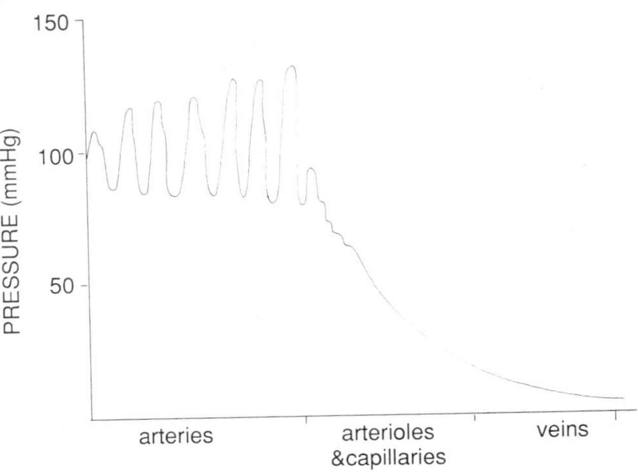

Fig. 2-8. As blood reaches the smaller arteries in the distal vessels, peak systolic blood pressure actually increases. Upon entering the arterioles and capillaries, the pressure drops dramatically.

Exchange of Nutrients and Wastes

Also discussed earlier was the importance of slow flow in the capillaries in order for the proper exchange of nutrients and wastes to take place. Once the deoxygenated blood leaves the capillaries, it enters the larger but less numerous venules. Because the total cardiac output is going from a region of larger total cross-sectional area (the capillaries) to a region of smaller total cross-sectional area (the venules), the velocity of the flow increases. This increase in velocity increases as the venous blood moves back toward the right atrium. Because of this factor, blood flow in the vena cava is much faster than blood flow in the venules.

If we measure the pressure and rate of flow as blood moves around the body, we will note that the blood pressure drops continually until it reaches the right atrium. On the other hand, the velocity of flow decreases until it reaches the venules, after which it increases until it reaches the right atrium.

Review Exercise

1. Flow refers to

   a. the amount of blood over time
   b. the speed of blood over time
   c. the quality of blood over time
   d. the movement of blood from one point to another

2. Flow = ______________ × ______________

3. Velocity refers to

   a. the amount of blood
   b. the speed of blood
   c. the quality of blood
   d. the movement of blood from one point to another

4. Velocity = ______________ × ______________

5. Flow is a much more accurate measurement of ______________.

6. Velocity and volume mean the same thing. True or False?

7. Although the average or mean velocity of blood flow continually ______________ as it moves to the extremities, like the pressure, the systolic velocity actually ______________________________ as flow moves distally.

8. The less ______________________________ blood meets, the greater its flow.

9. To obtain the equation for flow, ______________ both sides of the pressure equation (P = F × R) by resistance.

10. A larger vessel offers (more/less) resistance than a smaller vessel.

11. The ______________ blood pressure is greater in the aorta than in the capillaries.

12. Peak blood pressure actually ______________ until it reaches the distal arterial bed.

13. The importance of slow flow in the capillaries is for the proper exchange of ______________________________ and ______________.

14. Once the deoxygenated blood leaves the capillaries, it enters the

    a. arterioles
    b. arteries
    c. veins
    d. venules

15. If constant blood flow goes from a smaller diameter to a larger diameter vessel, the velocity of the flow ______________.

16. Blood flow velocity in the vena cava is much ______________ than blood flow in the venules.

17. If we measure the pressure and rate of flow as blood moves around the body, we will note that the blood pressure (increases/decreases) continually until it reaches the right atrium.

Pulsatile Flow Versus Steady Flow

The Cardiac Cycle

In a normal *cardiac cycle*, the two atria and two ventricles each contract and relax almost simultaneously. The term *systole* refers to the contraction of the heart, and the term *diastole* refers to the relaxation of the heart. A cardiac cycle consists of the systole and diastole of both atria and both ventricles.

Cardiac Output

The amount of blood ejected from the left ventricle per minute is called the *cardiac output*. Cardiac output is determined by two factors:

1. The *amount of blood* that is pumped by the left ventricle each beat
2. The *number of heartbeats* each minute

The amount of blood ejected in the average adult per minute is approximately 5,000 ml/min.

Pulsatile Flow

The impact of blood striking an artery as it surges out of the ventricle is transmitted along the length of the artery and can be felt at those points where the artery is close to the skin. This transmitted impact on the artery is known as a pulse. The pulse occurs during systole. Then, the arteries contract during the resting phase of diastole.

Being able to palpate, or feel, pulses usually indicates a healthy vessel. Conversely, the absence of a good pulse may indicate significant arterial disease. But don't be fooled! An occluded artery may transmit a palpable pulse even though there is no flow through it. This occurs when the entire vessel is being "thumped" by the blood attempting to enter a blocked vessel.

The velocity characteristics of *pulsatile flow* show an initial increase in velocity during systole and then a decrease during diastole. The more dramatic this rise and fall, the greater the pulsatility of the vessel.

Steady Flow

There is a tendency for pulsatile flow to become steadier the farther from the heart it travels. With the aid of a microscope one can view blood flow at the capillary level and observe that the cells appear to be moving very slowly at a steady rate. In the capillaries, *steady flow* is essential for reasons of nutrient and waste exchange, as was mentioned previously.

Significant disease in a vessel, however, will prohibit the normal expansion and contraction of an *artery*. This causes a nonpulsatile state. The Doppler signal and waveform will reflect that steady flow with a loss of the systolic and diastolic component of the blood flow.

Veins do not normally pulsate; however, because veins do follow the course of arteries, and often lie very close to them, the arterial pulse can be transmitted to the veins. Venous flow normally changes with respiration; that is, dampened with expiration and increased with inspiration.

Steady flow in a vein may indicate a deep venous obstruction shunting flow to the superficial system. Steady flow in an artery may indicate a high-grade stenosis.

Review Exercise

1. The two atria and ventricles each contract simultaneously in ______________, whereas they relax in ______________.

2. The term *systole* refers to the

   a. relaxation of the heart
   b. contraction of the heart
   c. opening of the one-way valves
   d. closing of the one-way valves

3. The term *diastole* refers to the

   a. relaxation of the heart
   b. contraction of the heart
   c. opening of the one-way valves
   d. closing of the one-way valves

4. A heart cycle consists of

   a. the systole and diastole of both atria and both ventricles
   b. the systole of both ventricles only
   c. the diastole of both ventricles only
   d. the systole of both ventricles and both atria

5. The amount of blood ejected from the left ventricle per minute is called

   a. cardiac output
   b. cardiac cycle
   c. ejection fraction
   d. blood pressure

6. Cardiac output is determined by which two factors?

   a. Blood pressure
   b. Heart rate
   c. The amount of blood pumped by the left ventricle each beat
   d. Resistance to the blood

7. The amount of blood ejected in the average adult per minute is approximately

   a. 5,000 ml/min
   b. 1,000 ml/min
   c. 50 ml/min
   d. 5 gal/minute

8. The transmitted impact on the artery from the systolic ejection of blood is known as a

   a. heartbeat
   b. pressure gradient
   c. pulse
   d. all of the above

9. The pulse occurs as the arteries ______________ to accept the increased load of blood into an already filled system.

10. The arteries contract during the resting phase of (diastole/systole).

11. Being able to palpate, or feel, pulses usually indicates

a. an aneurysm
b. an occlusion
c. a healthy vessel
d. none of the above

12. The velocity characteristics of pulsatile flow show an initial (increase/decrease) in velocity during systole and then an (increase/decrease) during diastole.

13. The greater the pulsatility of the vessel, the ______________________________ this rise and fall of the pulse.

14. There is a tendency for pulsatile flow to become _______________ the farther from the heart it travels.

15. In the capillaries, steady flow is essential for reasons of

a. nutrient and waste exchange
b. waste exchange
c. nutrient exchange
d. none of the above

16. Significant disease may prohibit ______________________________ and ______________________________ of an artery.

17. Veins _______________ pulsate. (Refers to frequency.)

18. Because veins follow the course of arteries, and often lie very close to them, the arterial pulse can be

a. anastomosed to the veins
b. circulated to the veins
c. transmitted to the veins
d. collateralized to the veins

19. Venous flow normally changes with

a. systole
b. diastole
c. blood pressure
d. respiration

20. Venous flow _______________ with inspiration and _______________ with expiration.

21. Steady flow in a vein is

a. suggestive of an obstruction
b. sometimes normal
c. always normal
d. never normal

22. Steady flow in an artery is

a. suggestive of stenosis
b. sometimes normal
c. always normal
d. never normal

EFFECTS OF STENOSIS ON FLOW CHARACTERISTICS

Up to this point, we have been studying normal blood flow and the factors that contribute to healthy circulation, but what happens to blood in an *abnormal* situation? In this section we will cover the various changes that occur when blood flow is altered by a flow-reducing lesion.

Key Terms

75% area reduction
Collateral blood flow
Conservation of energy
50% diameter reduction
Disturbed flow
Energy
Entrance/exit effect
Flow rate
Kinetic energy
Laminar flow
Midzone components
Occlusion
Parabolic flow
Parasympathetic nerves
Peripheral resistance
Potential energy
Pressure
Reynold's Number
Stenosis
Sympathetic nerves
Vasoconstriction
Vasodilation
Velocity

Energy Loss

How is blood flow affected by a *stenosis*? Figure 2-9 shows the turbulence a stenosis can create in blood flow. This turbulence is accompanied by a reduction in velocity and other effects. How does a stenosis produce these changes in the character of blood flow?

First of all, we must understand the law of the *conservation of energy*; that is, energy can be changed, but it cannot be created or destroyed. For example, you buy a tank of gasoline for your car. That gasoline is *potential energy*. Once you start driving, you convert that potential energy into *kinetic energy*, which moves the car down the road. So, what happened to the energy at the end of the trip, when you are out of gas and the car is not moving? Some was lost through inertial and frictional losses, but most of the energy was lost through heat.

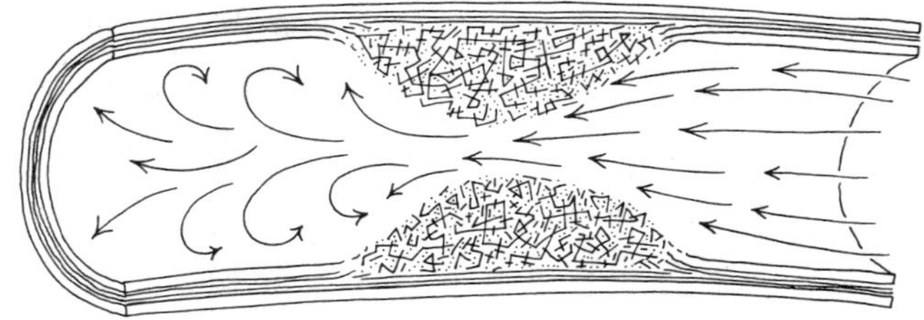

Fig. 2-9. Like water flow in a narrowing river, blood flow velocity will speed up through a stenosis (if > 50%) and will swirl and reverse its direction after exiting. This swirling and reversal of flow after a stenosis is called turbulence.

Let's assume that the *flow rate* (the amount of blood over a period of time) is constant. In other words, we are moving the same amount of blood through the vessel over the same period. If we are going to get the same amount of blood through a vessel that is reduced in size, however, we will have to increase the *velocity* of blood flow in order to ensure enough blood passes through.

When the velocity of blood flow is increased, it uses more *energy*. It takes that energy from the potential energy (*pressure*) and changes it to kinetic energy (velocity). So, while the velocity in the stenosis increases, the pressure actually drops a bit. In the meantime, energy is lost in the form of heat.

Once the flow exits the stenosis, a number of factors come into play. First, with the diameter of the vessel after the stenosis now equal to the diameter before the stenosis, blood velocity dramatically slows down. Subsequently, the reduction in velocity (kinetic energy) allows the pressure to return toward normal (an increase in potential energy). This explains how the pressure distal to the stenosis can be higher than pressure within the stenosis.

Diameter Reduction

In order for a stenosis to be hemodynamically significant, it must cause a

1. 50% diameter reduction
2. 75% area reduction

Figure 2-10 illustrates a stenosis that meets these criteria.

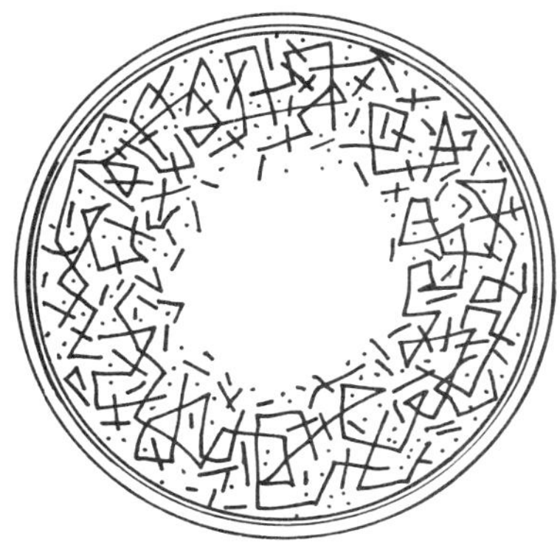

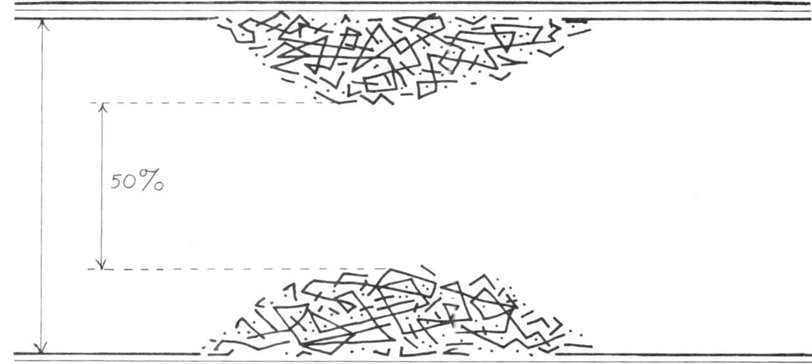

Fig. 2-10. A 75% area reduction is only equivalent to a 50% diameter reduction. When you are discussing percent stenosis, it is critical to be clear about how the vessel is being measured.

Velocity Acceleration

Poiseuille's law demonstrates how vessel length and radius, and the blood pressure and viscosity, affect blood flow. With a proper balance of inertial and viscous energy losses, blood velocity normally slows down until it reaches the capillaries.

Energy

Energy is defined as the capacity of doing work. Energy can be either potential or kinetic.

Gasoline has the potential for doing work by having the ability to make an engine move a truck. Therefore, gasoline may be said to represent potential energy. A moving truck has the capacity for doing work by the result of its motion and ability to move things. Therefore, a moving truck can represent kinetic energy.

We are told that in order to conserve energy (gasoline) we should drive at slower speeds. Although it may take us a little longer to get there, we waste less energy. Moving blood is subject to the same laws of energy. The potential energy from the heart, which provides the pressure to move blood, is greater when it is not required to move blood as great speeds.

The faster the blood moves, the more its potential energy (pressure) is converted into kinetic energy. In a stenosis of 50% diameter, the narrowing causes velocity to increase in order to move the same volume of blood through the stenosis. It is the same effect the narrowing of a river has on the velocity of the water.

Imagine you are floating down a river on a hot summer day. Suddenly, you hear some roaring water and you look up to notice you are floating into a narrowing of the river banks (Fig. 2-11). Why should you feel nervous? Because the narrowed river will undoubtedly cause the velocity of the water to increase. So you'd better hold on!

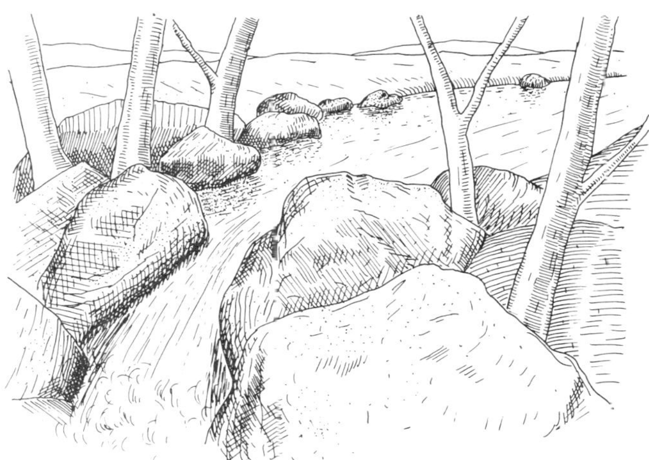

Fig. 2-11. "Get ready for the rapids!"

Entrance/Exit Effect

As blood enters from a normal diameter artery to a smaller diameter stenosis, two things occur.

1. The blood must change direction in order to enter the stenosis.
2. The blood must change direction again in order to exit the stenosis.

Because blood flow must change direction, energy is lost. This *entrance/exit* effect accelerates energy losses and therefore reduces pressure.

Review Exercise

1. Poiseuille's law demonstrates how vessel ______________ and ______________, and the blood ______________ and ____________________________, affect blood flow.

2. With a proper balance of inertial and viscous energy losses, blood velocity normally

   a. speeds up b. slows down
   c. remains steady d. fluctuates constantly

3. Name two types of energy associated with blood flow.

   a. ____

   b. ____

4. The faster blood flows the more ______________ is required.

5. Energy is the ability to perform ______________.

6. The ____________________________ energy from the heart, which provides the pressure to move blood, is greater when it is not required to move blood ____.

7. The faster blood moves, the

   a. more potential energy is required b. more kinetic energy is required
   c. less kinetic energy is required d. less potential energy is required

8. In a stenosis of greater than 50% diameter, the narrowing causes the velocity to

   a. increase b. decrease
   c. stay the same d. fluctuate

9. Once the flow exits the stenosis, blood velocity

   a. speeds up b. stays the same
   c. slows down d. none of the above

10. Pressure distal to the stenosis

    a. can be higher than pressure within the stenosis
    b. is always lower than within the stenosis
    c. is always the same as within the stenosis
    d. none of the above

11. For a stenosis to be hemodynamically significant, it causes

    a. 50% reduction in diameter b. 75% reduction in area
    c. 75% reduction in diameter d. a and b

12. The law concerning the conservation of energy states that

   a. energy can be changed, but it cannot be created or destroyed
   b. energy can be created but not destroyed
   c. energy can be destroyed but not created
   d. energy cannot be changed

13. When the velocity of blood flow is increased, it uses more

   a. oxygen b. energy
   c. red cells d. heat

14. While the velocity in the stenosis increases, the pressure (increases/decreases).

15. A ______________ ______________ is necessary to move blood from one part of the vessel to another.

16. Blood will flow only from a (low/high) pressure system to a (low/high) pressure system.

17. The decreased pressure from one point of the vessel to another is a result of ____.

Direction, Turbulence, and Disturbed Flow

Plug Flow

With the initial contraction of the left ventricle, the blood surges out into the aorta. At this early stage, there is little effect of resistance, as described in Poiseuille's law. That is, the cells have traveled through a wide vessel for a short period, with few branches or turns.

If you were able to look at the profile of blood cells as they exited through the *aortic valve*, you would see *plug flow*, as shown in Fig. 2-12A.

As the cells continue along the arch, effects of friction would begin to slow down the cells close to the vessel wall. Now your profile would show *laminar flow* (Fig. 2-12B).

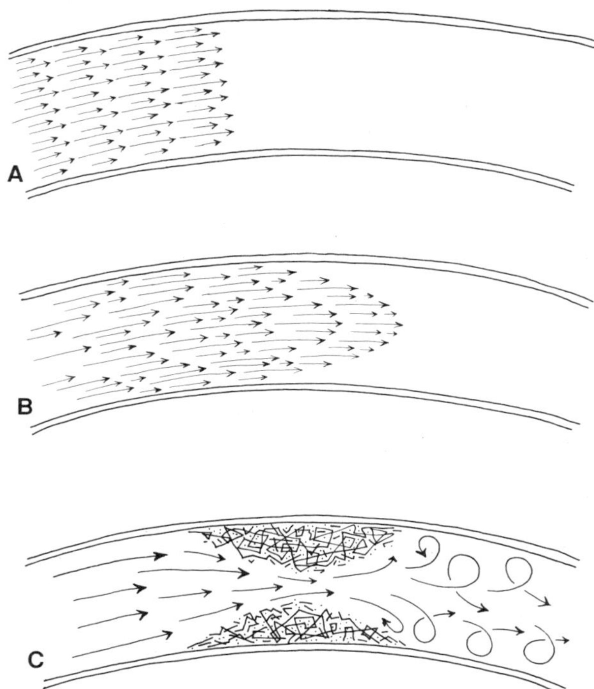

Fig. 2-12. Types of blood flow. (A) Plug flow. (B) Laminar flow. (C) Turbulent flow.

Disturbed and Turbulent Flow

As mentioned earlier, a stenosis affects flow in several different ways. First, the cells must change direction to enter the stenosis. Next, upon exiting the lesion, the cells change direction again amid a pressure drop and decreased velocity. All of this has a chaotic effect on the cells just beyond the stenosis, shown in Fig. 2-12C. Moderate changes in poststenotic flow is referred to as *disturbed flow*. Severely chaotic poststenotic flow can actually vibrate the vessel walls causing an audible bruit (noise) or palpable trill (vibration). This degree of disturbed flow is referred to as *turbulence*.

Reynold's Number

The elements that affect the development of turbulent blood flow are expressed in a term referred to as the *Reynold's Number*. When that number exceeds 2,000, turbulence tends to occur.

$$Re = \frac{v2rp}{n}$$

where Re = Reynold's Number, v = velocity, p = density, r = radius, and n = viscosity.

Keep in mind that any time blood flow changes direction, there is a subsequent loss of energy and therefore a drop in pressure.

Review Exercise

1. Blood surges out into the aorta with the initial contraction of the

   a. left ventricle
   b. right ventricle
   c. right atrium
   d. left atrium

2. At the early stage of blood flow profile in the aorta, there is little effect of

   a. inertia
   b. friction
   c. viscosity
   d. resistance

3. As the blood cells continue along the arch, what effects begin to slow down the cells close to the vessel wall?

   a. Inertia
   b. Friction
   c. Resistance
   d. All of the above

4. A stenosis affects flow as blood cells must change ______________________________ to enter the narrowing lesion.

5. Normal blood flow pattern in an artery is called

   a. laminar flow
   b. plug flow
   c. pulsatile flow
   d. arterial flow

6. Moderate directional changes in poststenotic flow are referred to as

   a. laminar flow
   b. plug flow
   c. disturbed flow
   d. turbulent flow

7. Severely chaotic poststenotic flow is referred to as

   a. laminar flow
   b. plug flow
   c. disturbed flow
   d. turbulent flow

8. The elements that affect the development of turbulent blood flow are expressed in a term referred to as the

   a. Raymonds Number
   b. Bernoulli effect
   c. Poiseuille's law
   d. Reynold's Number

9. Turbulence occurs when that number exceeds

   a. 2,000
   b. 1,000
   c. 3,000
   d. 5,000

10. In the following formula, define its components.

$$Re = \frac{v2rp}{n}$$

a. Re = ______________________________

b. v = ______________________________

c. p = ______________________________

d. r = ______________________________

e. n = ______________________________

11. Any time blood flow changes direction there is a subsequent loss of ____________ and therefore a drop in ____________.

12. In order to be hemodynamically significant a stenosis must be:

a. 75% diameter
b. 50% area
c. either a or b
d. none of the above

Peripheral Resistance

The force applied against the layers of the flowing blood is referred to as *resistance*. There are many ways in which resistance is exerted, and the body can control this resistance in order to increase or lower blood pressure.

The walls of the blood vessels offer the most important force of resistance to blood flow. As the least resistance is away from the contracting ventricles, blood is forced first against the walls of the arteries, then down to smaller and smaller branches. The smaller a blood vessel, the more resistance the blood flow meets (Fig. 2-13).

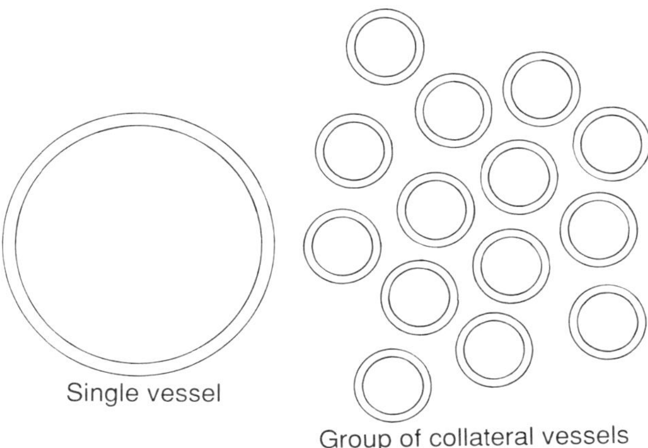

Fig. 2-13. Which vessel(s) will produce the higher resistant flow?

Control of Peripheral Vascular Resistance

An important function in the body is to control arterial blood pressure. The diameter of the arterioles can be changed by reflexes in the body in order to control peripheral resistance and therefore blood pressure. Changes in arteriole diameter increase or decrease peripheral resistance as required for this control. The change in arteriole diameter is controlled by the vasomotor center, which is located in the brain. Stimuli are transmitted to the smooth muscle of the vessel wall via the *sympathetic nervous system*.

The increase in vessel diameter causes a decrease in peripheral resistance; this is referred to as *vasodilation*. Under these circumstances, blood pressure will decrease. A decrease in vessel diameter causes an increase in *peripheral resistance*; this is referred to as *vasoconstriction*. Under these circumstances blood pressure will increase.

Parasympathetic Nerves

The *parasympathetic* division is concerned primarily with control of heart rate and activities that restore and conserve body energy. This activity includes impulses to digestive glands and smooth muscle of the digestive system, thus allowing energy-absorbing foods to be absorbed by the body.

Sympathetic Nerves

The *sympathetic* nerves are concerned primarily with control of heart rate, the force of contraction of the heart, the level of contraction in arteries and veins, and other processes involved with the expenditure of energy. The nerve impulses are conducted from the brain through the spinal cord to sympathetic ganglia and then through sympathetic nerves to the arterioles. Stimulation of the sympathetic nerves to the arterioles of all organs of the body, except those of the brain and the heart, causes vasoconstriction, a reduction in vessel diameter (Fig. 2-14). Normally, the sympathetic nerves to the smooth muscle of the arteriole are always active to some degree, which produces a tonic level of vessel contraction. When there is an increase in blood pressure, the vasoconstrictor area in the brain is inhibited (repressed). This causes a decrease in the signals (impulses) sent to the vasoconstrictor nerve fibers at the arterioles. This allows the arteriole to dilate (vasodilation) and blood pressure to fall.

Sympathetic nerve activity regulates the volume of blood in the digital arteries of the fingers. When one takes a deep breath, vasoconstriction reduces the volume of blood in the arterioles. When the breath is released, the volume of blood flow in the arterioles is increased through vasodilation.

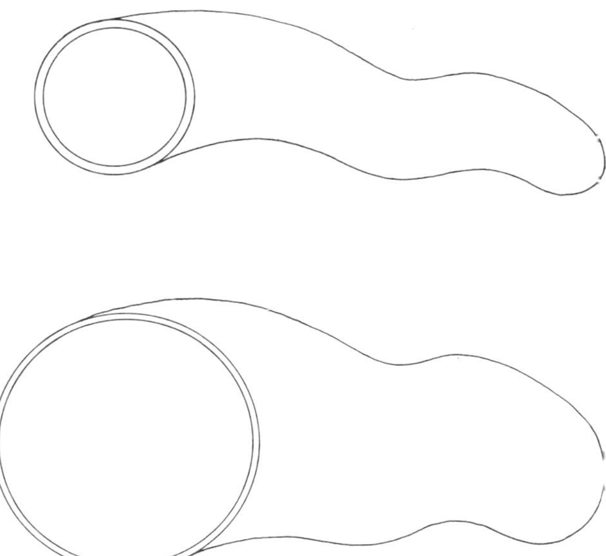

Fig. 2-14. A vessel may decrease its diameter (vasoconstrict) or increase its diameter (vasodilate).

Review Exercise

1. The force applied against the walls of the flowing blood is referred to as

   a. friction
   b. the Reynold's effect
   c. the Bernoulli effect
   d. resistance

2. Which of the following offers the most important force of resistance to blood flow?

   a. Heart muscle
   b. Heart valves
   d. Capillary resistance
   d. Vessel walls

3. The more surface contact the blood makes to the arterial walls, the more resistance the blood flow meets. True or False?

4. The body's ability to regulate blood pressure by changes in the vessel diameter occurs via changes in the activity of

   a. sympathetic nerves
   b. parasympathetic nerves
   c. metabolism
   d. vasocontrol center

5. An important function of the ____________________ __________ system is to control peripheral resistance and, therefore, blood pressure.

6. The change in arteriole ____________________ is an important control of peripheral resistance.

7. The change in arteriole diameter is controlled by the ____________________________, which is located in the medulla.

8. Stimuli are transmitted to the smooth muscle of the vessel wall via the

   a. autonomic nervous system
   b. autoregulation system
   c. parasympathetic nervous system
   d. sympathetic nervous system

9. The increase in vessel diameter causes

   a. an increase in blood pressure
   b. an increase in peripheral resistance
   c. a decrease in peripheral resistance
   d. no change in hemodynamics

10. Sympathetic-stimulated decrease in vessel diameter is referred to as

    a. hemodynamic control
    b. autoregulation
    c. vasoconstriction
    d. vasocontrol

11. A decrease in vessel diameter causes

a. an increase in blood pressure
b. an increase in peripheral resistance
c. a decrease in peripheral resistance
d. no change in hemodynamics

12. A sympathetic decrease in vessel diameter is referred to as

a. hemodynamic control
b. autoregulation
c. vasoconstriction
d. vasodilation

13. Nerve impulses are conducted from the medulla to the spinal cord through to the arterioles via the

a. autonomic nervous system
b. autoregulation system
c. parasympathetic nervous system
d. sympathetic nervous system

14. Sympathetic impulses reduce the diameter of the arterioles by stimulating

a. smooth muscle of the arterioles
b. fibrous tissue of the arteries
c. connective tissue of the arteries
d. all of the above

15. In normal regulation of blood pressure, when there is an increase in blood pressure, the vasoconstrictor stimuli from sympathetic nerves are inhibited. This causes the arterioles to dilate and blood pressure to

a. rise
b. fall
c. stay the same
d. fluctuate

16. Vasodilators bring about

a. an increase in blood pressure
b. an increase in peripheral resistance
c. a decrease in peripheral resistance
d. no change in hemodynamics

17. In normal blood pressure regulation, when blood pressure decreases, the ______________________________ nerves are stimulated and the vessel diameter decreases causing blood pressure to ______________.

Resistance and Collateral Blood Flow

You are driving down the main highway when you are stopped by a police officer. There's been an accident up ahead and all highway traffic has been diverted to a secondary road. You know you will be able to reach your destination, but you also know it is going to take you a lot longer to get there (Fig. 2-15).

The vascular system has some built-in contingencies for problems such as a severely stenotic or totally occluded artery. Although blood may not be able to go down the main road, there are secondary roads that blood flow can travel. Like traveling down secondary roads, however, blood gets slowed down due to the increased resistance of the vessel walls.

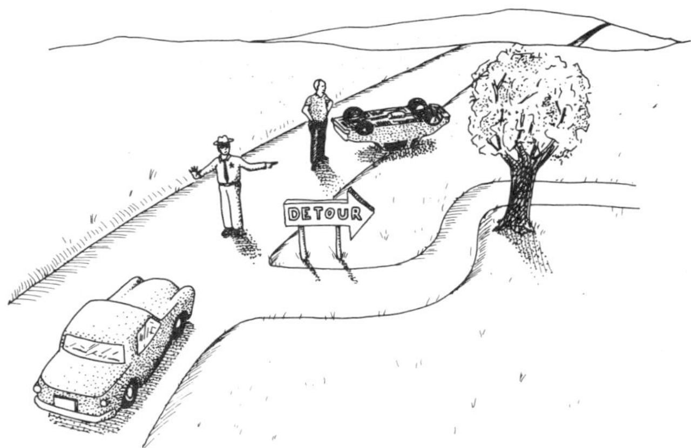

Fig. 2-15. Hope this car is not in a hurry!

Collateral Effects

When an artery develops a significant stenosis or narrowing or occlusion, the blood flow often seeks alternate routes. These alternate routes are termed *collateral pathways*; one such collateral is shown in Fig. 2-16. In the cerebrovascular system, we have seen how the external carotid artery serves as a collateral pathway or alternate route. When the superficial femoral artery is stenotic or occluded, a common collateral pathway is the profunda-geniculate route.

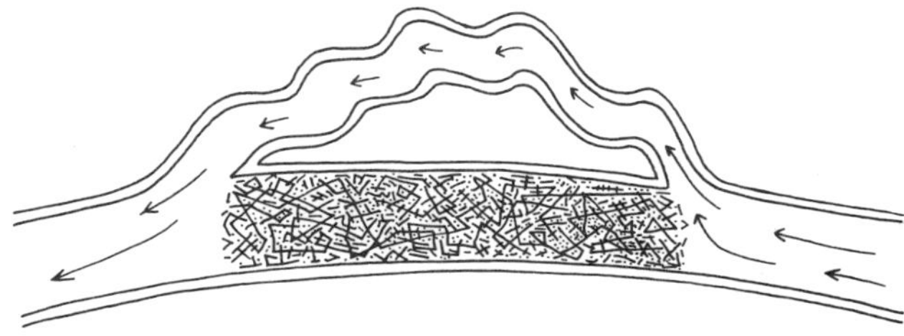

Fig. 2-16. A collateral vessel.

Midzone Components

As the arteries enter an organ, they divide and subdivide until they become small enough to be called arterioles. Then, each arteriole continues branching, leading to the capillaries, where nutrients are exchanged with the cells and waste products are removed. These cells are never supplied by just one branch of one major artery, however. Instead, they are fed by multiple arterioles of many branches from various arteries.

When there is a stenosis of the major arterial branches, the arteries and arterioles distal to the stenosis contain significantly lower pressure than normal. The decreased pressure is transmitted all the way down to the smaller branches where, in many cases, it causes the blood flow in other nearby arteries to reverse.

The profunda femoris, for example, will anastomose with the geniculate artery in the knee. When the pressure in the geniculate artery becomes lower than the pressure in the profunda, the flow in the geniculate will reroute, allowing flow to go around the stenosis. The area at which the arterioles reverse flow is referred to as the *midzone component.*

Resistance

Resistance is a term used to define the ratio of the pressure gradient across an arterial segment to the flow through the segment. It is important to keep in mind that pressure in a vessel can increase even when the vessel wall or stenosis stays the same. Or, in other words, the more traffic moving down the road, the bigger the backup. Like rush hour traffic, the highway width doesn't change, there are just more cars (Fig. 2-17).

In the arteries, we are looking for the change in pressure due to a stenosis. The longer the stenosis, the greater

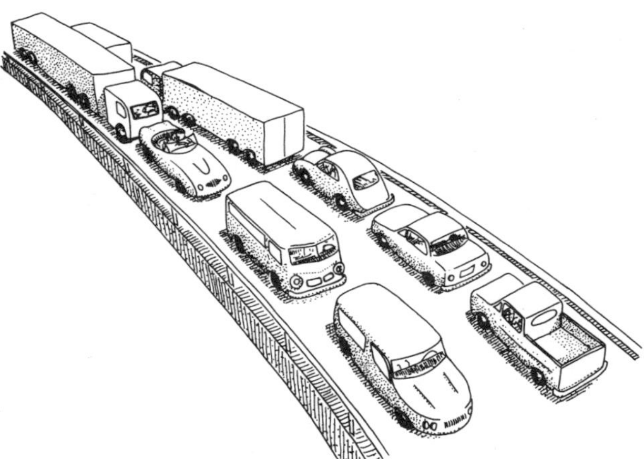

Fig. 2-17. Too many cars and not enough road.

the resistance. Now we can conclude two things: Pressure is affected by the length of the diseased section and how much blood is flowing through it. Expressed in a formula, this is

$$R_{seg} = \frac{P_1 - P_2}{Q}$$

This equation allows us to measure the resistance of flow (R_{seg}) by measuring the pressure before the stenosis (P_1), then subtracting the pressure after the stenosis (P_2) and dividing it by the flow (Q).

Illustration of Flow in Stenosis

Let's say that P_1 is 100 mmHg, P_2 is 50 mmHg, and Q is 10 ml/min.

$$100 \text{ mmHg} - 50 \text{ mmHg} = 50 \text{ mmHg}$$

$$\frac{50 \text{ mmHg}}{10 \text{ ml/min}} = 5\text{mmHg/ml/min}$$

So the resistance equals 5 mmHg/ml/min.

Effects of Exercise

Now let's put all of this into clinical terms. Mr. Jones has a stenosis of the superficial femoral artery. You take a resting Ankle/Brachial Index (a comparison between the arm blood pressure and the ankle blood pressure) and it is normal. Mr. Jones explains to you that his leg doesn't hurt when he's resting, only after he walks. So, you put him on a treadmill until he gets his symptoms and then check his Ankle/Brachial Index pressure again. This time it drops!

The pressure decreased for two reasons. First, the arterioles in the lower leg, anticipating a need for more blood, dilated (opened up). This increased flow across the stenosis causing a greater energy loss and thus decreased the pressure in the calf arteries. Second, energy was lost in the form of velocity (kinetic energy) and heat as blood tried to fight its way through the stenosis.

In sum, resistance to flow is affected by the diameter of the lumen. Also, the pressure drop across the resistance depends on the amount of flow going through it. Resistance will be increased by

1. decreasing the diameter
2. increasing the length of the stenosis

Occlusion

When there is a stenosis of a blood vessel, the body responds to deal with the diminished blood flow initially caused by the stenosis. One response is to reduce resistance downstream from the stenosis and therefore restore the original blood flow. If we look again at Poiseuille's law for resistance, we see there are several factors affecting resistance.

$$P = \frac{Q\ 8Ln}{\pi r^4}$$

We recall that there are several ways to reduce resistance. One of the more dramatic factors in Poiseuille's law is the change in radius. So, if we can increase the diameter of a vessel, we reduce the resistance and therefore increase the flow.

In response to ischemia (lack of oxygen) caused by low blood flow, smooth muscle of the arterioles relaxes and allows the vessel to dilate. The dilation increases the radius and therefore decreases the resistance. With a total *occlusion*, however, maximum benefit from vasodilation has usually occurred. The pressure proximal to the stenosis has allowed collaterals to dilate and bypass the occlusion. Because of diminished or absent flow, the vessel will most likely thrombose (clot off) distal to the last open vessel (Fig. 2-18).

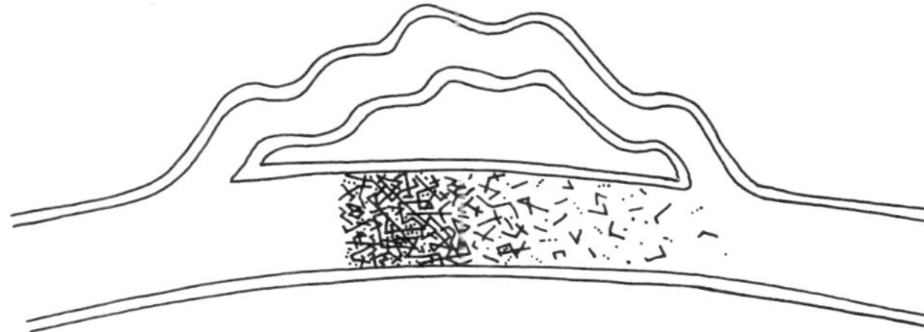

Fig. 2-18. This vessel is completely occluded, causing thrombus to develop at both ends.

Review Exercise

1. When an artery develops a significant stenosis or narrowing or occlusion, the blood flow often seeks an alternate route. This alternate route is referred to as

   a. bilateral circulation
   b. lateral circulation
   c. bifed circulation
   d. collateral circulation

2. The area where arterioles tend to reverse flow due to a significant stenosis is called the

   a. capillary zone
   b. endzone component
   c. midzone component
   d. ozone component

3. When the superficial femoral artery is stenotic or occluded, a common collateral pathway is the

   a. profunda femoris
   b. profunda-geniculate route
   c. saphenous vein
   d. superficial femoral vein

4. *Resistance* is a term used to define the _____________ of the pressure gradient across an arterial segment to the flow through the segment.

5. In the arteries, the longer the stenosis, the greater the

   a. velocity
   b. volume
   c. bruit
   d. resistance

6. Pressure drop across a stenosis is affected by which two factors?

   a. Length of the stenosis
   b. Amount of blood flowing through the stenosis
   c. Distance of stenosis from the heart
   d. Whether the plaque is soft or hard

7. Define the terms in this equation.

$$R_{seg} = \frac{P_1 - P_2}{Q}$$

   a. R_{seg} = ____
   b. P_1 = ____
   c. P_2 = ____
   d. Q = ____

8. The formula in question 7 states that the resistance of flow can be determined by measuring the pressure _____________ the stenosis, then subtracting the pressure _____________ the stenosis and dividing it by the _____________.

9. If P_1 is 200 mmHg, P_2 is 100 mmHg, and Q is 10 ml/min, the resistance is

a. 100 mmHg/ml/min
b. 1,000 mmHg/ml/min
c. 50 mmHg/ml/min
d. 10 mmHg/ml/min

10. Resistance will be increased by (increasing/decreasing)

a. ______________________________ the diameter

b. ______________________________ the velocity

c. ______________________________ the volume

d. ______________________________ the length of the stenosis

11. When there is a stenosis of a blood vessel, the body responds to deal with the diminished blood flow by reducing ______________________________ and therefore ______________________________ blood flow.

12. One of the best ways to reduce resistance, according to Poiseuille's law, is to change size of the vessel

a. diameter
b. area
c. radius
d. all of the above

13. If we can increase the diameter of a vessel, we increase the flow. True or False?

14. In response to ischemia, the smooth muscle of the arterioles ______________ and allows the vessel to dilate.

15. The dilation increases the ______________ and therefore decreases the ______________________________.

16. With a chronic total occlusion, maximum benefit from vasodilation has usually occurred. True or False?

17. The increased resistance caused by a stenosis allows which vessels to dilate and bypass the occlusion?

a. Capillaries
b. Venules
c. Arterioles
d. Collaterals

18. Because of diminished or absent flow, the vessel will most likely ______________________________ distal to the last open vessel.

VENOUS HEMODYNAMICS

In this section, we will cover the principles of *venous hemodynamics*. Arterial physiology described how blood flow gets from one point to another and what happens when normal flow enters a diseased artery. Venous hemodynamics deals mainly with how blood is returned back to the heart. The mechanisms are somewhat complicated when compared with the arterial system, however, but a thorough understanding of these principles is essential in order to understand the pathophysiology of the venous system.

Key Terms

Calf-muscle pump
Effects of inspiration and expiration
Hydrostatic pressure
Sinusoids
Transmural pressure
Veins
Vein wall distention
Venous valves
Venule

When studying the physiology of the arterial system, it seems logical to understand how blood that is pumped out of a left ventricle moves down the artery to the arterioles. However, when we attempt to understand how blood works its way *back* to the heart without assistance from a pump, and generally flowing "uphill" in the standing or sitting person, confusion arises. To better understand the somewhat complicated dynamics of venous physiology, let's review what we have already learned.

First of all, we know that a pressure gradient is necessary to move blood from one part of the vessel to another. Blood will flow only from a higher pressure system to a lower pressure system. The decreased pressure from one point of the vessel to another is a result of energy loss. In the prone patient, the loss of energy is due to the viscosity and volume of the blood, as well as the length and decreasing size of the vessel.

In the venous system, an energy gradient also exists. A 15 mmHg intraluminal (inside the vessel of the vein) venous pressure gradually and continually drops until it reaches the right atrium, which has an intraluminal pressure of 0 mmHg. Because the *venule* is larger than the capillary, and under no pressure from the heart (like the arteriole), blood flows to it. And because the vein is larger than the venule and offers less resistance, blood flows to it as well. But again, this all assumes the patient is prone. What happens when the patient stands up?

Effects of Inspiration and Expiration

Venous blood flow is also assisted back to the right atrium by the increase and decrease of intrathoracic pressure each time you inhale and exhale. Remember the spoiled brat who gets so angry he bears down and holds his breath until he's red in the face (Fig. 2-19)?

What is actually occurring is that the child is increasing his intrathoracic pressure by holding his breath and bearing down on his diaphragm. This pressure is so great that although arterial flow is able to flow out to the arteries, venous blood is meeting major resistance in the large veins in the chest. The result is a backup of blood in the veins and a red face!

In actuality, each time you take a breath, you decrease your intrathoracic pressure, causing the blood vessels in the chest to expand. This results in a pooling of blood to the pulmonary vessels and the right side of the heart. This reduces the quantity of blood returning to the left side of the heart and momentarily decreases cardiac output and blood pressure.

When you inspire, the diaphragm descends and this increases the pressure in your abdominal cavity. This impedes venous blood returning from the lower extremities (Fig. 2-20). As you exhale, intrathoracic pressure increases and blood is forced out of the pulmonary circuit and back to the left side of the heart. In addition, upon expiration, the diaphragm moves upward, which lowers abdominal pressure. This allows for the return of venous blood to the lower extremities (Fig. 2-21).

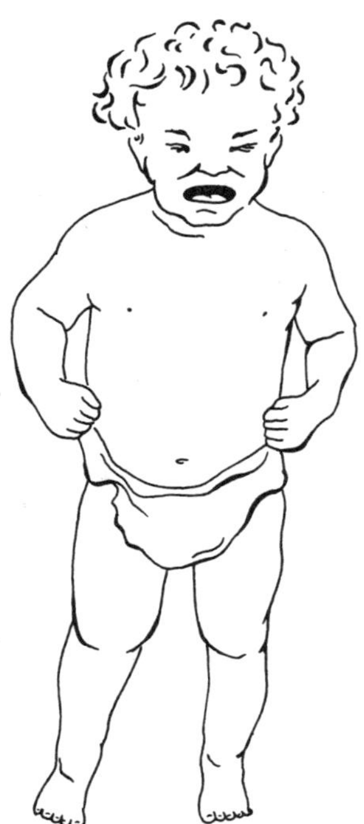

Fig. 2-19. Tantrums won't get this baby anything but a red face.

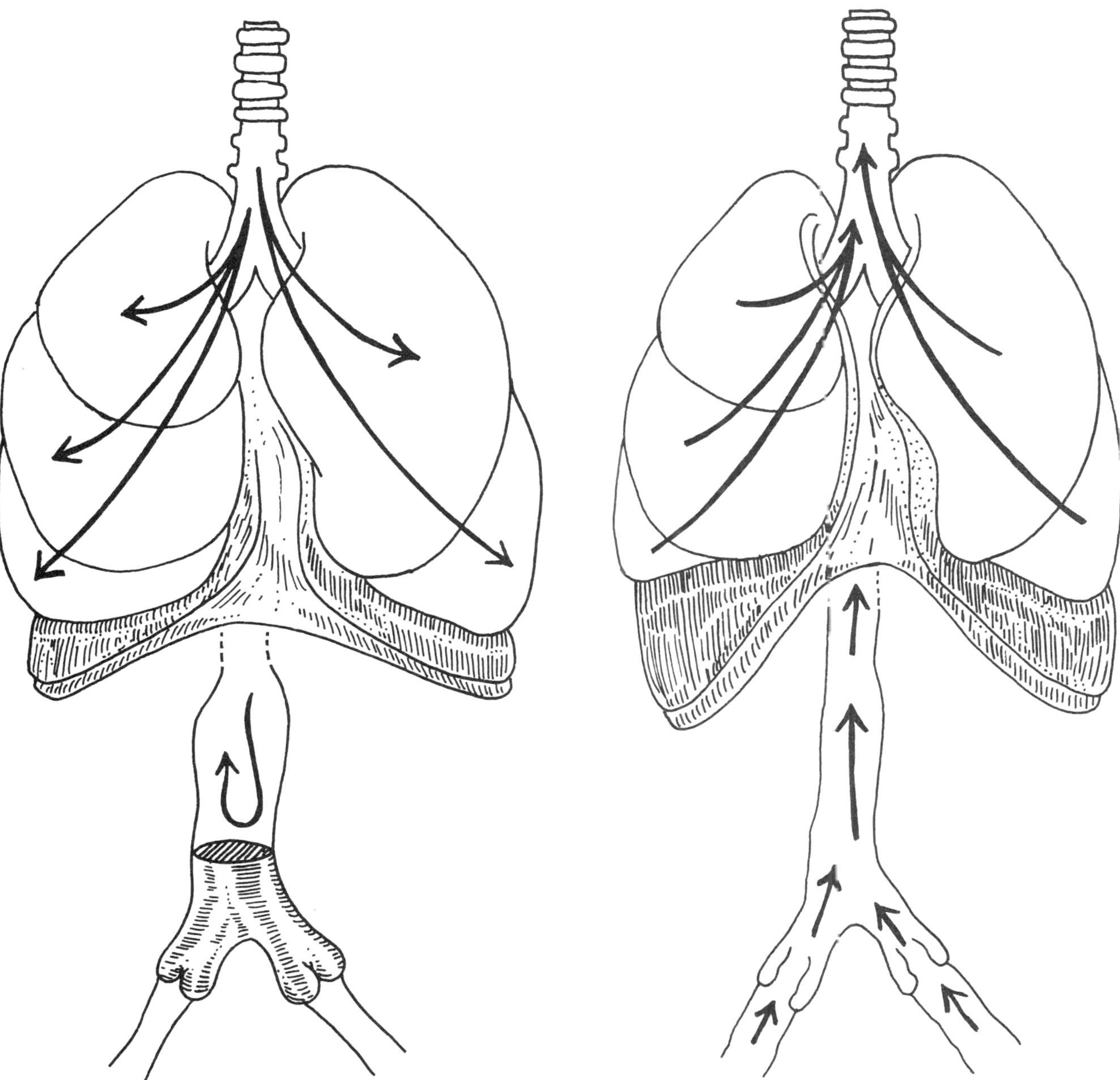

Fig. 2-20. Taking a deep breath increases intra-abdominal pressure and slows down the venous return to the right atrium of the heart.

Fig. 2-21. Exhaling decreases intraabdominal pressure and allows venous blood to return easily to the right atrium of the heart.

Venous Valves

Imagine trying to get to the second floor of a building without the benefit of stairs. Stairs allow the individual to move from one position to another with weight and energy expended and disbursed over a distance. *Venous valves* function pretty much the same way. They allow blood to be held at a point before it moves on to the next level. This is also like the jack of a car. It would be quite impossible to raise a car up a foot all in one effort. The jack provides incremental stops for the weight to rest on before it is raised to the next position.

Vein Wall Distention

Another difference between the veins and arteries is the thinness of the venous walls. This is because veins are not under the same amount of pressure as arteries. This serves as a particular advantage, too, and we can illustrate this by a simple maneuver. If you are sitting at your desk, lean over and let your hand dangle close to the floor. What do you see? Typically, the veins in the back of the hand distend and become easy to see.

The distention of the veins is a result of the increased hydrostatic pressure you have created in your veins because you have increased the distance of your hand from your heart. The result was the slowing down of venous return and the building up of venous blood and subsequent pressure. Now raise your hand up in the air. The veins collapse. Venous blood, with the assistance of gravity, pours down the brachial veins, which are assisted, not impeded, by gravity.

Review Exercise

1. Energy gradients only exist in the arterial system. True or False?

2. A 15 mmHg intraluminal venous pressure gradually and continually drops until it reaches the

   a. left ventricle
   b. right ventricle
   c. left atrium
   d. right atrium

3. The right atrium has an intraluminal pressure of

   a. 0 mmHg
   b. 2-3 mmHg
   c. 10 mmHg
   d. 100 mmHg

4. Blood flows from capillary to venule due to

   a. Poiseuille's law
   b. blood pressure
   c. gravity
   d. a pressure gradient

5. Venous blood flow is also assisted back to the right ventricle by the increase and decrease of

   a. intrathoracic pressure
   b. intraluminal pressure
   c. systole and diastole
   d. intracardiac pressure

6. Each time you take a breath, you decrease your intrathoracic pressure and

   a. increase the venous return back to the right side of your heart
   b. impede the venous return back to the right side of your heart
   c. both a and b
   d. neither a nor b

7. Veins have thinner walls than arteries. True or False?

8. The distention of veins can be a result of

   a. hydrostatic pressure
   b. gravity
   c. increased intrathoracic pressure
   d. all of the above

PRESSURE/VOLUME RELATIONSHIP

Transmural Pressure

The ability of veins to expand and collapse (collapse rather than contract) also serves an important function in the control of pressure. We have learned that arterioles expand to lower resistance, and therefore increase flow into the peripheral vascular bed during exercise.

During periods of low blood perfusion to the capillaries, the veins are rarely full. In fact, the more distal veins are almost completely collapsed. This is due to pressure against the outside of the vein being greater than the pressure in the vein. Thus the vein takes on an elliptical shape (Fig. 2-22).

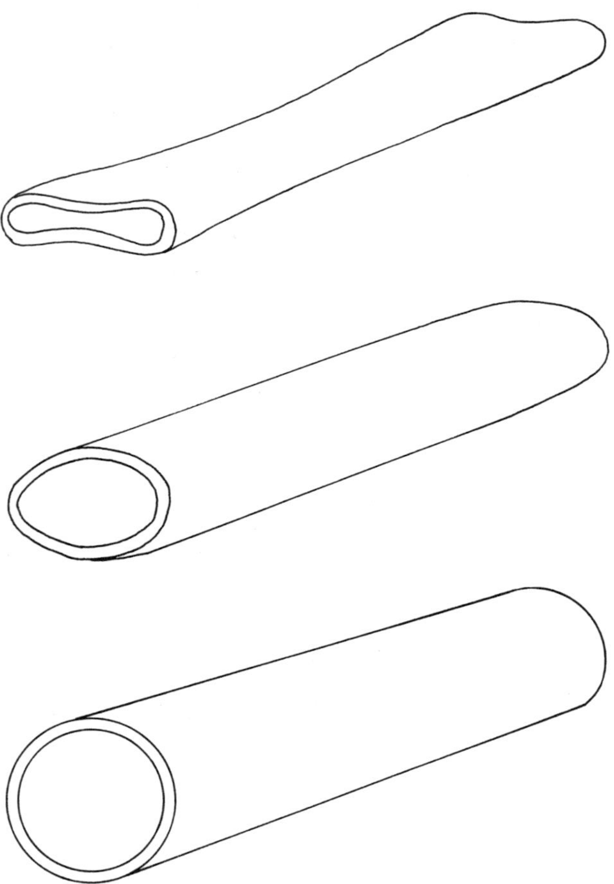

Fig. 2-22. Veins in the body change shape depending on how much blood is in the vessel. You can see this change by hanging your hand down below by your side for a few minutes. Now raise your hand above your head and watch your veins collapse as they empty of the venous blood.

When the cardiac output increases during exercise, and the arterioles dilate to accommodate the increased blood supply, the veins can also expand to contain the increased supply of blood. The veins become circular when they are full.

Hydrostatic Pressure

Hydrostatic pressure refers to the amount of force measured in the vein due to several factors:

1. Blood (density)
2. Acceleration due to gravity (standing versus lying)
3. Distance from the heart (how tall a person is)

Expressed mathematically:

$$P = pgh$$

where P = Pressure, p = density (approximately 1.065 g/cm^3), g = acceleration of blood flow (980 cm/sec^2), and h = distance from the heart.

Because the density of the blood and the acceleration of blood due to gravity normally do not change, the only variable that can change is the distance from the heart. So, in the standing patient, the farther the distance (h) from the heart, the greater the hydrostatic pressure (P) (Fig. 2-23). (Actually, hydrostatic pressure affects both the arterial and venous system, but because the veins are more flexible than the arteries it is more noticeable in the veins.)

Almost everyone recalls the poor soldier, who, after standing at a rigid attention for a while, faints and collapses on the ground. I think we have always believed it was from the heat or exhaustion. The real reason, however, is due to venous hemodynamics. This soldier illustrates the boundaries within which your venous system is able to function.

Let's put it this way. If you are on your feet all day, what is it you naturally want to do to relieve the achiness that occurs in your calves and feet? Perhaps doing some standing on your toes and then dropping back on your feet, or moving your foot around a large circle to stress your *calf muscle*. Better yet, sitting down with your feet up on a cushion (Fig. 2-24)!

These maneuvers are motions that assist your venous blood back to the right atrium. If you are not walking and have no benefit of the *calf-muscle pump* action, venous blood begins to pool in the lower leg. By rising from flat foot to toes or turning your foot around in a circle, you are engaging your calf-muscle pump even though you

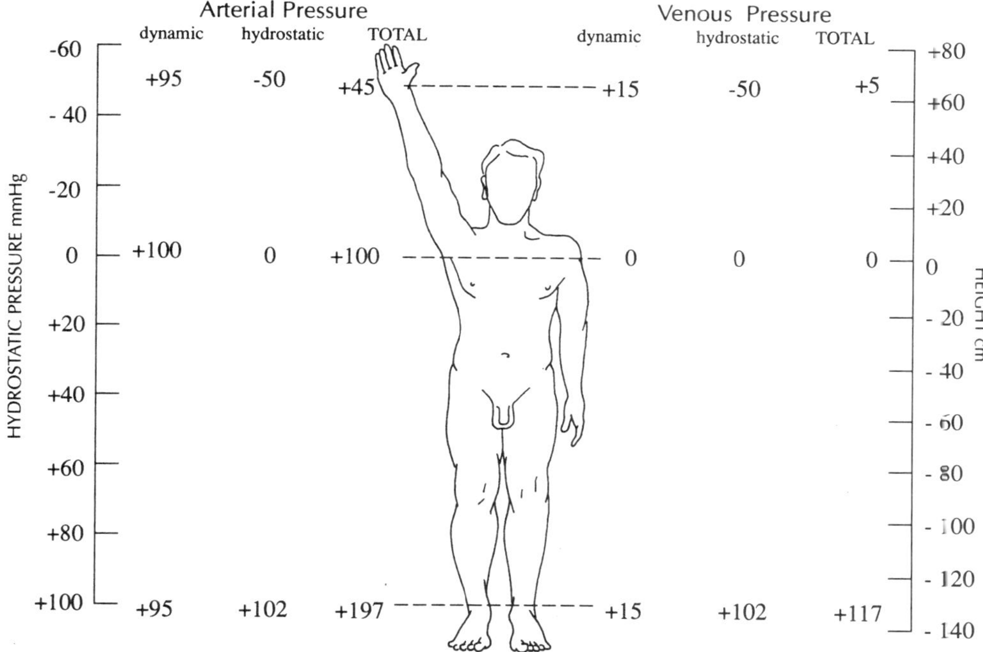

Fig. 2-23. Effects of hemodynamic pressure on the venous and arterial pressures. If this subject were lying flat (supine) on an examination table, the total intravascular pressure would be very close to the hydrostatic pressure. Note that the reference point for venous pressure is 0 and is located at the right atrium.

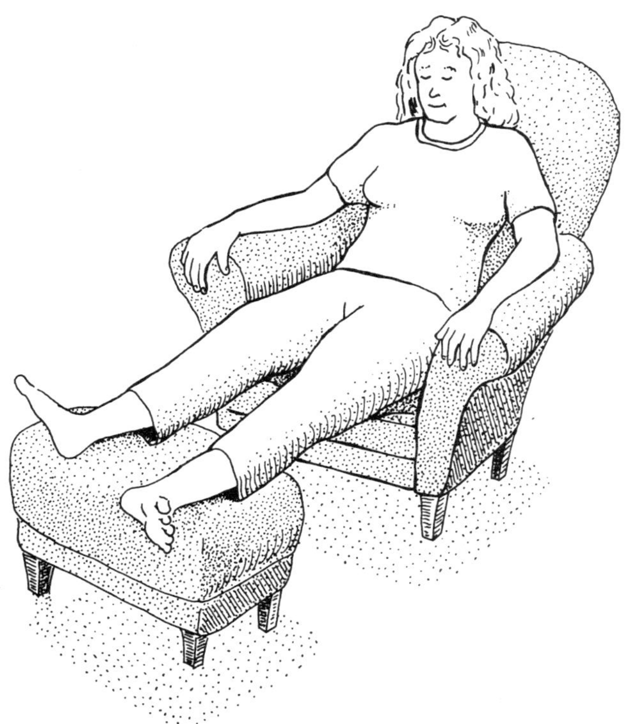

Fig. 2-24. There is nothing like propping your feet up to relieve swelling and pressure.

are not walking. Clearly, by lying down with your feet up, you gain the greatest benefit from gravity-assisted venous return.

Unfortunately soldiers who are standing at attention cannot fidget or do "toe ups" and certainly are not allowed to take a break just because their feet get tired. They are forced to stand with gravity pulling the venous blood down and nothing to help the blood go back up. The result is that blood is leaving the heart but not enough is returning back. There is one mechanism that will come into play when all else fails, though. The brain, lacking some of the blood that is pooling up in the feet, says, "Enough's enough," and the soldier faints! This puts the soldier horizontal—a much better position for venous return.

Soldiers are not the only victims of poor venous hemodynamics. Surgeons, shopkeepers, traffic officers, and any other group of people who are not at liberty to move around or rest at will are subject to the adverse effects of venous hemodynamics. Later, we will discuss some apparatus available to assist the vertically bound vascular specialist.

Calf-Muscle Pump

The return of the blood from the legs back to the right atrium is also facilitated by the calf-muscle pump mechanism. The muscles of the calf act as the power source for squeezing the veins, and the venous sinusoids act as the "rubber bulbs" from which the venous blood is squeezed. Finally, the one-way *venous valves* act to propel the blood in one direction only (Fig 2-25).

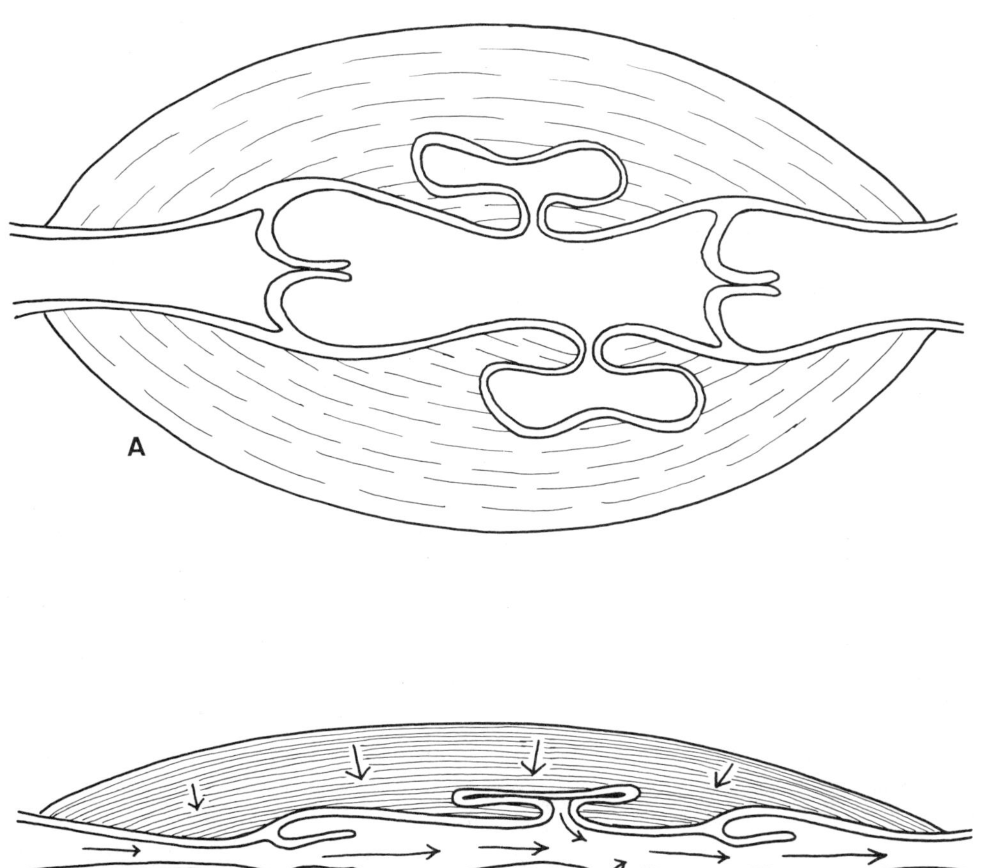

Fig. 2-25. Calf muscles contract during exercise. The effect of one-way valves forces the blood up the leg and in one direction only.

Review Exercise

1. Intraluminal venule pressure is about

   a. 50 mmHg
   b. 100 mmHg
   c. 5-10 mmHg
   d. 75 mmHg

2. Pressure of the right atrium is about

   a. 50 mmHg
   b. 100 mmHg
   c. 0-5 mmHg
   d. 75 mmHg

3. The venule is ______________________________ when compared with the capillary. (Refers to size.)

4. Venous blood flow is also assisted back to the

   a. right ventricle
   b. right atrium
   c. left atrium
   d. left ventricle

5. Blood flow is assisted back to the heart by the __________ and __________ of intrathoracic pressure.

6. Each time you take a breath, you (select two)

   a. decrease intrathoracic pressure
   b. increase intrathoracic pressure
   c. impede venous blood flow back to the right side of your heart
   d. assist venous blood flow back to the right side of your heart

7. ____________________ allow venous blood to be held at a point before it moves on to the next level.

8. The walls of the veins and the walls of arteries are about the same size. True or False?

9. The structure of venous walls allows veins to ____________________ or ____________________, depending on the different phases of venous blood flow.

10. During periods of low blood perfusion to the capillaries, the veins are rarely full. True or False?

11. Change in vein wall shape is due to an increase or decrease in

    a. barometric pressure
    b. systolic pressure
    c. diastolic pressure
    d. hydrostatic pressure

12. Hydrostatic pressure in the veins of a standing person is due to the amount of

a. blood in a vein
b. distention in a vein
c. force in a vein
d. valves in the vein

13. Hydrostatic pressure is due to three primary factors:

a. ______________________

b. ______________________

c. ______________________

14. The hydrostatic pressure formula is P = pgh. Define the components.

a. P = ______________________

b. p = ______________________

c. g = ______________________

d. h = ______________________

15. Because ____________ and ____________________ of blood normally do not change, the only variable that can change is the ______________________.

16. In the standing patient, the farther the distance from the heart, the

a. lower the hydrostatic pressure
b. higher the hydrostatic pressure
c. both a and b
d. neither a nor b

17. The return of the blood from the legs back to the right atrium is facilitated by

a. decreasing intrathoracic pressure
b. calf-muscle pump mechanism
c. venous valves
d. all of the above

18. The ____________________ of the calf act as the power source for squeezing the veins.

19. Which of the following act as the "rubber bulbs" from which the venous blood is squeezed?

a. coronary sinuses
b. maxillary sinuses
c. venous sinusoids
d. pump sinuses

20. The one-way ____________________ act to propel the blood in one direction only.

3
Pathophysiology

ARTERIOSCLEROTIC DISEASE

The major cause of death in the United States and most industrial nations is vascular insufficiency of the cardiovascular system. Cerebrovascular disease is the third leading cause of death in this country. Most of this arterial insufficiency is attributed to *arteriosclerosis*, which literally means the thickening and *induration* (hardening) or overall degeneration of the arteries. In this section, we will learn about the major causes of this disease and how the disease develops.

Key Terms

Adventitia
Arteriosclerosis
Atherosclerosis
Calcification
Capillaries
Collagen fibers
Emboli
Embolus
Endothelial cells
Hemorrhage
Induration
Intima
Media
Plaque
Platelets
Shear effect
Thrombus
Turbulent
Ulceration
Vasa vasorum

Atherosclerosis

Arteriosclerosis is characterized by hardening and loss of elasticity of the arterial walls. *Atherosclerosis* is a common form of arteriosclerosis in which deposits of yellowish plaque (atheroma) containing cholesterol and other lipid material are formed within the intima and inner media of large- and medium-sized arteries (Fig. 3-1). Arteriosclerosis is responsible for atherosclerotic and coronary heart disease, as well as cerebrovascular disease.

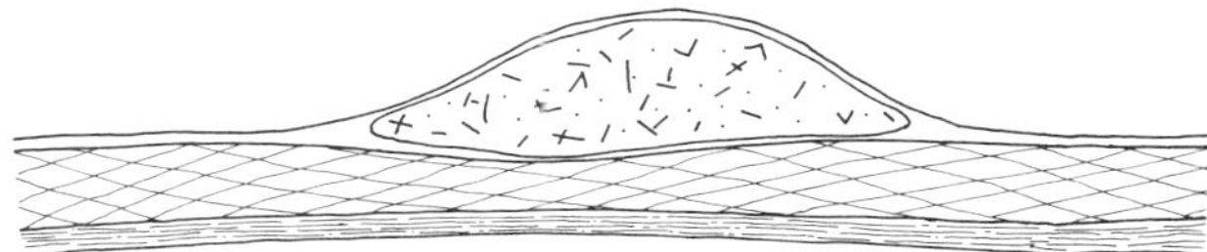

Fig. 3-1. Atherosclerotic plaque of an artery.

Vessel Anatomy Review

Recall that the blood vessel is comprised of three primary layers: the intima (inner lining), the media (middle layer), and the adventitia (outer layer).

The Intima

The *intima* is a thin lining consisting of *endothelial* and elastic fibers. The intima is present in all vessels (arteries, capillaries, venules, and veins) with the exception of the sinusoids. Of the three layers, the intima has the closest contact with the blood flow and is therefore most susceptible to initial damage of its very thin wall.

The Media

The *media* consists of smooth-muscle cells and elastic fibers arranged in concentric spirals. In the major branches, such as the aorta, subclavian, and the beginning of the common carotid arteries, the media is especially prominent. This is due to the enormous expansion and contraction that the vessel's wall is exposed to so close to the heart. Also, the smooth-muscle layer of the media assists the arteries in passively contracting with each diastolic component of the cardiac cycle in order to propel blood toward the smaller and terminal vessels away from the heart.

The Adventitia

The *adventitia* is the outermost layer of the vessel. This layer consists of longitudinally directed bundles of *collagen fibers*. Collagen fibers are the *fibrous component* of cartilage, bone, and smooth muscle that provide that tissue with its strength. Also in the adventitial layer are elastic fibers, nerve bundles, and a source of blood supply to the vessel itself via small blood vessels called the *vasa vasorum*.

Metabolism and Nutrition of the Vessel Wall

One of the important aspects in the development of vascular disease stems from the method by which the blood vessel is nourished. The exchange of oxygen and wastes within the blood vessel occurs both from the adventitial side as well as the lumen. There is a midpoint in the vessel, however, where the vasa vasorum cannot reach. At this point, the vessel is dependent on nourishment from the direction of the inner endothelial lining. If there is an interruption to this avenue of nourishment, the vessel becomes a target for tissue damage and subsequent disease—atherosclerosis.

Endothelial Response to Injury

Certain sections of blood vessels, particularly areas just distal to bifurcations (sections where the vessel divides in two), are susceptible to the constant *turbulent* force of blood flow. The fragile endothelium, only a single cell-layer deep, is being eroded continuously; therefore, the body is constantly making new endothelial layer.

The Shear Effect

The trauma of the force of blood flow on the endothelial lining is referred to as the *shear effect*. The shear effect develops in areas where the vessel turns, forcing the blood away from the inner arterial wall (Fig. 3-2). In some cases, the healing process does not result in normal endothelium but may develop a thickening. In time, these areas of abnormal healing can develop accumulations of lipids (or fatty deposits), and progress to the early stages of *plaque* (Fig. 3-3). Leukocytes (white cells) are also attracted to the damaged intima, which results in an inflammatory response. As plaque organizes and enlarges, fibrosis and calcification occur.

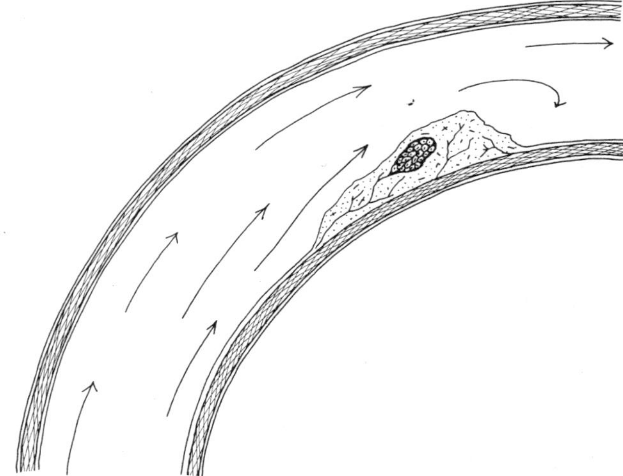

Fig. 3-2. The "shear" effect further damaging atherosclerotic plaque.

Simple Plaque

As *plaque* becomes more organized, it develops into a fibrous plaque. While the damaged endothelial wall attempts to "patch itself," the same way the skin would, by bringing in *platelets* and *thrombi*, the plaque grows still further (Fig. 3-3).

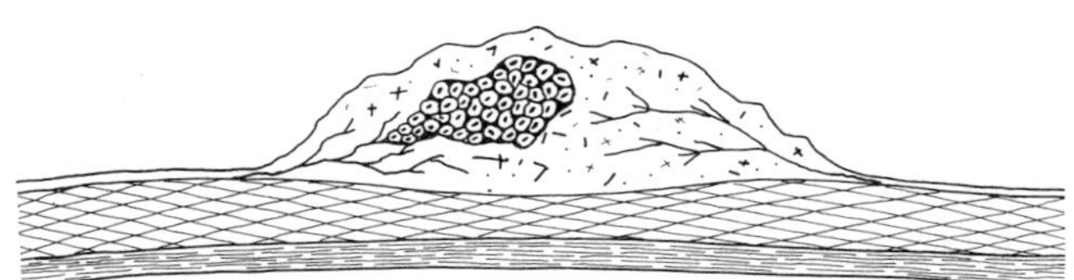

Fig. 3-3. Tissue damage within the atherosclerotic plaque.

Complex Plaque

In addition to the formation of thrombus and plaque, capillaries develop to transport oxygen and nutrients from the vessel lumen to the inner layers (Fig. 3-3). These tiny capillaries can rupture inside the vessel wall and result in an intraplaque hemorrhage. After a while, the intraplaque hemorrhage may erupt and bleed into the lumen, resulting in multiple small, or a few large, emboli.

This whole process of "tugging" and revascularization, combined with the constant building up of platelet and thrombus, adds to the problem. The plaque causes more turbulent (swirling) blood flow, which results in a greater shearing effect. Small areas on the surface of the plaque, which become eroded, form small *ulcerations* (little craters on the plaque surface). As new platelets attempt to "patch" the damaged areas, they can become dislodged by the force of the blood, causing them to break away. This dislodged material floating in the blood stream is called an *embolus* (Fig. 3-4).

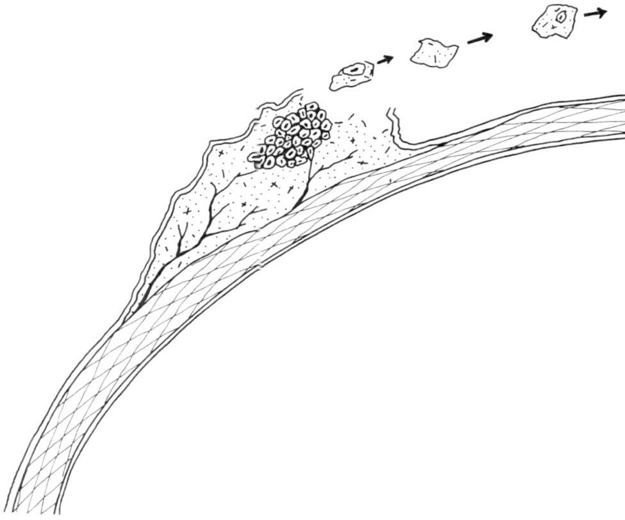

Fig. 3-4. Emboli erupting from damaged atherosclerotic plaque.

Review Exercise

1. The major cause of death in the United States and most industrial nations is

   a. stroke
   b. cardiovascular disease
   c. cancer
   d. pulmonary disease

2. Most arterial insufficiency is attributed to

   a. trauma
   b. thrombosis of the artery
   c. diabetes mellitus
   d. arteriosclerosis

3. *Atherosclerosis* refers to

   a. thickening and hardening of the artery
   b. rupture of the artery
   c. clotting of the artery
   d. obstruction of the artery

4. One typical form of arteriosclerosis is ______________________________, which is responsible for cerebrovascular and coronary artery disease.

5. Atherosclerosis is

   a. rare
   b. non-existent
   c. common
   d. present in everyone

6. Atherosclerosis in general affects

   a. capillaries
   b. arterioles
   c. small arteries
   d. medium- and large-sized arteries

7. The blood vessel is comprised of three primary layers:

   a. ______________________________

   b. ______________________________

   c. ______________________________

8. The adventitia is vessel layer closest to the blood flow. True or False?

9. Intima is present in

   a. arteries
   b. veins
   c. capillaries
   d. all of the above

10. The intima has close contact with the blood flow and is therefore

    a. the most protected from damage
    b. the least protected from damage
    c. not influenced by flow damage
    d. irrelevant

11. The media consists of

a. smooth-muscle cells and elastic fibers
b. endothelial tissue
c. fibrous tissue
d. collagen cells

12. The smooth-muscle layer of the media assists the arteries in contracting with each ________________________ component of the cardiac cycle in order to propel blood toward the smaller and terminal vessels away from the heart.

13. The adventitia is the

a. entire layer of the vessel
b. inner layer of the vessel
c. middle layer of the vessel
d. outer layer of the vessel

14. The adventitia consists of longitudinally directed bundles of

a. smooth muscle and elastic fibers
b. endothelial tissue
c. collagen fibers
d. none of the above

15. Collagen fibers are the fibrous component of

a. cartilage
b. bone
c. smooth muscle
d. all of the above

16. Collagen fibers provide tissue with its strength. True or False?

17. The adventitial layer is elastic fibers, nerve bundles, and a source of blood supply to the vessel itself via small blood vessels called the

a. vena cava
b. vas deferens
c. vasa vasorum
d. none of the above

18. One of the important aspects in the development of vascular disease stems from the method in which the blood vessel is

a. developed
b. nourished
c. traumatized
d. all of the above

19. The vasa vasorum has difficulty nourishing

a. the endothelium
b. the thickness of the vessel wall
c. the adventitia
d. the intima

20. The ________________________ plays a major role in nourishing the vessel wall.

21. If there is an interruption to the avenue of nourishment mentioned in question 20, the vessel becomes a target for

a. arteriosclerosis
b. embolus
c. atherosclerosis
d. all of the above

22. Certain sections of blood vessels, particularly areas distal to bifurcations, are protected by the turbulent force of the blood. True or False?

23. The fragile endothelium is being eroded continuously; therefore, the body is constantly making new

    a. adventitia
    b. media
    c. endothelial tissue
    d. all of the above

24. The "rebuilding" of damaged intima may lead to atherosclerosis. True or False?

25. As plaque organizes and enlarges, fibrosis decreases. True or False?

26. The damaged intimal layer *initially* "scabs" over with a layer of

    a. fatty deposits
    b. lipid deposits
    c. fibrin deposits
    d. platelet deposits

27. This patching is fragile; therefore, platelets and clots

    a. dissolve over time
    b. strengthen the vessel
    c. weaken the vessel
    d. can break off and travel distally

28. In addition to the formation of thrombus and plaque, new ______________________________ develop within the vessel.

29. The intraplaque hemorrhage may erupt and bleed into the lumen, resulting in

    a. new vessel growth
    b. low blood pressure
    c. turbulent blood flow
    d. multiple emboli

30. A small crater in a blood vessel or plaque is called

    a. a fibrous plaque
    b. a calcific plaque
    c. a thrombus
    d. an ulceration

31. The dislodged material from plaque floating in the blood stream is called

    a. a subintimal hemorrhage
    b. a homogeneous plaque
    c. a thrombus
    d. an embolus

CEREBROVASCULAR DISEASE

As vascular specialists, it is extremely important that we understand the various terms used to classify cerebrovascular disease. What is meant by amaurosis fugax? Can a stroke clear up, leaving no symptoms? And how can we use this knowledge to help guide us in noninvasive vascular examinations?

Key Terms

Amaurosis fugax
Aphasia
Asymptomatic
Atherothrombotic
Auscultation
Brain infarction
Bruit
Cardioembolic
Cerebrovascular accident
Dysarthria
Dysphasia
Embolic infarction
Hemodynamically significant infarction
Infarction
Lacunar infarct
Paresthesia
Resolving ischemic neurological deficit
Stroke
Subarachnoid hemorrhage
Thrombotic infarction
Transient ischemic attack
Transient monocular blindness
Vertebrobasilar symptoms

Asymptomatic

The *asymptomatic* category includes patients with no cerebral (brain) or retinal (eye) symptoms of vascular disease. This is a relatively common indication for a duplex study when the referring physician has discovered a bruit on routine physical examination.

Auscultation of Bruits

A *bruit* is a term meaning sound or murmur heard in *auscultation* (using a stethoscope to listen). It is most usually caused by the abnormal flow of blood in an arterial narrowing (stenosis). When the physician listens to the heart, he or she will bring the stethoscope up to the neck and listen for any sound in the carotid bifurcation area (Fig. 3-5). Normally, there should be no sound,

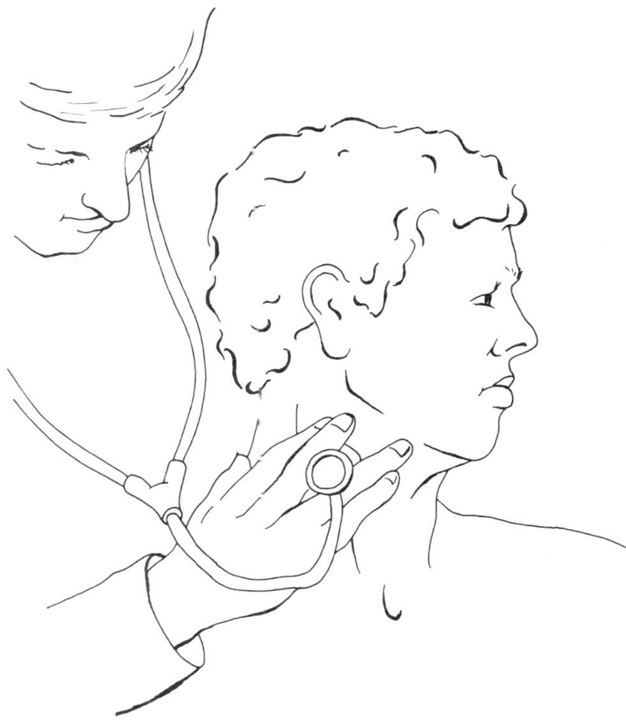

Fig. 3-5. Proper placement of a stethoscope to listen for a bruit.

although some young healthy people will have a "soft" bruit in the presence of no vessel pathology. In addition, certain types of heart murmurs, especially aortic stenosis, transmit sound up into the neck. In other cases, a bruit may be transmitted to the opposite side of the neck. As a general rule, the bruit is loudest at the point of origin.

It is not always easy for the physician to distinguish the transmitted murmur of valvular disease from that associated with the turbulence of carotid stenosis. Subsequently, the physician will refer the patient to the vascular lab for evaluation of an asymptomatic bruit to determine the source of the murmur in the neck.

Transient Ischemic Attack

A *transient ischemic attack* (TIA) is defined as a brief loss of brain function due to a temporary loss of blood supply to a particular area in the brain supplied by one vascular system. By definition, symptoms of a TIA last less than 24 hours, but most episodes last only a few minutes. The longer a TIA lasts, the more likely a *brain infarction* (irreversible damage) will be found by CAT scan or magnetic resonance imaging (MRI).

An infarction refers to necrosis (the death of tissue or cells) secondary to loss of blood supply to a particular area. For example, a *myocardial infarction* refers to the necrosis of heart muscle due to a blocked coronary artery. Blockage of blood supply to the brain results in necrosis as well (Fig. 3-6). The important distinction to make, however, is that a TIA does not usually cause brain infarction.

Most often, TIAs last just a few minutes (between 5 and 15 minutes). Symptoms most often occur in fewer than 2 minutes and very rarely in only a few seconds (symptoms *that* brief are probably not a real TIA).

The diagnosis of TIA is dependent on the circumstances, the pattern, and the timing surrounding the attack. Symptoms of numbness and dizziness are common complaints and do not necessarily indicate a TIA. A carefully documented patient history from the referring physician should clarify whether the symptoms are related to a TIA.

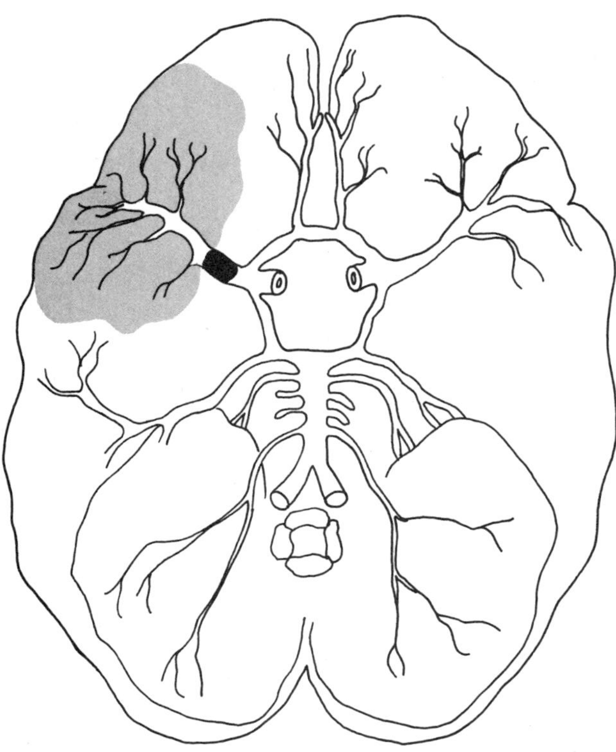

Fig. 3-6. Blocked midcerebral artery, with brain damage shown in the shaded area.

Left Carotid System TIA

The left carotid system supplies the left hemisphere with blood. TIAs in this distribution typically have a rapid onset (fewer than 2 minutes) to maximum symptoms. These include one or more of the following:

1. Motor dysfunctions such as *dysarthria* (difficulty articulating speech), weakness, paralysis, or clumsiness of the right extremities and/or face.
2. Loss of vision in the left eye (*amaurosis fugax*) or, rarely, the right field of vision.
3. Sensory symptoms such as numbness, including *paresthesia* (loss of sensation involving the right upper and lower extremity and/or face).
4. *Dysphasia* (difficulty saying words in their proper order).

Amaurosis Fugax

Amaurosis fugax (fleeting blindness) refers to a temporary loss of vision of one eye. Patients will explain this disorder as, "It was like a shade being pulled over my eye" (Fig. 3-7). Symptoms usually last for just a few minutes. Access to a thorough patient history should

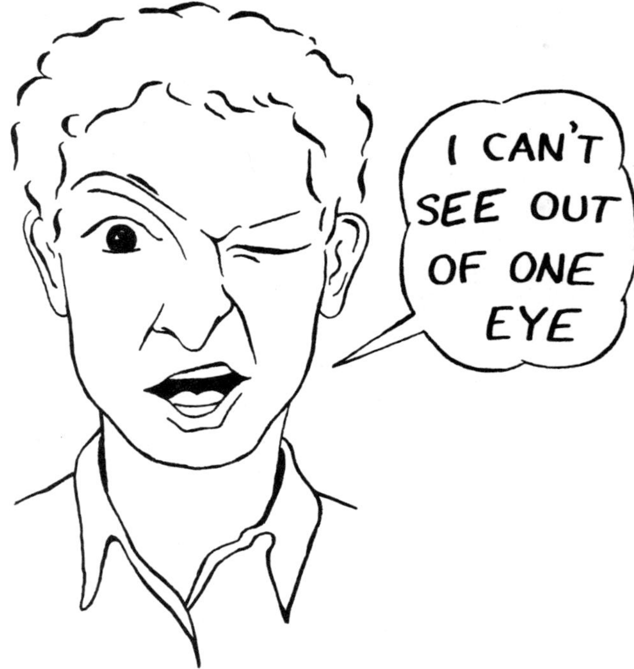

Fig. 3-7. Patients may need to close one eye to realize they have lost the vision from the other eye. This helps to differentiate bilateral blurry vision from loss of vision in one eye only.

indicate a clear distinction between general deteriorating vision and the transient loss of vision in one eye. This condition is also known as *transient monocular blindness* (TMB).

Right Carotid System TIA

The right carotid system feeds the right hemisphere with blood. TIAs in this distribution usually produce similar symptoms on the opposite side of the body. Aphasia (inability to speak), however, occurs only when the right hemisphere is dominant for speech.

Vertebrobasilar System TIA

The *vertebrobasilar system* feeds primarily the posterior brain structures. TIAs in this distribution may cause symptoms that are sometimes referred to as "drop attacks" and are characterized by the rapid onset of symptoms, including

1. motor dysfunction, which includes weakness, paralysis, or clumsiness of any combination of upper and lower extremities and face, left and/or right
2. sensory symptoms, which include loss of feeling, numbness, or paresthesia (abnormal sensation) involving the left, right, or both sides
3. loss of vision in one or both visual fields
4. loss of balance, vertigo, unsteadiness or disequilibrium, diplopia (double vision), dysphagia (trouble swallowing), or dysarthria (difficulty saying words clearly), which are generally characteristic but should not be considered as a TIA if one of these symptoms occurs alone; for example, dysarthria may occur with either carotid or vertebral artery symptoms.

Most patients have TIAs that include some type of motor (affecting movement) symptoms. Sensory (affecting sensation) symptoms involving only part of one extremity or only one side of the face during a single attack and not accompanied by other symptoms are difficult to interpret with certainty. It is common to experience amaurosis fugax without other symptoms. Some patients will have only episodes of aphasia.

Possible TIA

One beneficial concept is the diagnosis of *possible TIA*. Many patients have some symptoms that can be seen in TIAs, but there is insufficient evidence to make the diagnosis. The patient may have additional uncharacteristic symptoms, the symptoms may occur in unusual circumstances, or the description may be too vague to make a specific diagnosis of TIA. Instead of making or omitting the diagnosis of TIA when it is still suspected, a preliminary diagnosis of possible TIA may ensure that the patient still gets appropriate evaluation and care until the symptoms can be clarified.

Stroke Versus Reversible Ischemic Neurological Deficit

Stroke is defined as a neurological deficit that lasts longer than 24 hours. However, there are a number of patients who develop symptoms of a stroke that last more than 24 hours yet clear up in 1 to 3 weeks. Because some physicians consider this a more limited stroke, they identify it as a *reversible ischemic neurological deficit* (RIND).

Vertebrobasilar Disease

Symptoms of transient vertigo (a sense that the room is spinning), sudden nausea or vomiting, and ataxia (imbalance) may suggest disease of the posterior or vertebral artery system. It is also important to remember that many patients with these symptoms have other problems, such as inner ear disturbances. Symptoms of vertebrobasilar arterial system distribution include

1. motor dysfunction (weakness, paralysis, or clumsiness) of any combination of arms or legs, left or right (e.g., left arm and right leg weakness)
2. sensory dysfunction (numbness or paralysis) involving any combination of arms or legs, left or right (e.g., left arm and right leg numbness)
3. cerebellar symptoms, including loss of balance, vertigo, diplopia, or dysarthria

Review Exercise

1. Asymptomatic includes patients with

   a. no cerebral symptoms
   b. no retinal symptoms
   c. a or b
   d. neither a nor b

2. A relatively common indication for a duplex study is when the referring physician has discovered a ____________ on routine physical examination.

3. A *bruit* is a term meaning

   a. stenosis
   b. turbulence
   c. occlusion
   d. sound or murmur

4. One common condition that may mimic a bruit in the neck is

   a. asthma
   b. atheroma
   c. a stroke
   d. aortic stenosis

5. It is relatively easy for the astute physician to distinguish the transmitted murmur of valvular disease from that associated with the turbulence of carotid stenosis. True or False?

6. Symptoms of a transient ischemic attack usually last less than

   a. 24 hours
   b. 12 hours
   c. 1 hour
   d. a few minutes

7. The longer a transient ischemic attack lasts, the more likely a ________________________________ will occur.

8. An infarction refers to

   a. pain
   b. temporary loss of blood supply
   c. loss of vision in one eye
   d. necrosis of tissue

9. Ischemia refers to

   a. pain
   b. temporary loss of blood supply
   c. loss of vision in one eye
   d. necrosis of tissue

10. Transient ischemic attack, by definition, means a brain infarction has occurred. True or False?

11. Match the terms with the correct definitions:

a. Dysarthria	____ Sense the room is spinning
b. Amaurosis fugax	____ Difficulty talking
c. Aphasia	____ Abnormal sensation in the extremity
d. Dysphagia	____ Inability to talk
e. Paresthesia	____ Temporary loss of vision in one eye
f. Vertigo	____ Difficulty swallowing

12. Left carotid system TIAs typically have a rapid onset (fewer than 2 minutes) to maximum symptoms of one or more of the following. Which is not one of the symptoms?

    a. Motor dysfunction such as dysarthria, weakness, paralysis, or clumsiness of the right extremities and/or face
    b. Loss of vision in the left eye (amaurosis fugax) or, rarely, the right field of vision
    c. Sensory symptoms such as numbness, including loss of sensation (or paresthesia) involving the right upper and/lower extremity and/or face.
    d. Dizziness alone

13. Right carotid system TIAs produce similar symptoms on the opposite side except that aphasia occurs only when the right hemisphere is

    ________________________________.

14. Vertebrobasilar system TIAs are characterized by the rapid onset of symptoms. Which of the following is not a symptom?

    a. motor dysfunction, which includes weakness, paralysis, or clumsiness of any combination of upper and lower extremities and face, left and/or right
    b. sensory symptoms, which include loss of feeling, numbness, or paresthesia (abnormal sensation) involving the left, right, or both sides
    c. unconsciousness alone

15. Loss of balance, vertigo, unsteadiness or disequilibrium, diplopia, dysphagia, or dysarthria are generally characteristic of

    ________________________________.

16. Dysarthria refers to difficulty in

    ____.

17. Dysarthria occurs only with carotid TIAs. True or False?

18. It is uncommon for a patient to experience a TIA without either a motor defect, visual loss, or aphasia. True or False?

19. Temporary loss of vision in one eye is referred to as ______________

    ______________.

Stroke (Cerebrovascular Accident)

Stroke is the third leading cause of death in the United States, and this rate is increasing as the population gets older. The prognosis (forecast of the probable outcome) of stroke suggests that 80% of individuals will survive the initial event; however, 70% of those that survive will have some type of residual dysfunction, 65% will not be able to return to work, 20% will be unable to take care of themselves, and almost 5% will require total custodial care. In sum, stroke is a condition with significant ramifications.

The term *cerebrovascular accident* (CVA) includes:

1. infarction (death of tissue due to interruption of blood supply)
2. hemorrhage within the brain
3. subarachnoid hemorrhage (SAH), a hemorrhage below the lining of the brain.

Initial Assessment Categories in Stroke

One of the first assessments made of a stroke patient is whether or not the patient has the condition of improving stroke, stable stroke, or worsening stroke.

Improving Stroke

The patients with improving stroke show a steady improvement in the symptoms that have developed since the initial evaluation.

Stable Stroke

Stable stroke refers to a patient with stroke who has shown little change in deficit over a period of time, which should be specified (e.g., stroke with a stable deficit for 24 hours). The term *stable stroke* is preferred over *completed stroke* due to confusion over the latter's definition. One interpretation of completed stroke means the stroke stopped worsening, while the other meaning suggests that the stroke has resulted in maximum impairment.

Worsening Stroke

Stroke patients can worsen for a variety of reasons but the most common reason is *progressing* stroke, or what is referred to as *stroke in evolution*. Almost 50% of all stroke patients show worsening during the first few minutes or hours after the onset of the stroke. In almost 25% of patients, worsening occurs after the patient is hospitalized. Worsening stroke can be either smooth, as in gradual; step-like, as when symptoms develop after which there is a period of no worsening, followed by another increase in symptoms; and finally, fluctuating worsening.

Diagnosis of Cause of Stroke

Determination of the etiology, or cause, of a stroke can be essential to treatment and prognosis of the patient. Through various diagnostic methods, including MRI, computer tomography (CT), lumbar puncture, and noninvasive vascular and cardiac ultrasound, sources of disease and the subsequent treatment of those sources can be determined.

Common Causes

Brain Hemorrhage

Approximately 10% of all strokes are due to a brain hemorrhage. A brain hemorrhage is defined by bleeding into the brain from a vessel that has essentially ruptured. Hypertension is the leading condition associated with brain hemorrhage. The other conditions include ruptured aneurysm, arteriovenous malformations, drug abuse (with cocaine, amphetamines, or alcohol), anticoagulant therapy, and brain tumor. The process of a brain hemorrhage is usually acute and rarely preceded by a TIA. Patients will complain of a severe headache followed by a decreased level of consciousness. Symptoms and signs of brain hemorrhage may not distinguish it from other types of stroke, however.

Subarachnoid Hemorrhage

The typical characteristic clinical picture of primary subarachnoid hemorrhage (SAH) (in which the initial bleeding is into the subarachnoid space) begins with a sudden onset of a severe headache. The suddenness of the onset and the severity of the pain are usually dramatic. The headache is so severe that it interferes with the patient's activity, and vomiting is common. Patients with SAH may be younger and less likely to have underlying hypertension and other diseases before the onset of the stroke than patients with other types of stroke.

Intracranial Hemorrhage from an Arteriovenous Malformation

Subarachnoid hemorrhage, intracerebral hemorrhage, or a combination of both may occur from arteriovenous malformation (AVM). An AVM is an abnormal connection between an artery and vein where blood is inefficiently shunted between the two systems prior to the capillary level. Because of the excessive pressure of arterial flow in this sometimes fragile connection, the vessel may rupture and bleed into the brain. It is characteristic that the hemorrhage has fewer pronounced symptoms and may be less severe than SAH. There may be a history of seizures and sometimes focal cerebral symptoms and signs. In some patients, a bruit over the head may be heard.

Ischemic Stroke or Vascular Stroke

Patients with brain infarction generally have a medical history that includes one or more risk factors for the stroke; that is, patients are unlikely to have been completely healthy before the stroke. Although many of the patients have hypertension, diabetes, and heart disease, previous TIAs and strokes are also common. Neurological symptoms usually develop rapidly and may continue to worsen over hours and days. There are rarely severe headaches and vomiting associated with the onset of these symptoms. There are numerous mechanisms that result in ischemic infarction.

Thrombotic infarction usually occurs when a thrombus is superimposed on atherosclerotic plaque. In some circumstances, thrombotic infarction may be predicted by an abnormality in blood clotting.

Embolic infarction is due to occlusion of an artery by an embolus distal to a point where adequate collateral blood flow is available. The most common source of embolic infarction is from the heart. Most carotid disease causes stroke by emboli.

Hemodynamically determined infarction most commonly occurs when there is a severe stenosis (50% diameter or 75% area) or occlusion proximal to a portion of the brain and collateral circulation is inadequate to bypass the stenotic area. Most commonly, the stenosis or occlusion involves the extracranial carotid system, particularly the carotid bifurcation, although stenosis may occur at any one section (or several sections) of the vessels.

Subclavian Steal Syndrome

Subclavian steal syndrome is a result of collateral circulatory redistribution. When the origin of the subclavian artery becomes stenosed or occluded, the vertebral artery, being a significant branch of the subclavian artery, can become a major collateral vessel for the distribution of blood flow to the upper extremity. This, however, creates a problem for two reasons.

First, because of the obstruction of the subclavian artery, blood flow to the ipsilateral (same) side vertebral artery becomes compromised. Second, the diminished blood flow and pressure of the arteries of the upper extremity may siphon (suck away) blood from the basilar artery back down the vertebral artery (Fig. 3-8). This is especially true during exercise of the upper extremity when the demand for blood flow of that artery is significantly increased. The classic symptoms of subclavian steal include vertigo and presyncope following exercise of the upper extremity on the same side as the subclavian artery occlusion.

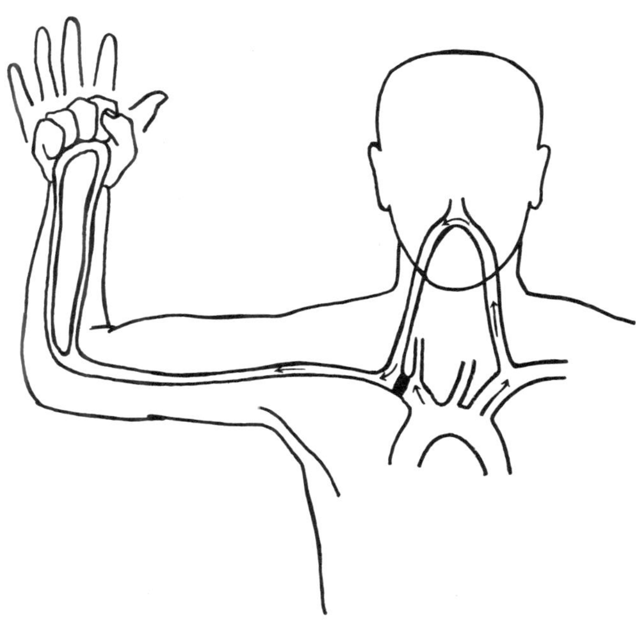

Fig. 3-8. Blocked right subclavian artery. Note blood flow in the right vertebral artery is reversed in order to supply the right arm with blood.

Clinical Categories

Vascular stroke is commonly categorized as

1. atherothrombotic-embolic
2. cardioembolic
3. lacunar

Atherothrombotic-Embolic

There are two primary mechanisms by which atherosclerosis produces infarction. First, the extracranial arteries develop plaque, which enlarges to either narrow or totally obstruct the lumen of the vessel. Second, a more common condition is the development of a superimposed thrombus. This thrombus tends to attach to plaque material and use the atherosclerosis as kind of "anchor" from which the thrombus continues to grow.

The thrombus may grow to a point at which it occludes the entire artery. In very rare cases, the thrombus may progress distally as a "stagnation clot."

The fragile thrombus that develops often breaks up, sending pieces of thrombus distally where it occludes in the narrow vessels of the brain. This condition is also known as an artery-to-artery embolus (Fig. 3-9).

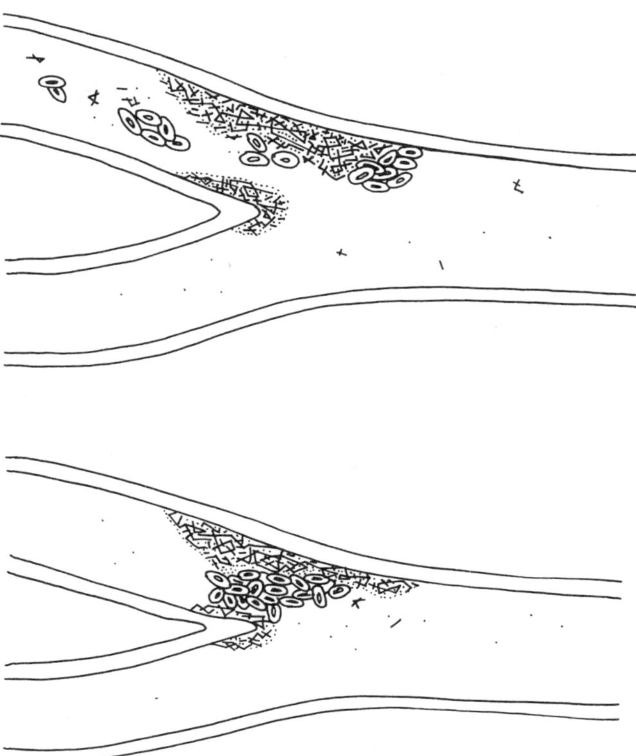

Fig. 3-9. Thrombus that forms on plaque may break away, resulting in emboli to a distal artery (A) or progress to an occlusion (B).

Cardioembolic

As the name might imply, *cardioembolic* refers to the heart as being the source of the brain infarction (Fig. 3-10). The basis for clinical diagnosis is the demonstration of cardiac disease in the absence of any other source. Cardiac conditions that may produce emboli include intermittent or continuous atrial fibrillation or flutter, recent myocardial infarction, congestive heart failure, and mitral and/or aortic valve disease. The diagnosis of cardioembolic infarction may be suggested by evidence of multiple brain or systemic infarctions in different arterial distributions. This is different from carotid artery disease, which usually causes multiple small infarcts in the same distribution.

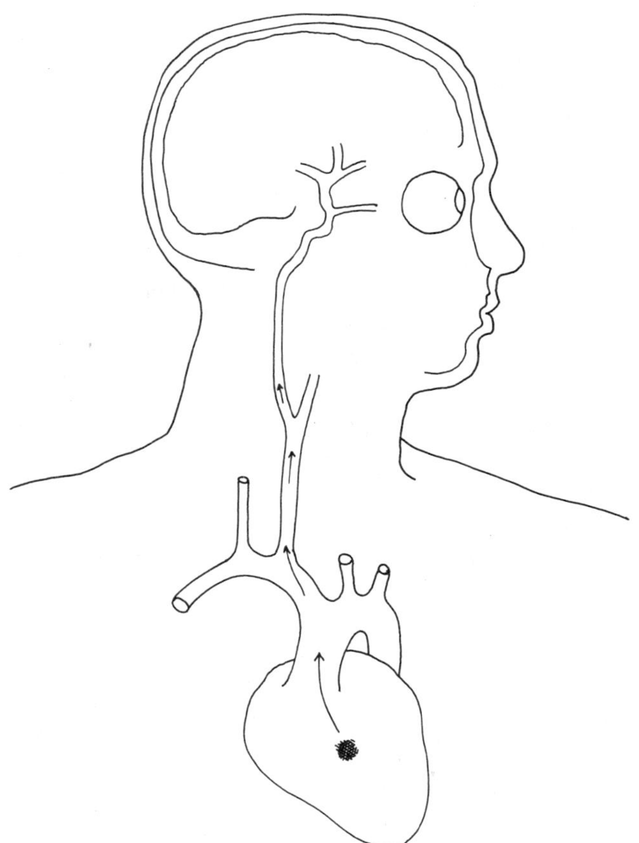

Fig. 3-10. Cardioemboli. The heart is a common source of thrombotic emboli to the brain.

Lacunar

Although *lacunar infarction* is a pathological term, it is commonly used as a clinical category for small lesions that result from the involvement of deep, small, and penetrating arteries (Fig. 3-11). There is some question as to whether lacunar infarcts may actually be thromboembolic in origin.

Lacunar arteries tend to branch deep inside the brain at 90 degrees from the main intracerebral vessels that supply the deep penetrating arteries of the white and gray matter of the cerebral hemispheres. Because these arteries typically have poor collateral connections, obstruction of blood flow by arterial disease, thrombus, or embolus leads to infarction in the limited distribution of these arteries. Over a period of time, these infarctions become cystic and filled with fluid and surrounded by normal tissue, giving a lake-like appearance (lacunar means "lake").

Diagnosis is usually made by brain imaging, which typically shows a small (less than 1.5 cm in diameter) lesion consistent with the distribution of the deficit. Prognosis is generally good for recovery of function.

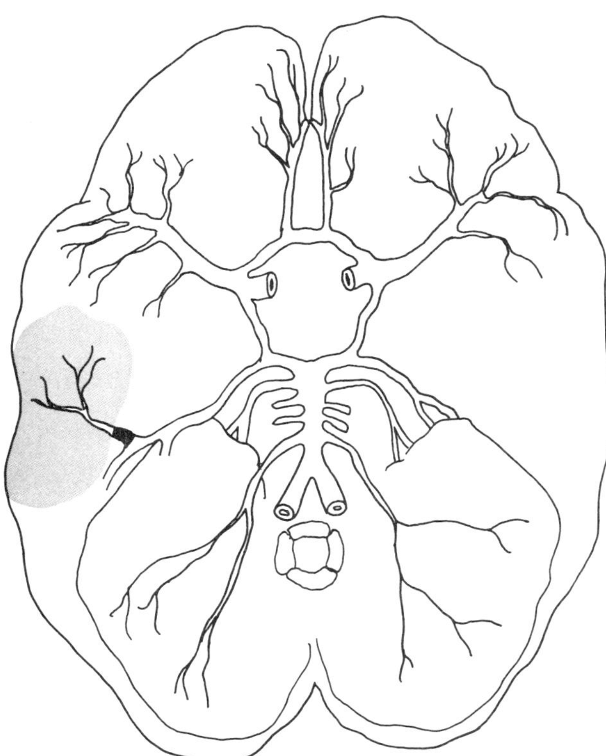

Fig. 3-11. Lacunar infarcts stem from deep branches inside the brain.

Symptoms by Site (Arterial Distribution)

Another method in describing cerebrovascular disease is by describing the symptoms by site. Although much of this information may sound repetitive, it will help to further enhance your understanding of both the pathology and terms used to describe various conditions.

When a patient is referred for a noninvasive vascular study, the referring physician may already have a fairly good idea where the stroke *originated*, depending on the site and size of the brain damage. To be certain, one must look at the particular area affected and know the vascular anatomy of that area. The usual practice is to think of the brain as being divided into two major categories:

1. The carotid system
2. The vertebrobasilar system

The Carotid System

The Internal Carotid Artery

The clinical picture of symptoms originating from carotid artery system disease includes

1. monoparesis (weakness of a single limb)
2. hemiparesis (weakness of one half of the body)
3. transient monocular blindness
4. sensory losses (numbness)
5. paresthesias (burning or prickling sensations)

Although *transient monocular blindness*, or amaurosis fugax (loss of vision in one eye) is commonly associated with carotid artery disease, permanent monocular blindness is rare with total occlusion of the vessel.

Occlusion of a carotid artery may result in anything from no symptoms at all to a slight TIA or a devastating stroke. In the presence of an adequate collateral system, occlusion of the internal carotid artery in the neck may not produce any characteristic clinical picture. Carotid artery stenosis may also cause stroke by artery-to-artery embolism or propagation of a stagnation clot distally into the stem of the middle cerebral artery.

Middle Cerebral Artery

The *middle cerebral artery* begins at the bifurcation of the internal carotid artery. Occlusion of the first portion of the middle cerebral artery most often produces a neurological deficit. Because an occlusion of the middle cerebral artery is distal to the circle of Willis, opportunities for collateralization are limited.

Occlusion of the middle cerebral artery may result in a significant deficit, including hemiplegia (paralysis of half the body, usually the contralateral arm and leg), hemisensory deficit (loss of feeling of half the body, usually the contralateral arm and leg), visual changes, and if the infarction occurs on the dominant side of the brain, aphasia. Severe stenosis of the middle cerebral artery may also be associated with infarction of the portions of the hemisphere supplied by the artery or its major branches.

Anterior Cerebral Artery
The most common symptom associated with occlusion or severe stenosis of the anterior cerebral artery is weakness of the opposite leg. Loss of sensation may also accompany the weakness and aphasia (difficulty in expressing speech), and cognitive impairment may also occur. Frontal lobe infarcts may produce "soft symptoms" such as personality change or memory loss.

Vertebrobasilar System

Severe stenosis or occlusion of one or both vertebral arteries may cause ischemia or infarction of the posterior sections of the brain. These symptoms are characterized by severe vertigo, nausea, vomiting, dysphagia, and decreased pain and temperature discrimination. Severe stenosis or occlusion of the left subclavian artery or the brachiocephalic artery may cause a reversal of blood flow of the ipsilateral vertebral artery; however, as previously mentioned, it does not always cause symptoms.

Basilar Artery
Occlusion of the basilar artery may result in infarction of the brain stem or sometimes TIAs, but on rare occasions, there are no symptoms at all. Dizziness and vertigo are frequent symptoms and nystagmus (jumpy eye movements with looking to the left or right) is a common finding.

Posterior Cerebral Artery
The basilar artery terminates in the two posterior cerebral arteries. Severe stenosis or occlusion of these arteries may result in visual defects, unremitting body pain, and behavior disorders.

Intracranial Hemorrhage from an Arteriovenous Malformation

Occasionally, an artery and vein may connect inside the brain, causing blood to shunt back and forth between the two vessels. Subsequently, these vessels may burst and hemorrhage. Although the symptoms may mimic those of a subarachnoid or intracerebral hemorrhage, the development of those symptoms usually occurs more slowly.

Review Exercise

1. Stroke is the ______________ leading cause of death in the United States.

2. There are two primary mechanisms by which atherosclerosis produces infarction. First, the extracranial arteries develop plaque, which enlarges to either ____________________________blood flow or totally ____________________________ the lumen of the vessel.

3. What condition may occur once a thrombus grows to a point that it occludes the artery?

   a. Ulceration
   b. Cerebral vascular accident
   c. Atherosclerosis
   d. Pulmonary embolus

4. An arterial thrombus that breaks up, sending pieces of thrombus distally where it occludes in the narrow vessels of the brain, is referred to as

   a. transmural thrombus
   b. artery-to-artery embolus
   c. atherosclerosis
   d. stagnation clot

5. The basis for clinical diagnosis of a cardioembolic stroke is the demonstration of

   a. cardiac disease in the absence of any other source
   b. MRI
   c. CT
   d. duplex ultrasound

6. The diagnosis of cardioembolic infarction may be suggested by evidence of multiple brain or systemic infarctions. True or False?

7. Lacunar infarction is used as a clinical category for lesions that result from the involvement of

   a. large cerebral arteries
   b. small superficial arteries
   c. circle of Willis
   d. deep, small, and penetrating arteries of the brain

8. Lacunar infarctions are lesions usually

   a. hemispheric
   b. variable
   c. less than 1.5 cm in diameter
   d. greater than 1.5 cm in diameter

9. Once the diagnosis of lacunar infarct is made, prognosis is generally (good/poor) for recovery of function.

10. In regard to cerebrovascular disease it is helpful to think of the brain as being divided into two major vascular systems: the ____________________________ and ____.

11. Which of the following conditions is *not* a typical symptom originating from internal carotid artery system disease?

a. Monoparesis
b. Hemiparesis
c. Visual and speech problems
d. Vertigo

12. Transient monocular blindness is commonly associated with _______________ artery disease.

13. Permanent monocular blindness is common with total occlusion of the carotid artery. True or False?

14. The middle cerebral artery begins at the

a. bifurcation of the internal carotid artery
b. circle of Willis
c. bifurcation of the anterior cerebral artery
d. bifurcation of the anterior communication artery

15. Occlusion of the first portion of the middle cerebral artery most often produces

a. transient monocular blindness
b. a neurological deficit
c. instant death
d. no symptoms at all

16. With an occlusion of the middle cerebral artery opportunities for collateralization are _______________

17. Typically, occlusion of the middle cerebral artery results in significant deficit, including all the following symptoms *except*

a. transient monocular blindness
b. vertigo
c. hemisensory deficit
d. hemiplegia

18. If an infarction of the middle cerebral artery occurs on the dominant side of the brain,

a. aphasia occurs
b. aphasia never occurs
c. ataxia occurs
d. ataxia never occurs

19. The most common symptom associated with occlusion or severe stenosis of the anterior cerebral artery is

a. weakness of the ipsilateral (opposite) leg
b. weakness of the contralateral (same) leg
c. weakness of both legs
d. none of the above

20. Severe stenosis or occlusion of the left subclavian artery or the brachiocephalic artery may cause a _______________ of blood flow on the same side.

21. Severe stenosis or occlusion of one or both vertebral arteries may likely cause ischemia or infarction of the

a. anterior part of the brain
b. posterior parts of the brain
c. lateral sides of the brain
d. entire brain

22. Symptoms of vertebral artery disease are characterized by which of the following?

a. Transient monocular blindness
b. Hemiparesis
c. Severe vertigo, nausea, and vomiting
d. Dysarthria

23. It is common for an occlusion of the basilar artery to cause no symptoms at all. True or False?

24. Which are typical symptoms of basilar or vertebral artery stenosis?

a. Transient monocular blindness
b. Hemiparesis
c. Dysarthria
d. Dizziness and vertigo

25. Subclavian steal syndrome is a result of collateral circulatory

a. distribution
b. redistribution
c. development
d. none of the above

26. When the origin of the ____ becomes stenosed or occluded, the vertebral artery can become a major collateral vessel for the distribution of blood flow to the upper extremity.

27. Ipsilateral refers to the _____________ side

28. Contralateral refers to the __________________________ side.

29. When blood flow of the subclavian artery is obstructed, flow to the ipsilateral side

a. increases
b. becomes compromised
c. fluctuates
d. stays the same

30. The diminished blood flow and pressure of the arteries of the upper extremity may _____________ blood from the basilar artery back down the vertebral artery.

31. Symptoms of subclavian steal are actually increased during

a. sexual activity
b. walking
c. valsalva
d. arm exercising

32. The classic symptoms of subclavian steal include _____________ and __________________________ after exercising the upper extremity on the same side as the subclavian artery occlusion.

PERIPHERAL ARTERIAL DISEASE

Peripheral arterial disease (PAD) is an extremely common disorder in the United States. Unlike cerebrovascular disease, symptoms might be less dramatic or life threatening and the patient may not seek medical help until the level of disease has advanced significantly. It is important for the vascular specialist to be aware of the various symptoms associated with this disorder and the mechanisms for developing the disease.

Key Terms

Abductor hiatus
Aneurysm
Aortoiliac disease
Bruit
Buerger's disease
Diabetes
Claudication
Femoropopliteal disease
Gangrene
Hunter's canal
In-flow disease
Ischemia
Peripheral vascular disease
Popliteal artery entrapment
Pseudoaneurysm
Rest pain
Raynaud's disease
Run-off
Thoracic outlet syndrome
Thromboangiitis obliterans
Tibioperoneal disease

Mechanism for Disease

Peripheral refers to the area outside or away from the central area, or in this case, outside or away from the heart. It is a term used to distinguish between the general categories of vascular disease, either cerebrovascular or venous. The peripheral arteries are generally the main arteries to the upper and lower extremities.

The mechanisms of PAD, including aortoiliac disease, are primarily hemodynamic in nature. PAD is typically atherosclerosis of the large- and medium-sized arteries. Diabetic vascular disease, on the other hand, usually affects small vessels of the feet and, less commonly, the hands. Because of clinical considerations, lower extremity disease is categorized as

1. inflow or aortoiliac disease
2. outflow or femoropopliteal disease
3. run-off or tibioperoneal disease

Aortoiliac Disease or Inflow Disease

Aortoiliac disease involves the abdominal aorta and iliac arteries. As with most parts of arterial circulation, the point at which the common iliac arteries bifurcate from the abdominal aorta is a common site for A-I stenosis. Patients with significant disease at the aortoiliac level may complain of buttocks pain when exercising. Impotence may also be a complaint of A-I disease in that the blood supply to the penis can be affected.

Femoropopliteal or Outflow Disease

Femoropopliteal disease includes disease of the common femoral, superficial femoral, and popliteal arteries. The bifurcation of the profunda and superficial femoral artery is a common site for stenosis. The most common site for disease is the section of the superficial femoral artery that passes through the *adductor hiatus*, also known as *Hunter's Canal*, located at the distal third of the thigh. Although bifurcations and bends in any artery are common sites for stenosis, significant plaque may occur anywhere in the vessel.

Tibioperoneal or Run-off Disease

The distal vessels of the lower extremity—the anterior tibial, the posterior tibial, and the peroneal artery—are the major branches that supply the lower extremity. Like the superficial femoral artery, disease may occur at the bifurcations and take-off (or the origin) of these vessels or occur in isolated segments. Again, the most common cause of significant *tibioperoneal disease* is diabetes mellitus.

Common Symptoms

Claudication

When one exercises, the increased demands of the muscles in the legs require a greater blood flow to maintain the oxygen and nutritional needs. In fact, that demand can exceed four to five times the blood flow at rest. That is an enormous increase in demand! To meet that demand, the blood vessels, especially in the calf, dilate in order to lower the arterial resistance and increase the necessary amount of blood flow to the muscle. In the normal vessel, this is precisely what happens. This dilation occurs at the precapillary level but not in the main conduit arteries.

With a stenosis in one or more of the major arteries, however, it becomes more difficult for the increased amount of blood to get through the diseased vessel. Subsequently, the muscle is unable to receive the blood it requires. The muscle lets the brain know of the problem by "sending a message" indicating the lack of blood to that muscle. This message may be interpreted as "weakness," "aching" or "cramping." This condition is called *claudication* (from the Greek word meaning "to limp").

As with cerebrovascular disease, a good patient history will help suggest where the offending lesion is located. For example, if a patient complains of right-calf claudication, it is likely that the vessel in question is the right iliac, femoral, or popliteal artery. If, on the other hand, the patient complains of bilateral buttocks pain with walking, the vascular specialist would likely suspect the aortoiliac system. Most patients with aortoiliac disease, who complain of proximal (buttock or thigh) symptoms also have calf claudication, which may be of worse severity. It is also extremely important to distinguish neurological or orthopedic type symptoms from those of a vascular origin.

Rest Pain

The patient with claudication has adequate blood flow at rest and only becomes symptomatic when the demands of exercise exceed the limited blood flow. What happens when a blood vessel is so diseased that the blood flow has difficulty supplying the tissue at rest? This condition may present initially at night when the blood pressure drops during sleep and the leg is lying horizontal (as opposed to dependent in a standing position).

The patient will wake from sleep with a "burning" or "dull aching pain" in the foot, which is only relieved when he gets up from bed and either dangles the leg over the edge of the bed (dependency) or gets up out of bed and walks around. The reason for relief of symptoms is that blood pressure improves just enough with walking, in combination of the dependence of the foot, to increase the pressure to get blood through the lesion.

It is important to distinguish the difference between rest pain and night leg cramps. Charlie horses or muscle cramps are common among elderly patients and it is important to ask the patient particular questions that will clarify between the two. Night muscle cramps often will be described as a "knot" in the muscle, which the patient needs to rub or massage in order to get relief. Rest pain is more typically burning in nature and releived by foot dependency.

Gangrene

The most severe form of arterial insufficiency occurs when the patient is not able to relieve the symptoms by any means available, such as resting after exercise or walking at night. At this point, the blood vessel is so diseased that blood supply cannot meet even the minimal demands of the muscle tissue. Subsequently, that tissue that is most distal to the leg (usually the toes or the heel) becomes extremely painful and dies. *Gangrene* is characterized by the loss of tissue associated with the loss of vascular supply. This is usually followed by bacterial invasion and putrification (production of foul-smelling compounds due to the breakdown of organic material).

Functional Impairment as a Measure of Severity of Disease

The severity of the restriction to blood flow is reflected in how far the patient can walk. It is important to inquire how far the patient *must* walk before the symptoms occur and how long it takes before the symptoms go away. Most often, distance references are in blocks (as in "city blocks"); because not everyone lives in a city, however, it is important to determine the distance by other measurements (i.e., feet or yards).

Review Exercise

1. The mechanisms of peripheral arterial disease, including aortoiliac disease, are primarily ______________________________ in nature.

2. The major clinical categories of peripheral arterial disease include

   a. ______________________________

   b. ______________________________

   c. ______________________________

3. Aortoiliac disease includes disease of the

   a. abdominal aorta
   b. common iliac arteries
   c. external iliac arteries
   d. all the above

4. The aortic ______________________________ is a common site for aortoiliac disease.

5. Pain associated with vascular disease, which is made worse with exercise and relieved with rest, is called

   a. rest pain
   b. calf cramps
   c. ischemia
   d. claudication

6. When one exercises, the increased demands of the muscles in the legs require an even greater ______________________________ to maintain the oxygen and nutritional needs.

7. To meet that demand, the blood vessels _______________ in order to lower the arterial resistance and increase the necessary amount of blood flow.

8. When there is an ______________________________ or severe ______________________________in one or more of the major arteries, it becomes more difficult for the increased amount of blood to get through the vessel, and the exercising muscle is unable to receive the blood it requires.

9. Initially, a good ______________________________ will help suggest where the offending lesion of peripheral arterial disease is located.

10. If a patient complains of right-calf claudication, it is likely that one of the vessels in question is the:

    a. the peroneal artery
    b. right anterior tibial artery
    c. right posterior tibial artery
    d. right superficial femoral artery

11. If a patient complains of bilateral buttocks pain with walking, the vascular specialist would likely suspect the

    a. aortoiliac arteries
    b. right internal iliac artery
    c. right posterior tibial artery
    d. right superficial femoral-popliteal artery

12. In regard to functional impairment, it is important to inquire ______________________________ before the symptoms occur and ______________________________ before the symptoms go away.

13. The next stage of arterial disease after claudication is typically

    a. non-healing foot ulcers
    b. rest pain
    c. pseudoclaudication
    d. surgery

14. Rest pain typically occurs

    a. after exercising
    b. during the day
    c. day or night
    d. at night

15. A patient who wakes from sleep with a burning or aching pain in the leg associated with ischemic rest pain will typically get some relief by

    a. taking aspirin
    b. elevating the foot
    c. massaging the calf
    d. hanging the foot over the edge of the bed

16. The most severe form of arterial insufficiency occurs when the patient is unable to relieve symptoms by any means available, such as resting after exercise or hanging the foot over the edge of the bed. True or False?

17. Ischemic rest pain suggests that the blood supply cannot meet even the ______________ demands of the muscle tissue.

18. Ischemic tissue that is most distal to the leg (usually the toes or the heel) may become

    a. necrotic
    b. painful
    c. cold
    d. all of the above

19. The condition of dead tissue associated with severe vascular insufficiency is referred to as

    a. claudication
    b. gangrene
    c. edema
    d. diabetic neuropathy

Aneurysms

Arterial *aneurysms* are a relatively common disorder that affect as many as 4% of the adult population in the United States. Although the most common type of aneurysm is the abdominal aortic aneurysm (AAA), they may be found in any arterial segment, including femoral, popliteal, and cerebral arteries.

Enlarged aneurysms may compress nearby nerves, resulting in paresthesia or paralysis of extremities. In addition, the enlarged vessel causes turbulent blood flow increasing the possibility of thrombus and emboli. Finally, a ruptured aneurysm most often has devastating consequences because enormous quantities of blood are pumped out of the vessel in a very brief time.

An aneurysm generally is defined as a permanent localized dilatation of an artery. This dilatation is most often due to the degenerative changes in the arterial wall. However, it is also believed to be a result of the nutritive changes in the arterial wall due to blockages of the small vessels that feed the vasa vasorum. This process causes a weakening of all three layers of the vessel wall, which causes a bubble to extend outside of the vascular wall segment (Fig. 3-12). The weakness of the vessel wall is considered to be genetic in that almost 50% of all popliteal arteries are bilateral and 30% are associated with an aortic aneurysm. It is essential to carefully monitor the abdominal aortic aneurysm's size, which affects the surgeon's decision regarding whether to operate.

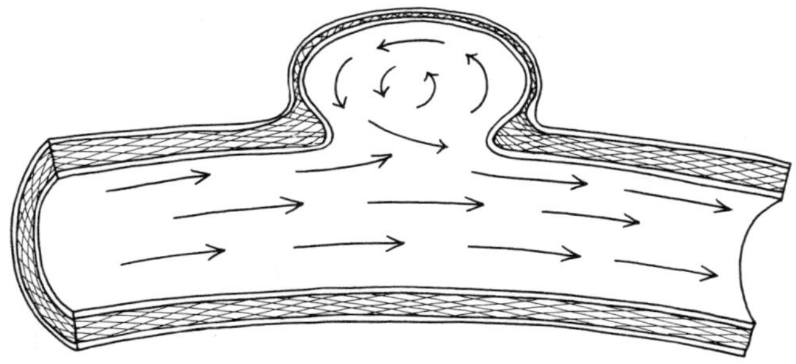

Fig. 3-12. A true aneurysm involves all three layers of an arterial wall.

False Aneurysm

Clinically, false aneurysms (*pseudoaneurysms*) may appear similar to a true aneurysm. The patient history, however, will suggest that either trauma or recent vascular surgery may be the cause. False aneurysms occur when there has been a rupture of all three layers of the arterial wall. Blood escaping from the artery forms a sac outside the vessel wall. Flow between the sac and the artery results in a pulsating mass that typically feels like a true aneurysm (Fig. 3-13).

The most common source for a pseudoaneurysm is trauma. Patients usually complain of a severe blow or penetrating injury to an extremity, after which a pulsating mass is noticed. Hospitalized patients undergoing invasive arteriography procedures are also at increased risk. As many as 0.5% to 1% of patients undergoing cardiac catheterization report an incidence of complication in the form of a pseudoaneurysm. These induced aneurysms are the unfortunate result of a needle at the puncture site. The subsequent leak of blood into the adjacent tissue results in a small pocket of blood that moves freely in and out of the vessel with each cardiac cycle. The risk of the pseudoaneurysm is possible rupture and hemorrhage.

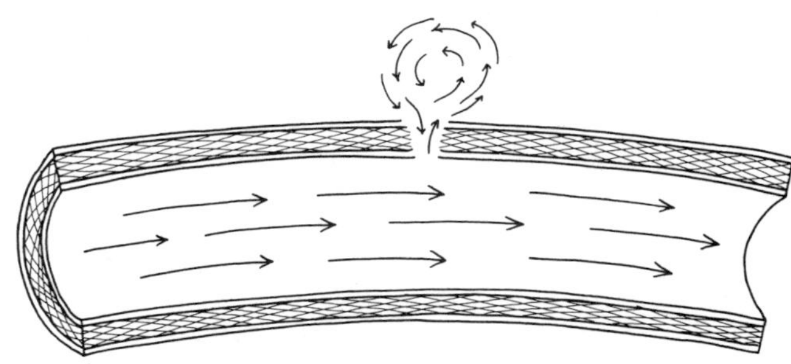

Fig. 3-13. A false aneurysm.

Abdominal Aortic Aneurysm

Abdominal aortic aneurysms (AAAs) most often arise below the level of the renal arteries (Fig. 3-14). In most cases, they are a result of atherosclerosis. Most patients present with an asymptomatic pulsatile mass that has been discovered by themselves, their primary physician, or inadvertently by ultrasound, CT, or x-ray done for other reasons. In general, AAAs larger than 5 cm in diameter should be electively repaired. Smaller aneurysms should be followed every 3 to 6 months by ultrasound, which is considered to be 95% accurate within 0.5 cm.

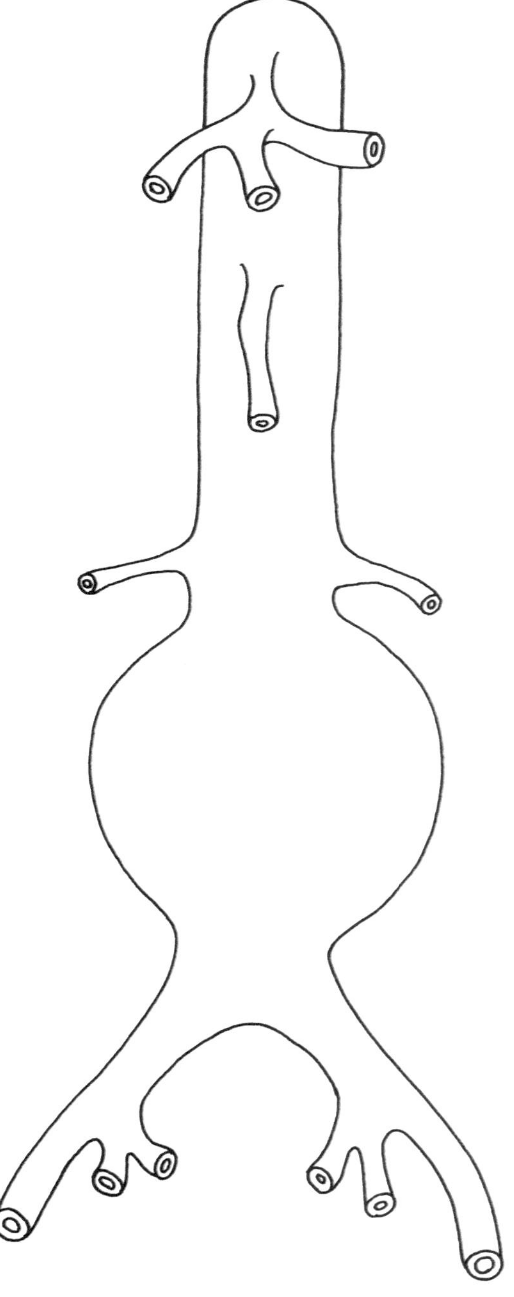

Fig. 3-14. An abdominal aortic aneurysm.

Popliteal Artery Entrapment Syndrome

Popliteal artery entrapment is a condition that may be responsible for the complaint by younger patients of unilateral claudication in the lower extremity. This condition develops as a result of a compression of the gastrocnemius muscle on the popliteal artery. Twenty-five percent of the time, the opposite leg is affected as well, although the actual number may be higher because few angiographic studies are performed bilaterally. This condition is relatively rare, but it must be considered in young adults who present with unilateral calf claudication. The usual feature of this syndrome is normal pedal pulses at rest that diminish when the calf contracts.

Buerger's Disease

Thromboangiitis obliterans, also known as Buerger's disease, is an occlusive disease of the medium-sized and small arteries chiefly of the upper extremities and lower limbs of young adult male smokers. The annual incidence of this disease is rare—only about 8 in 100,000—and occurs in males more often than in females.

Raynaud's Disease

Raynaud's disease and Raynaud's phenomenon are described as a bilateral paroxysmal (sudden) contraction of the arterioles and arteries in the digits. The condition is usually brought on by cold or emotion and is relieved by warming the affected digits. The classic sign of Raynaud's disease is that the color in the hands changes with the vasoconstriction from white to blue to red.

Diagnosis of Raynaud's disease is made from the following points:

1. Women are much more commonly affected than are men.
2. It is a disease that is less common before puberty and after age 40, although it may occur at any age.
3. Symptoms involve bilateral and symmetrical involvement of the digits. The hands are much more commonly affected than are the feet.
4. Pallor (waxy whiteness) of the digits can be reproduced by immersion of the digits into cold water or by emotional arousal. The fingers turn blue if the smaller vessels remain dilated or pale if they contract. Upon warming, hyperemia (excess of blood flow) causes the digits to turn red.

Review Exercise

1. Aneurysms have been described as a weakening of

   a. the intima b. the media
   c. the adventitia d. all of the above

2. List three complications of an arterial aneurysm.

   a. ______________________________

   b. ______________________________

   c. ______________________________

3. The most common causes of a pseudoaneurysm are ______________ or ______________________________.

4. The most common site for aneurysms is

   a. aorta b. femoral arteries
   c. popliteal arteries d. all of the above

5. The weakness of the vessel wall is considered to be genetic. True or False?

6. Bilateral popliteal artery aneurysms are rare. True or False?

7. Estimation of the aneurysm ______________ is important in clinical decisions regarding the need for treatment.

8. The most common source for a pseudoaneurysm is

   a. genetic b. infection
   c. atherosclerosis d. trauma

9. With a pseudoaneurysm, patients usually describe a history of trauma and develop

   a. a painful extremity b. an ischemic ulcer
   c. a pulsating mass d. claudication

10. Hospitalized patients undergoing ______________________________ are also at high risk for pseudoaneurysm.

11. As many as ______________% to ______________% of patients undergoing cardiac catheterization report an incidence of complication in the form of a pseudoaneurysm.

12. The most likely cause of a *pseudoaneurysm* during cardiac catheterization is

    a. hypertension
    b. needle puncture during angiography
    c. hyperlipidemia
    d. all of the above

13. The leakage of blood from a pseudoaneurysm often moves freely in and out of the vessel with each cardiac cycle. True or False?

14. List two risks of the untreated pseudoaneurysm:

    a. ______________________________

    b. ______________________________

15. Popliteal artery entrapment syndrome is more common among

    a. diabetics
    b. hospitalized patients
    c. older patients
    d. younger patients

16. Typical symptoms of popliteal artery entrapment syndrome are

    a. calf claudication
    b. non-healing ulcers
    c. bilateral calf pain
    d. unilateral calf pain

17. Popliteal artery entrapment is a result of a compression of the ______________________________ on the popliteal artery.

18. Thromboangiitis obliterans is an occlusive disease of the

    a. digits of the hands and feet
    b. abdominal vessels
    c. medium-sized vessels of the upper and lower extremities
    d. small-sized vessels of the upper and lower extremities

19. Buerger's disease is chiefly a disease of:

    a. young adult male smokers
    b. young adult female smokers
    c. older patients
    d. diabetics

20. Buerger's disease is more common in young men than in young women. True or False?

21. Raynaud's disease and Raynaud's phenomenon are described as a bilateral paroxysmal (sudden) contraction of the arteries and arterioles in the

    a. upper extremities
    b. lower extremities
    c. extremities and digits
    d. digits

22. Raynaud's syndrome is usually brought on by

a. cold
b. emotion
c. infection
d. a and b

23. The symptoms of Raynaud's disease are relieved by

a. massaging the affected area
b. taking blood thinners
c. elevating the affected digits
d. warming the affected digits

24. Diagnosis of Raynaud's disease is made from the following points:

a. Women are (more/less) affected than are men.
b. It is a disease that is less common before ____________ and after ____________
c. The (hands/feet) are much more commonly affected than are the (hands/feet).
d. Pallor (waxy whiteness) of the digits can be reproduced by immersion of the digits into ________________________ or by ________________________________.

25. In Raynaud's phenomenon, the fingers turn ____________ if the smaller vessels remain dilated.

26. In Raynaud's disease, the fingers turn ____________ if the smaller vessels contract.

27. In Raynaud's disease, the fingers turn ____________ when they are warmed.

Arterio-Venous Fistulas

An *arteriovenous fistula* (AV fistula) is an abnormal communication between an artery and a vein (Fig. 3-15). Although congenital arteriovenous fistulas are relatively rare, the noninvasive vascular lab is seeing more trauma-related conditions. Any object that penetrates the skin and injures both artery and vein may cause a traumatic arteriovenous fistula. Venipuncture and catheterization occasionally cause AV fistula, but bullets and knife wounds are more often the causes found in inner city medical centers.

Arterioventricular fistulas, if large, may cause varicosities (enlarged veins), edema (swelling), and a local mass that may press on adjacent nerves. Traumatic fistulas are almost always accompanied by a bruit, and a thrill (palpable bruit) may also be felt.

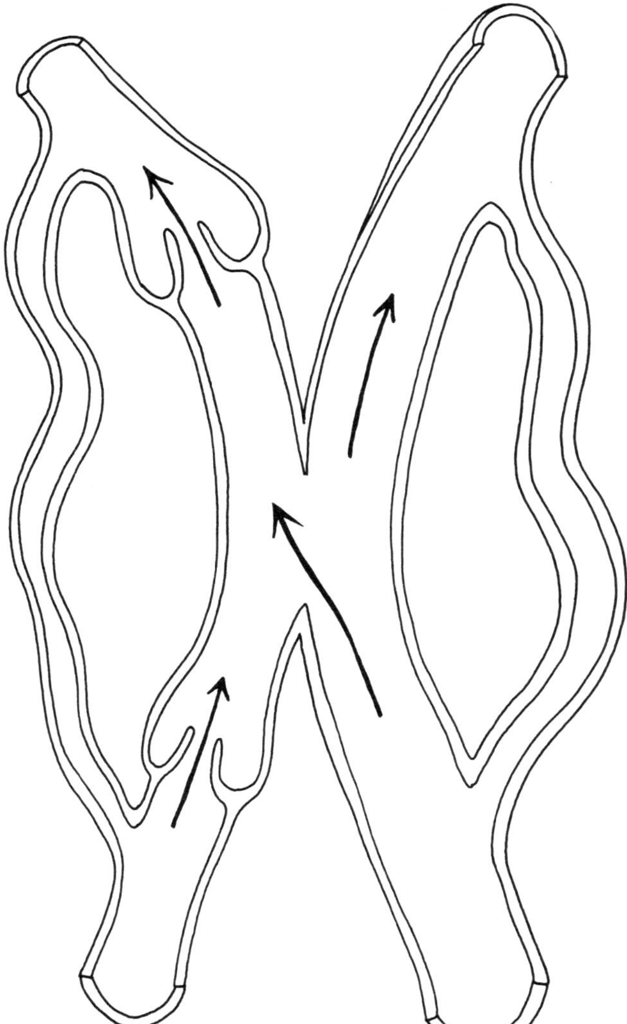

Fig. 3-15. Abnormal connection between the artery and vein. High-pressure arterial blood will flow into the low-pressure venous system. This results in abnormally high venous flow velocities in the venous system.

Thoracic Outlet Syndrome

Thoracic outlet syndrome (TOS) is a relatively rare condition that affects the shoulder and upper extremity in young and middle-aged adults. This condition is caused by a congenital abnormality of the muscle bands in the axilla where the network of arteries, veins, and nerves comes together (Fig. 3-16). TOS may also be caused by trauma.

Symptoms of TOS consist of aching discomfort, which usually radiates down the forearm to the hand. Paresthesia (numbness and tingling) are usually present due to compression of the nerves. The most common arterial problem of TOS is arterial embolism from a constricted axillary artery. Patients with stenotic lesions most often develop arm *claudication*. Sometimes patients will complain that the whole arm "goes to sleep," and in more severe cases the hand may lose muscle strength and coordination.

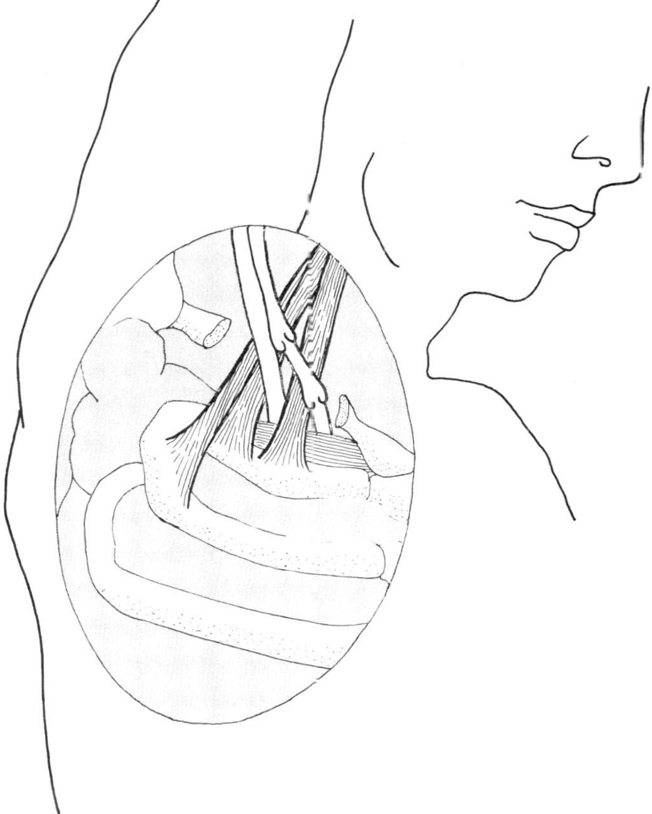

Fig. 3-16. Axillary artery and vein between the muscular bands of the shoulder. These muscular bands may cause constriction of blood flow to or from the upper extremity.

Review Exercise

1. An arteriovenous fistula (AV fistula) is an abnormal ______________________________ between an artery and a vein.

2. Congenital arteriovenous fistulas are relatively rare. True or False?

3. Any object that punctures the skin and injures both artery and vein may cause

   a. an aneurysm b. a pseudoaneurysm
   c. an AV fistula d. b and c

4. What two situations may cause an AV fistula or pseudoaneurysm?

   a. diabetes mellitus b. venipuncture
   c. cardiac catheterization d. cardioembolus

5. Traumatic fistulas are almost always accompanied by a

   a. pulsating mass b. hemorrhage
   c. aneurysm d. bruit

6. A palpable bruit is referred to as a

   a. fistula b. thrill
   c. venous hum d. murmur

7. Thoracic outlet syndrome (TOS) is an affliction of the:

   a. chest cavity b. lungs
   c. upper extremities d. vertebrobasilar system

8. TOS is caused by an abnormality of the muscle bands in the axilla where the network of ____ comes together.

9. The area where the above structures come together is referred to as the

   a. solar plexus b. brachial plexus
   c. axilla d. none of the above

10. TOS rarely involves the

    a. subclavian artery b. axillary artery
    c. subclavian vein d. a and c

11. TOS is a rare disorder usually seen in

    a. young and middle-aged adults b. older females
    c. older males d. Asians

12. Symptoms of TOS typically radiate down

    a. the chest wall b. the back
    c. the arm d. all of the above

VENOUS DISEASE

The noninvasive vascular testing has become a reliable and accurate screening technique for deep vein thrombophlebitis. In many vascular labs, over half of all the studies performed are to rule out deep vein thrombosis. As with other noninvasive studies, it is extremely important that the vascular specialist be fully knowledgeable of the physiology associated with venous disease in order to best perform the study and interpret the findings.

Key Terms

Calf-muscle pump
Chronic stasis ulcer
Chronic venous thrombosis
Deep vein thrombosis
Dorsiflexion
Erythrocytes
Edema
Fibrin
Gaiter distribution
Homan's sign
Leukocytes
Platelet
Postphlebitic syndrome
Pulmonary emboli
Recurrent deep vein thrombosis
Stasis dermatitis
Tachycardia
Valve cusp
Virchow's triad

One of the most common and life-threatening conditions is acute deep venous thrombosis (DVT). In the United States, there are more than 2.5 million cases of DVT reported each year, resulting in approximately 600,000 cases of *pulmonary embolus* and 200,000 deaths. Despite these grim statistics, the clinical diagnosis of DVT is difficult to make.

Venous Disease Syndromes

There are six recognized syndromes of venous disease:

1. Deep venous thrombosis
2. Recurrent deep vein thrombosis
3. Superficial thrombophlebitis
4. Pulmonary embolism
5. Postthrombotic syndrome
6. Varicose veins

These syndromes are interrelated by their common origin in thrombotic disease processes. Thus, it is not uncommon to find several of these syndromes coexistent in the same patient.

Thrombus Formation

A newly developed venous thrombus consists of a mixture of red blood cells (RBCs) and *platelets*. Due to a rapid series of clotting factors, thrombus actually begins to form within just a few hours. After a few days, some of the RBCs are destroyed through a normal process known as *lysis*, but the remnants of the RBCs and *fibrin* remain. Because the evolution of the thrombus is an ongoing process, new fibrin and platelet are being formed at either end of the thrombus structure while the older thrombus at the center is being destroyed. For this reason, ultrasound imaging of a thrombus may give the appearance of heterogeneous thrombus.

The first step in thrombus formation is the aggregation (coming together) of platelet in the stagnant portion of the venous sinus just behind one of the *valve cusps* (Fig. 3-17). Fibrin layer coats aggregated platelets which attract large quantities of *erythrocytes* (red cells) or *leukocytes* (white cells) (Fig. 3-18). Platelets further aggregate on the surface of RBCs and WBCs, which sustains the process (Fig. 3-19). Thrombus propagates antegrade or retrograde to the next connecting point. The proximal segment may be free-floating (Fig. 3-20).

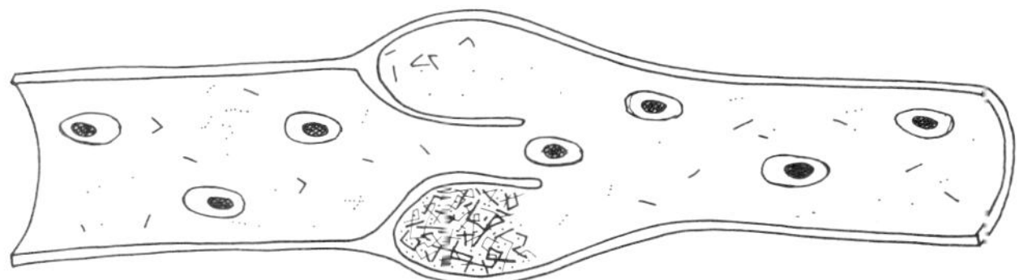

Fig. 3-17. The first stage in thrombus formation is the aggregation (coming together) of platelets in the stagnant portion of the venous sinus just behind the valve cusps.

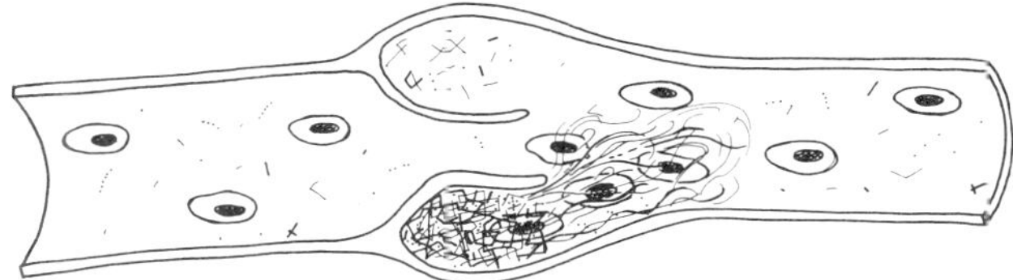

Fig. 3-18. Fibrin layer coats aggregated platelets, which attract large quantities of red and white cells.

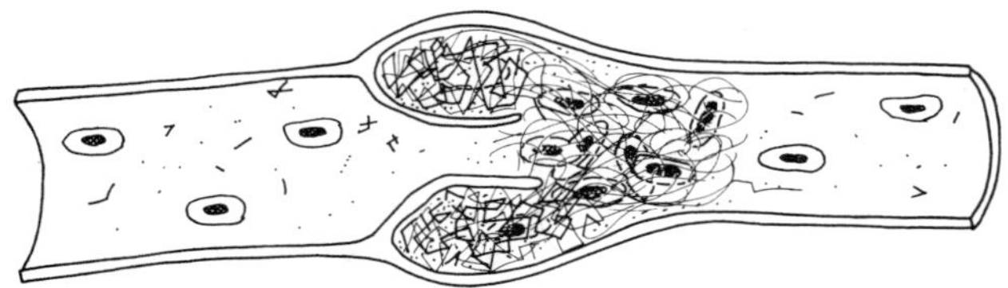

Fig. 3-19. Platelets further aggregate on the surface of RBCs and WBCs, which sustains the process.

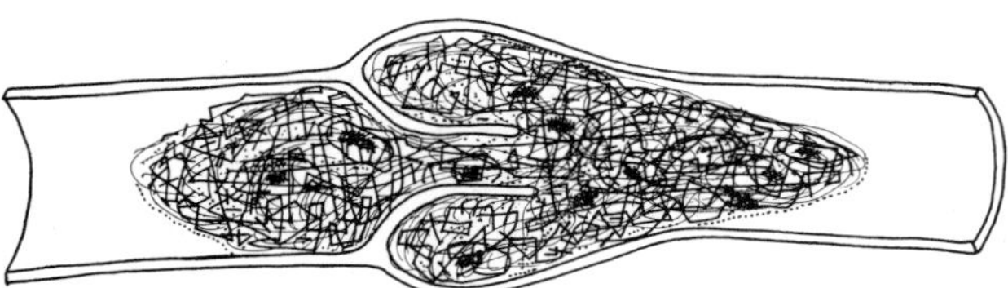

Fig. 3-20. Thrombus propagates antegrade or retrograde to the next vein branch. The proximal portion of the thrombus may be free-floating, which is quite unstable.

Deep Vein Thrombosis

The early stage of thrombus formation is believed to form at the hemodynamically stagnant portion of the vein sinus behind the venous valve. This zone of the vein is also ideal for thrombus development because it is able to form in this somewhat protected zone by the shielding of the valve.

Within 3 to 5 days, the thrombus will either lyse (dissolve) on its own or begin to adhere to the vein wall. Once it adheres, the thrombus is less likely to break off and result in an embolus. In about 20% of all patients with calf vein thrombosis, the thrombus will spread to the popliteal and superficial femoral and common femoral veins. Few thrombi will continue to spread to the iliac veins.

The classic signs of DVT are pain, swelling, and warmth. Unfortunately, about 50% of patients presenting with these symptoms will have no evidence of DVT by either venogram or ultrasound. Yet, some patients at risk with none of the classic signs of DVT will show positive for DVT with either venogram or ultrasound. The point to be made is that the clinical diagnosis of DVT is very difficult; some would even say it's a flip of the coin whether a patient with the symptoms is positive or negative for DVT.

The most common symptom is pain in the extremity. There may be some calf pain induced upon *dorsiflexion*, which is pulling the toes up and therefore stretching the tissues deep in the calf. This is called a positive *Homan's sign* (Fig. 3-21). This test, however, is nonspecific for deep venous disease because any inflammation of the muscle tissue will elicit the same response. Swelling and redness may also be present, but again, these are nonspecific signs for DVT because any *superficial* inflammation will present with the same symptoms.

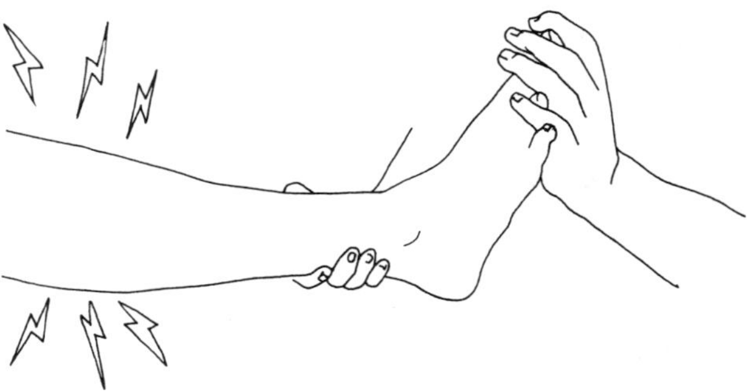

Fig. 3-21. The Homan's sign. Stressed dorsiflexion of the foot may cause pain in the calf muscle in deep vein thrombophlebitis.

Risk Factors: Virchow's Triad

Risk factors play an important role in recognizing patients with DVT. Virchow's triad, first described in 1856, lists the primary risk factors that predispose patients to DVT:

1. Increased coagulability
2. Endothelial damage
3. Venous stasis

Increased Coagulability

Increased coagulability is a condition in which blood is more prone to thrombus than is normal blood. Hypercoagulability plays a major role in the formation of venous thrombus, but it still must be considered as a cause of DVT. The more common mechanisms responsible for this condition include

1. trauma
2. cigarette smoking
3. birth control pills
4. malignancies
5. severe medical illness
6. systemic infection

Endothelial Damage

Anytime there is endothelial damage to the venous wall, the natural healing process of that injury increases the potential for DVT. As you recall, damage to the endothelial lining brings in platelet and fibrin, which attempt to "patch" the injury. This condition continues to the stage of thrombus development.

Stasis

The development of the early stages of thrombus development occurs in the low-flow areas in the venous sinus, behind a venous valve cusp. While venous blood flow is moving freely (e.g., during exercise), thrombus has little chance to organize and attract platelet aggregation, but imagine the opportunity within a patient who has had major pelvic or lower extremity surgery and who has likely been paralyzed during long periods of anesthesia.

The surgical patient is at risk for several reasons. Not only is blood flow particularly stagnant during surgery but also during the painful postoperative period when the patient is at bed rest. It is difficult to encourage early ambulation in order to activate the venous pump mechanisms. Subsequently, this low-flow state of the postoperative surgical patient promotes an ideal condition for the development of DVT. In this high-risk group, as many as 20% to 50% of patients have developed calf DVT.

Previous History of Deep Venous Thrombosis

One of the greatest predisposing factors for DVT is a history of that disease. Because the manifestations of DVT essentially destroy venous valves, normal venous return is hindered. Calf-muscle pumping becomes less effective in that blood is unchecked by valves, is propelled in both directions during ambulation. Subsequently, blood remains static in the calf, increasing the risk for another acute DVT.

Collateral Pathways

Once the development of the thrombus enlarges to the stage where it totally obstructs the vein, the process of thrombus development accelerates. This is due to the further stagnation of blood flow from the thrombus. The venous system attempts to compensate for this obstruction in two ways. First, collateral pathways of veins that are *not* affected dilate to assist the return of blood back to the heart. Second, the back-up pressure forces greater amounts of blood through the perforator veins and to the superficial system, thus allowing venous return to bypass the obstruction.

Pulmonary Embolus

Pulmonary embolism, refers to the obstruction of one of the main branches of the pulmonary artery due to an embolus from the deep venous system (Fig. 3-22). It is interesting to note that patients may be completely asymptomatic even with a 20% obstruction of the pulmonary arteries. However, once more than 20% of the pulmonary vasculature is obstructed, the patient will experience

1. anxiety
2. hyperventilation (rapid breathing)
3. tachycardia (rapid heart rate)

Once more than 50% of the pulmonary vasculature is obstructed, the patient will have dyspnea (difficult breathing) and likely go into shock.

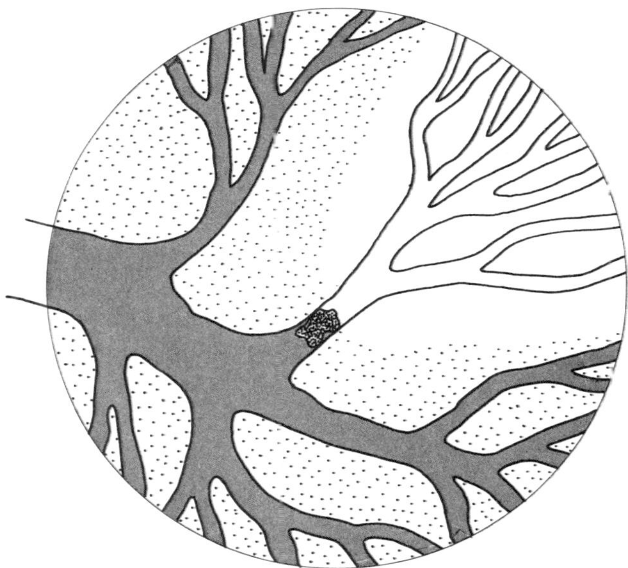

Fig. 3-22. A thrombus of the pulmonary artery prevents blood flow from reaching the distal section of the lungs where oxygen and carbon dioxide are normally exchanged.

Risk Factors

One of the most important factors for the diagnosis of DVT is based on a high degree of suspicion. Because people at risk are likely candidates for developing deep venous thrombus, it is essential to be aggressive in diagnostic studies with anyone at risk who develops even vague symptoms of calf tenderness or swelling redness. By diagnosing DVT early on, the clinician can limit the risk of pulmonary embolus and postthrombotic syndrome. The risk factors for DVT are

1. pregnancy
2. major surgical procedures, especially in the pelvis
3. past history of DVT
4. obesity
5. cancer
6. paralysis, prolonged bed rest, and immobility
7. trauma, especially to the lower extremities
8. cardiac disease, especially low-flow cardiac output state

Superficial Thrombophlebitis

Superficial thrombophlebitis is a condition of thrombus and inflammation of the superficial veins. This condition most often affects the greater or lesser saphenous veins or their branches in the lower leg. At times, patients may present with symptoms similar to DVT; however, for the most part, complaints will be localized to a superficial surface of the skin at or near the superficial venous system. Superficial thrombophlebitis may occur in the upper extremities following intravenous injection or trauma. It is sometimes difficult clinically to distinguish deep vein thrombosis from superficial phlebitis (inflammation of the vein).

Chronic Venous Thrombosis and Postphlebitic Syndrome

One of the common complications of acute deep venous thrombophlebitis is the damage or destruction of the valves that assist in preventing blood flow from flowing backward. Once the valves are damaged, the hydrostatic pressure of the deep venous system is increased due to the weight of the column of venous blood unchecked by the valves. To best understand the fluid mechanics that occur in the postphlebitic leg, let's review some basic hemodynamics at the capillary level.

As blood passes through the capillary, fluid escapes into the interstitial spaces on the arteriolar level and is reabsorbed at the venule level. Because the pressure of the arteriole level is greater than that of the tissue and less than that of the venule, a sufficient pressure gradient exists in order to move blood from arterial to venous system. At the center of the capillary, the forces are balanced so that there is very little fluid loss into the lymphatic system (Fig. 3-23).

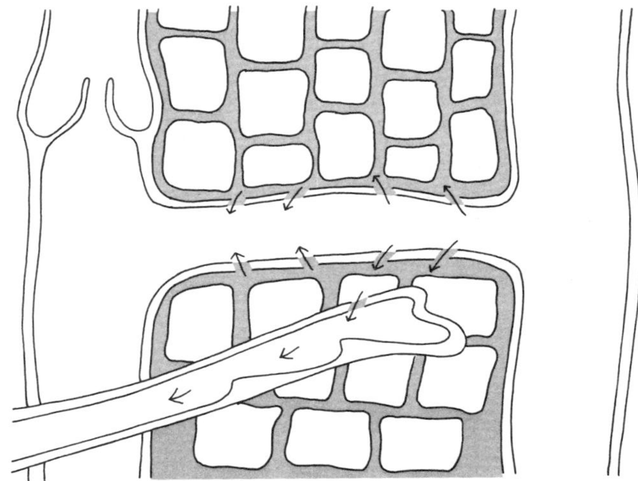

Fig. 3-23. Forces involved with fluid exchange across the capillary bed.

When venous pressure is elevated due to increased hydrostatic pressure, the necessary pressure gradient for flow from arteriole to venule becomes more difficult. Subsequently, fluid is "squeezed out" of the blood into the tissue and reabsorbed by the lymphatic system (Fig. 3-24). The result is increased fluid in the leg or *edema* (swelling).

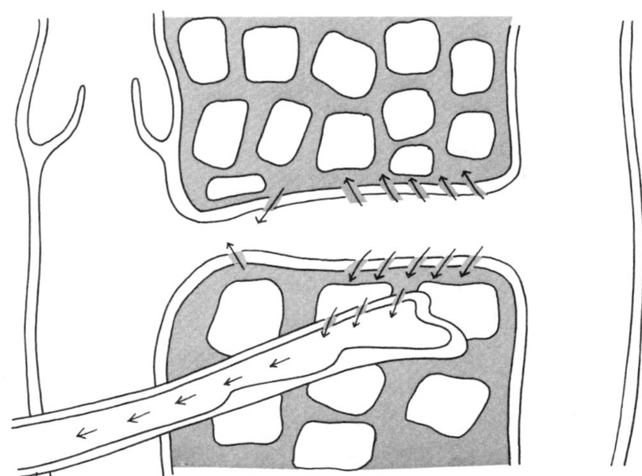

Fig. 3-24. With increased venous hypertension, more fluid is forced into the tissue (illustrated by increased number of arrows), and edema of the leg results.

This increased fluid in the tissue ends up strangulating the delicate capillaries and reducing blood supply to the local tissue. This results in ischemia of the tissue at the local area and the development of skin ulcers. These *chronic stasis ulcers* form around the ankle at what is referred to as *gaiter distribution* (Fig. 3-25). (A gaiter is a type of ankle protector used by mountaineers and skiers to keep snow from entering the boots.) This is a term used to define an anatomical area that is generally around the level of the ankle.

Postphlebitic syndrome also causes *stasis dermatitis*, a drying and scaling of the skin that may resemble eczema. This is often accompanied by hyperpigmentation around the circumference of the lower leg.

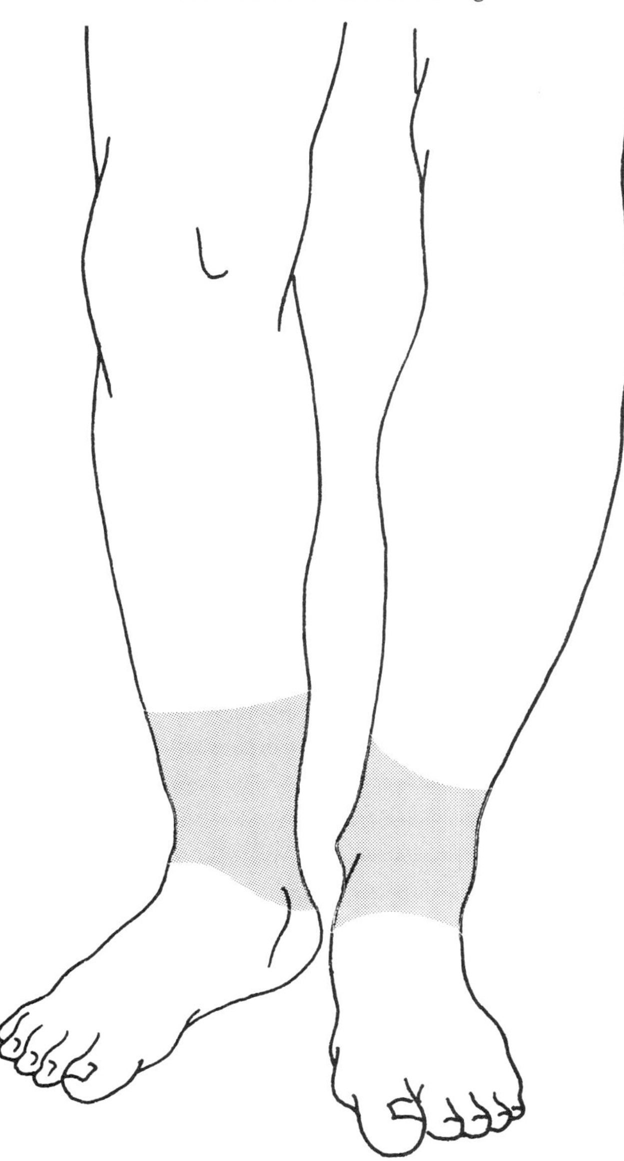

Fig. 3-25. The gaiter area of the lower extremities where, most often, venous ulcers occur.

The Ulcerated Leg

One of the most common conditions for which a patient is referred to a vascular surgeon is the evaluation of leg ulcers. Those of vascular origin include ischemic and stasis ulcers.

Ischemic Ulcers

Ischemic ulcers are typically quite painful lesions associated with arterial insufficiency. They usually are associated with symptoms of severe peripheral vascular disease, such as rest pain. Ischemic ulcers have a "punched-out" characteristic and are commonly located at the dorsum of the toes or on the heel of the foot.

Stasis Ulcers

Stasis ulcers are from venous insufficiency and are more commonly located on the gaiter area of the ankle. They can be painful but less so than ischemic ulcers. Stasis ulcers are normally larger and shallower than ischemic ulcers and present with a constant ooze.

Recurrent Deep Vein Thrombosis

Recurrent deep vein thrombosis refers to the recurrence of DVT after the initial episode. Patients present with warmth, swelling, and pain of the lower extremity. These symptoms, however, often mimic postphlebitic syndrome, a condition resulting from the destruction of valves from the initial DVT described earlier. Because recurrent DVT can lead to a pulmonary embolus, as can an acute DVT, care must be taken to ensure proper diagnosis.

Review Exercise

1. In the United States, there are approximately ______________________________ cases of pulmonary emboli reported each year.

2. Almost ______________% of pulmonary emboli are fatal.

3. Nearly 50% of pulmonary emboli, a condition of a blood clot that travels from a vein to the lung, are associated with:

   a. chronic venous insufficiency
   b. acute venous thrombosis
   c. postphlebitic syndrome
   d. pulmonary embolism

4. Almost ______________________________ deaths occur each year as a direct result of pulmonary emboli associated with DVT.

5. Noninvasive vascular testing has become an accurate and reliable screening technique for deep vein thrombophlebitis. True or False?

6. List the six recognized syndromes of venous disease:

   a. ____

   b. ____

   c. ____

   d. ____

   e. ____

   f. ____

7. Acute deep vein thrombosis implies the thrombotic obstruction of one or more veins of the

   a. superficial system
   b. vena cava
   c. deep venous system
   d. b and c

8. Most often, thrombus will initially form in the

   a. popliteal vein
   b. superficial femoral veins
   c. femoral veins
   d. venous plexi

9. Once the thrombus begins in the calf, it will most often spread to the

   a. tibial veins
   b. peroneal veins
   c. vena cava
   d. a and b

10. The early stage of thrombus formation is believed to form at the hemodynamically stagnant portion of the

   a. perforating veins
   b. superficial veins
   c. a and b
   d. venous sinuses

11. The most common site for thrombus formation is behind the ______________ ______________

12. The zone of the vein referred to in question 11 is also ideal for thrombus development because it is able to form in this somewhat protected zone by the shielding of the

   a. vein walls
   b. calf-muscle pump
   c. valve cusps
   d. none of the above

13. Within 3 to 5 days, the thrombus will begin to adhere to the vein wall and therefore be less likely to break off and

   a. cause an embolus
   b. thrombose
   c. obstruct the vein
   d. disintegrate

14. In about ______________ % of all patients with calf vein thrombosis, the thrombus will spread to the popliteal and superficial femoral and common femoral veins.

15. Few thrombi will continue to spread to the iliac veins. True or False?

16. List the steps of thrombus formation in chronological order

   a. formation of a fibrin layer
   b. entrapment of RBIs
   c. propagation of thrombus
   d. aggregation of platelet

17. A newly developed venous thrombus consists of a mixture of

   a. red cells and white cells
   b. red cells and platelet
   c. platelet and calcium
   d. fibrin and platelet

18. Due to a rapid series of clotting factors, thrombus actually begins to form within just a few

   a. minutes
   b. days
   c. hours
   d. less than one minute

19. After a few days, some of the red cells are destroyed through a normal process known as

   a. electrolysis
   b. paracentesis
   c. thrombosis
   d. lysis

20. The remnants of the red cells and fibrin disperse entirely after lysis. True or False?

21. Because the evolution of the thrombus is an ongoing process, new fibrin and platelet are being formed at the

   a. center of the thrombus structure
   b. circumference of the thrombus structure
   c. center and edges of the thrombus structure
   d. ends of the thrombus structure

22. Due to the ongoing development and lyses of thrombus, ultrasound imaging of a thrombus may give the appearance of a

   a. homogeneous mixture
   b. heterogeneous mixture
   c. calcific
   d. hypoechoic

23. Once the development of the thrombus enlarges to the stage where it totally obstructs the vein, the process of thrombus development

   a. comes to an abrupt halt
   b. accelerates
   c. decelerates
   d. stays the same

24. The process stated above is due to the further

   a. lysis of the clot
   b. collection of platelet
   c. collection of fibrin
   d. obstruction of blood flow

25. ______________________________ of veins that are not affected by thrombus, dilate and assist the return of venous blood back to the heart.

26. Back-up pressure forces greater amounts of blood through the ____________________ veins and to the superficial system, thus allowing venous return to bypass the obstruction.

27. Pulmonary embolism refers to the obstruction of one of the main branches of the ______________________________ due to an embolus from the deep venous system.

28. Patients are always symptomatic with pulmonary emboli. True or False?

29. List three symptoms of pulmonary embolism.

   a. ______________________________
   b. ______________________________
   c. ______________________________

30. Once more than __________% of the pulmonary vasculature is obstructed, the patient will likely have dyspnea and go into shock.

31. ______________________________ refers to the recurrence of DVT after the initial episode.

32. "Classic" symptoms of DVT include

a. ______________________________

b. ______________________________

c. ______________________________

33. Acute DVT symptoms may mimic chronic DVT. True or False?

34. A recurrent DVT, unlike acute DVT, will never lead to a pulmonary embolus. True or False?

35. Superficial thrombophlebitis is a condition of thrombus and inflammation of the

a. superficial and deep venous system
b. superficial system only
c. superficial or deep system
d. veins of the upper extremities

36. Superficial thrombophlebitis most often affects the

a. posterior tibial veins
b. anterior tibial veins
c. peroneal veins
d. saphenous veins

37. At times, patients may present with symptoms that are indistinguishable from deep vein thrombosis. True or False?

38. Complaints of superficial thrombophlebitis are most often:

a. asymptomatic
b. exactly the same for DVT
c. localized to the skin surface
d. equally as dangerous as a DVT

39. Superficial thrombophlebitis may occur in the upper extremities following ______________________________ or ______________.

40. One of the common complications of acute deep venous thrombophlebitis is the damage of the

a. tricuspid valves
b. perforator veins
c. venous sinusoid
d. bicuspid valves

41. Once the valves are damaged, the pressure of the deep venous system is increased due to the column of venous blood's

a. having increased viscosity
b. having a clot that is heavier than blood
c. having more blood, filling a larger space
d. being unchecked by valves

42. As blood passes through the capillary, fluid escapes into the interstitial spaces on the arteriolar level and is reabsorbed at the venule level. True or False?

43. At the center of the capillary, the forces of venous and arterial blood are normally ______________________________ so that there is very little fluid loss into the lymphatic system.

44. When venous pressure is elevated due to increased ____, the necessary pressure gradient for flow from arteriole to venule becomes more difficult.

45. With increase intraluminal pressure, fluid is "squeezed out" of the blood into the tissue and reabsorbed by the

a. digestive system
b. lymphatic system
c. superficial venous system
d. arterial system

46. The result of increased swelling in the leg due to extra fluid in the lymphatic system is called

a. phlebitis
b. portal hypertension
c. lymphedema
d. edema

47. The increased fluid in the tissue ends up strangulating the delicate ______________________________ and reducing blood supply to the local tissue.

48. This results in death of the tissue at the local area and the development of

a. thrombosis
b. chronic DVT
c. ulcers
d. pulmonary emboli

49. Venous ulcers form around the ankle at what is referred to as _______________ distribution.

50. Draw the gaiter distribution.

51. Postphlebitic syndrome causes ____, which is a drying and scaling of the skin that may resemble eczema.

52. This skin condition is often accompanied by

a. hypopigmentation
b. a severe rash
c. numbness and tingling
d. hyperpigmentation

53. Risk factors play an important role in recognizing patients with deep vein thrombosis. Virchow's Triad, first described in 1856, lists the primary risk factors that predispose patients to DVT. They are

a. ______________________________

b. ______________________________

c. ______________________________

54. Hypercoagulability plays a ____________ role in the formation of venous thrombus.

55. The more common mechanisms responsible for hypercoagulability are:

a. ______________________________

b. ______________________________

c. ______________________________

d. ______________________________

e. ______________________________

f. ______________________________

56. At any time in which there is intimal damage to the venous wall, the natural healing process of that injury decreases the potential for DVT. True or False?

57. Damage to the endothelial lining brings in

a. fatty deposits
b. lipids
c. fibrin and platelet
d. all of the above

58. A patient with an injured extremity is less likely to

a. develop platelet and fibrin
b. have a normal clotting process
c. be aware of a thrombosis
d. ambulate

59. Venous blood that is ____________________ is an ideal breeding ground for DVT.

60. Large bone fractures are a classic condition for the development of DVT. True or False?

61. While venous blood flow is moving freely during exercise, thrombus has a better chance to organize and attract platelet aggregation. True or False?

62. The patient who has had major pelvic or lower extremity surgery and who has likely been paralyzed during long periods of anesthesia is at ______________ risk for DVT.

63. After surgery, it may be difficult to encourage early ambulation in order to activate the

a. antithrombus mechanisms
b. antiplatelet mechanisms
c. a and b
d. calf-muscle pump mechanisms

64. In postoperative patients who have had major surgery, as many as ______________% to ______________% of patients have developed calf DVT.

65. One of the greatest predisposing factors for deep vein thrombosis is

a. history of cigarette smoking
b. history of previous DVT
c. history of taking birth control pills
d. history of trauma

66. One of the most significant manifestations of DVT is

a. pulmonary embolus
b. ischemic pain
c. skin discoloration
d. muscle cramps

67. What percentage of patients presenting with "classic symptoms" of deep vein thrombosis will have no evidence of DVT by either venogram or ultrasound?

a. 90%
b. 50%
c. 10%
d. less than 5%

68. The clinical diagnosis of DVT is in general

a. easy and reliable
b. 99% accurate
c. difficult to make
d. dependent on which leg is affected

69. The most common symptom is

a. swollen legs
b. redness over the area of phlebitis
c. numbness in the extremity
d. pain in the extremity

70. Dorsiflexion of the foot, which causes pain in the calf, is called the

a. Homan's sign
b. Hoffman's sign
c. Babinski's sign
d. dorsiflexion sign

71. Dorsiflexion of the foot as a test for deep venous disease is a ______________________________ sign.

72. Although there are different types of leg ulcers, those of vascular origin include either ______________ or ______________ ulcers.

73. Ischemic ulcers are typically

a. numb and tingly
b. itchy
c. asymptomatic
d. painful

74. Ischemic arterial ulcers are commonly located at the

a. ankles (gaiter distribution)
b. toes or on the heel
c. arch of the foot
d. all of the above

75. Stasis ulcers are more commonly located at the

a. ankles (gaiter distribution)
b. toes or on the heel
c. arch of the foot
d. all of the above

76. Stasis ulcers are normally ______________ and ______________ than ischemic ulcers of arterial origin.

ABDOMINAL VASCULAR DISEASE

In this section we will review some of the more common medical and surgical conditions for which the vascular laboratory may be asked to obtain information for diagnosis.

Key Terms

Acute intestinal ischemia
Ascites
Budd-Chiari syndrome
Chronic intestinal ischemia
Chronic renal failure
Hydronephrosis
Portal hypertension
Portal veins
Splenomegaly
Renal hypertension
Renal transplant
Transplant rejection
Vena cava filter

Inferior Vena Cava Conditions

Venous conditions of the vena cava, which the vascular specialist may be required to evaluate, are

1. presence or absence of a venous thrombus
2. patency of a filter
3. congenital abnormalities

A filter is a device that is placed in the vena cava to "trap" blood clots that may enter the vessel from thrombosis in the lower extremities.

Portal Venous System Conditions

Indications for noninvasive evaluation of the portal venous system include

1. hepatic transplant patients
2. portal hypertension
3. portal vein occlusion
4. primary hepatic malignancies
5. unexpected ascites
6. splenomegaly
7. pancreatic disease

Portal Hypertension

Portal hypertension occurs when venous flow returning to the liver is impeded. The most common cause of portal hypertension is disease of the liver, most commonly cirrhosis, which causes an obstruction of the venous return. Portal hypertension also may be the result of a thrombosis in the portal vein or narrowing/obstruction of the hepatic veins. This obstruction of venous blood flow results in the engorgement of the venous system proximal to the obstruction.

Veins in the esophagus may become enlarged and may bleed (*esophageal varices*), due to increased pressure that develops in the impedance of venous flow to the liver. Fluid is forced out of the other major veins in the abdomen much like fluid from chronic venous obstruction in the lower extremities forces fluid out into the legs. In the abdomen this condition is called *ascites*, which is a collection of fluid in the abdominal cavity. Finally, portal hypertension can result in increased venous resistance in the highly vascular spleen, causing it to enlarge (*splenomegaly*).

Hepatic Veins

Indications for noninvasive evaluation of the hepatic venous system include

1. Budd-Chiari syndrome
2. suspected portal vein/hepatic vein fistula (rare)
3. constrictive pericarditis

Mesenteric Artery System Conditions

You will recall that the superior mesenteric artery supplies blood to the small intestine and the first portion of the large intestine. When the small intestine requires an increase of blood flow, typically for the digestive demands after eating, blood flow is increased through the superior mesenteric artery. If the vessels have a stenosis in the artery and the supply of blood cannot meet that demand, pain most often occurs. This ongoing condition is referred to as *chronic intestinal ischemia.* If the superior mesenteric artery is suddenly occluded, as with an embolus, *acute intestinal ischemia* may occur.

The pain of chronic intestinal ischemia typically is located on the mid-abdomen and may radiate to the back. The pain usually occurs postprandial (after eating) and varies from a continuous dull ache to a colicky (crampy) type of pain. The pain usually lasts for less than an hour and is associated with the amount of food digested. The typical pattern for patients with intestinal ischemia is a history of reduced meal size and a loss of weight. This has resulted in the terms *small-meal syndrome* and *food fear*.

Budd-Chiari Syndrome

Budd-Chiari syndrome is an obstruction of the hepatic veins associated with ascites and liver failure. Constrictive pericarditis increases pressure on the right side of the heart due to the presence of inflammation and fluid. This condition impedes the returning venous blood flow, which is reflected back to the hepatic veins.

Review Exercise

1. Venous conditions of the vena cava, which the vascular specialist may be required to evaluate, are

   a. ______________________________

   b. ______________________________

   c. ______________________________

2. Indications for noninvasive evaluation of the celiac and mesenteric arteries include

   a. ______________________________

   b. ______________________________

3. The superior mesenteric artery supplies blood to the

   a. liver
   b. small intestine
   c. small intestine and first part of the large intestine
   d. small intestine and spleen

4. When blood flow is compromised in the mesenteric artery, the result is

   a. ascites
   b. liver failure
   c. diarrhea
   d. abdominal pain

5. After eating, blood flow in the mesenteric artery usually

   a. does not change at all
   b. decreases
   c. increases
   d. fluctuates

6. Which symptom is the most common physical finding in patients with intestinal ischemia?

   a. Ascites
   b. Weight loss
   c. Diarrhea
   d. Abdominal pain

7. Pain from intestinal ischemia is typically located in the

   a. right upper quadrant
   b. mid-abdomen
   c. left upper quadrant
   d. back

8. The pain of intestinal ischemia usually occurs after ______________ and varies from a continuous dull ache to a colicky type of pain.

9. The pain usually lasts for less than an hour and is associated with

a. the type of food
b. the time of day
c. how much food
d. stress

10. The typical condition for patients with intestinal ischemia is a history of

a. psychological problems
b. obesity
c. stomach ulcer
d. reduced meal size and weight loss

11. List three indications for noninvasive evaluation of the portal venous system.

a. ____________________

b. ____________________

c. ____________________

12. Portal hypertension occurs when the blood flow returning to the right side of the heart is

a. increased
b. decreased
c. impeded
d. absent

13. The most common cause of portal hypertension is disease of the

a. right ventricle
b. liver
c. spleen
d. esophagus

14. One of the most common reasons for the liver to function poorly is

a. Budd-Chiari syndrome
b. cholelithiasis
c. AAA
d. cirrhosis

15. With severe liver disease, veins in the ____________________ become enlarged and may bleed.

16. In severe portal hypertension, ____________________ is forced out of the major veins in the abdomen.

17. The condition of fluid forced into the abdominal cavity is called

a. portal hypertension
b. esophageal varices
c. intestinal ischemia
d. ascites

18. Portal hypertension can result in increased venous resistance in the

a. spleen
b. left ventricle
c. lower extremities
d. all of the above

19. The enlargement of the organ named in question 18 is referred to as

a. organomegaly
b. ventriculomegaly
c. splenomegaly
d. varicose veins

20. Indications for noninvasive evaluation of the hepatic venous system include

a. ______________________________

b. ______________________________

c. ______________________________

21. Budd-Chiari syndrome is obstruction of the

a. renal veins
b. hepatic veins
c. iliac veins
d. the vena cava

22. Budd-Chiari syndrome is associated with

a. ascites
b. liver failure
c. constrictive pericarditis
d. a and b

23. Constrictive pericarditis increases pressure on the

a. portal vein
b. superior vena cava
c. right side of the heart
d. all of the above

24. Pericarditis impedes the returning venous blood flow, which is reflected back to the

a. hepatic arteries
b. renal arteries
c. splenic arteries
d. hepatic veins

Renal Vascular Hypertension

Of the 20 to 30 million Americans with hypertension, approximately 5% to 10% of the patients have renal artery stenosis (Fig. 3-26). Because of the great arterial demands of the kidneys, the renal arteries carry a significant amount of blood flow to these organs. With a stenosis of the renal arteries leading off the abdominal aorta, the subsequent increase in arterial pressure can lead to significant *renal vascular hypertension.*

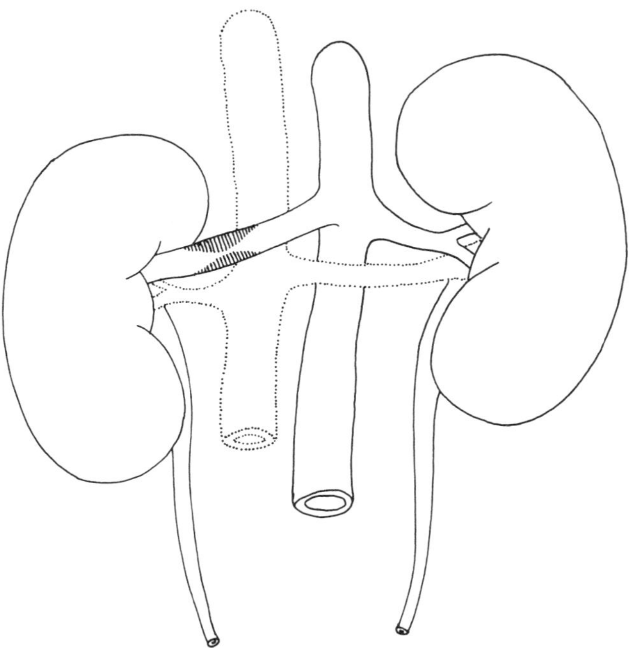

Fig. 3-26. Stenosis of the right renal artery.

Renal Transplant

Within the past 20 years renal transplantation has become the usual long-term treatment for *chronic renal failure*. Most of the many complications that follow renal transplantation can be assessed usefully by ultrasound. The most common indication for examination of *renal transplant* by ultrasound is the worsening renal failure. Possible explanations include *hydronephrosis*, *transplant rejection*, acute tubular necrosis, and vascular problems, including focal infarct or venous thrombosis.

A renal transplant is usually placed in the iliac fossa or just above the groin. The ureter of the donor kidney is anastomosed to the bladder. Sometimes the patient's own ureter is left intact. The rejected kidney transplant usually occurs within the first few months after the operation.

Review Exercise

1. Of the 20 to 30 million Americans with hypertension, approximately ______________% to ______________% of the patients have renal artery stenosis.

2. With a significant stenosis of the ______________ arteries leading off the abdominal aorta, the subsequent increase in arterial pressure can lead to hypertension.

3. Within the past 20 years, renal transplantation has become the usual long-term treatment for

   a. renal hypertension
   b. Bright's disease
   c. chronic renal infections
   d. chronic renal failure

4. Most of the complications that follow renal transplantation cannot be adequately assessed by ultrasound. True or False?

5. The most common indication for examination of renal transplant by ultrasound is

   a. evaluation of urine output
   b. tubule function
   c. transplant position
   d. worsening renal failure

6. A renal transplant is usually placed in the

   a. retroperitoneum
   b. abdominal cavity
   c. iliac fossa
   d. right upper quadrant

7. A rejected kidney transplant usually occurs within the ______________________________ after the operation.

4
The Physics of Imaging

SOUND VERSUS ULTRASOUND

What is sound? How does it move through tissue and what happens to those signals when it interacts with tissue? In this section, the basic principles of sound will be discussed. Special attention will be paid to the interaction of ultrasound in tissue and how those changes benefit the vascular specialist in interpreting normal and abnormal conditions.

Key Terms

Absorption
Acoustic impedance
Amplitude
Artifacts
Attenuation
Band width
Center operating frequency
Compressibility
Decibels
Density
Frequency
Hertz
Horizontal waves
Intensity
Kilohertz
Longitudinal waves
Medium
Megahertz
Propagation velocity
Pulse-echo
Pulse length
Reflection
Refraction
Resolution
Scattering
Sound
Sound waves
Source
Specular reflectors
Transverse waves
Ultrasound
Waveform
Wavelength

THE ULTRASOUND MYTH

One of the basic misunderstandings concerning *ultrasound* is that something is actually emitted out of the transducer, like a bullet out of a gun, and that something penetrates tissue after it hits a target and then bounces back to the transducer. This is simply not true. Nothing but mechanical energy actually leaves the transducer. The transducer vibrates very quickly in short pulses, causing the tissue near the transducer to vibrate also. That vibration is then transmitted into the body as an ultrasound wave where it (the wave) bounces off different tissues before returning to the transducer.

The Pulse-Echo Principle

Have you ever tried to find a stud in the wall in order to hang a picture? By firmly tapping on the wall, one can listen to the different sounds produced in order to determine whether there is wood or empty space behind the plaster (Fig. 4-1). The tapping is the pulse and what you hear back is the echo. You don't actually touch the stud with your hand nor can you see it, but by listening to the subtle changes that are produced as you tap on the wall, you can make determinations as to where your nail is going to end up.

Diagnostic ultrasound, in a way, is like tapping on the body's wall and listening to the returning signal in order to determine what is inside and where it is located. Of course, ultrasound is far more sensitive to the tissue structure. The tapping, or pulsing, of ultrasound is done at thousands of times a second. The molecules in the tissue respond to that pulse and echo back the signal. By understanding how this sound travels and how different tissues respond to the tapping, the vascular specialist can obtain a great deal of information about what is inside the body.

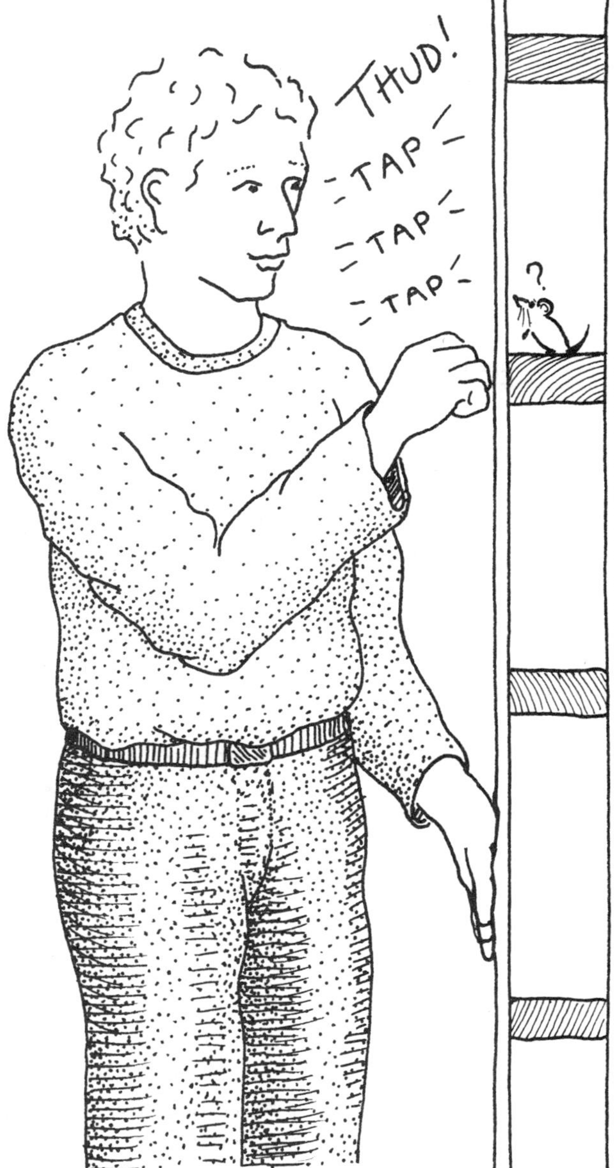

Fig. 4-1. The pulse-echo principle. By tapping on the wall and listening to the returning signals, one can tell whether there is space or a stud behind the plaster.

Before we discuss specific transducer technology, we will look carefully at how sound is created, how it travels, how it interacts with the molecules in the tissue, and what the echoes received tell us about the tissue inside.

What Is Sound

The perception of *sound* is, in a way, a "feeling" that something is moving. That "feeling" is movement or pressure sensed by the tympanic membrane (ear drum), which in turn transmits those vibrations to the auditory nerves in the inner ear. The auditory nerve then translates those vibrations into volume and tone. But how does this pressure get transmitted from its source to your ear?

Sound Source

First of all, sound must come from a *source*. If you strike a large bell briskly with a hammer, you will create a source (the bell) for sound (Fig. 4-2).

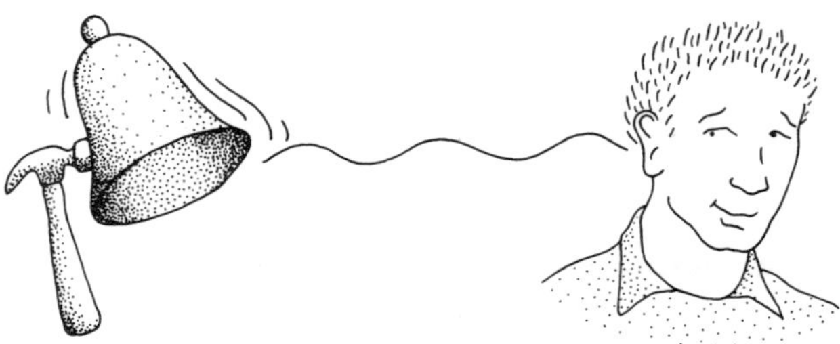

Fig. 4-2. The bell is the source of the sound.

Sound starts as the sudden disturbance of molecules in the bell. When the bell is first struck with the hammer, the molecules in the metal don't just fire off in the air like little rockets into space; they vibrate or oscillate like a pendulum swinging back and forth (Fig. 4-3).

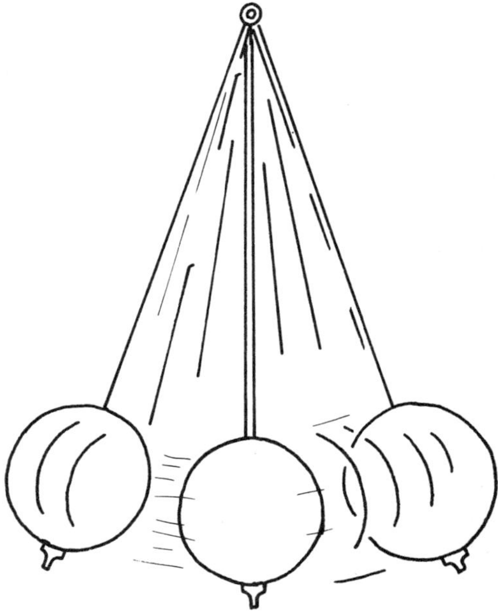

Fig. 4-3. Molecules vibrate in a back-and-forth motion like a swinging pendulum.

The molecules in the bell are densely packed. When stimulated, they start oscillating or vibrating for a while, which causes other molecules near them to start vibrating. Then those vibrating molecules start banging into neighboring molecules on down the line until they reach the air molecules on the surface of the bell. Then *those* air molecules start vibrating one another in the air until the transmitted vibration finally reaches your ear. At this point, the vibrating molecules on the ear drum transmit to your auditory nerves, which interpret the vibration as sound (Fig. 4-4).

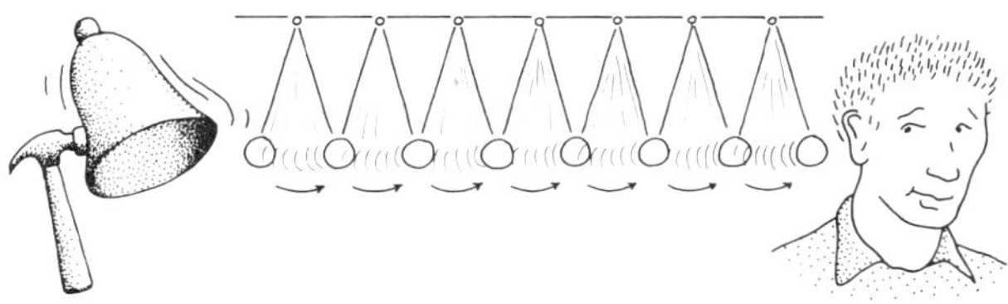

Fig. 4-4. Sound is transmitted through the air by molecules interacting with each other.

Resonance Frequency

Also like a pendulum, the molecules in the bell like to oscillate at their own characteristic pace, which is characteristic of the sound *source* and varies depending on the type of source from which the sound originates. The source for ultrasound is a crystal that, when charged with electricity, vibrates or oscillates at a specific pace or frequency. This pace is called the *resonance frequency*. In other words, the oscillating pace of molecules in wood is much different from the oscillating pace of molecules in the metal bell. Generally speaking, the sound source likes to oscillate at its own resonance frequency.

Medium

Sound is generated by hitting the bell with a hammer; the bell is the source of sound. But to move sound from one point to another, the sound must move through a *medium*. In the case of the sound generated by the bell, metal, air, and tissue all serve as media.

A medium contains molecules; no molecules, no medium, no transmission. That is why sound cannot be transmitted in a vacuum. In the case of the ringing bell, the metal in the bell is the medium that transmits sound to the air. The air is the medium that transmits sound from the bell to the ear, and the ear drum is the medium that transmits sound from the air to the auditory nerve.

Sound is therefore mechanical in nature. It requires the physical interaction of one molecule with another. If you attempt to move sound through molecules that cannot move, the transmitted vibration stops and sound cannot propagate further.

Elastic and Deformable Medium

The material that contains molecules that can move is referred to as elastic and deformable, but don't misunderstand the definition of elastic and deformable as something that you can physically stretch or deform with a poke of your finger. Even the bell has material that is elastic and deformable, otherwise it could not transmit sound. Elastic and deformable means that the molecules on the substance are able to move around enough to knock into other molecules, therefore causing a type of chain reaction and thus the propagation of sound.

Propagation Velocity

Sound propagates, or reproduces itself, through a material at a certain speed. This is called *propagation velocity*. The propagation velocity depends on the mechanical properties of the medium, namely, density and stiffness. *Note*: The opposite of stiffness is *compressibility*.

In general, the denser the medium, or the less stiff (more compressible) the medium, the slower the propagation of sound waves. Conversely, the less dense, or more stiff, the medium (less compressible), the faster the propagation of ultrasound.

Higher Velocity	Lower Velocity
Decreased density	Increased density
Increased stiffness	Decreased stiffness

In general, material like the bell is both stiff and dense; therefore, these properties tend to compete with each other. For example, the density of air is less than the density of water, but air is less stiff (much easier to compress) than water. The second effect (stiffness) dominates the first effect (density). Thus, the speed of sound in air is slower than that in water.

In sum, the more densely packed the molecules or the more compressible the medium, the more difficult it will be to move one molecule into the other. This is why sound propagates slowly through dense objects such as metal or less stiff (compressible) material such as foam rubber. Again, sound is mechanical in nature; without this interaction of molecule to molecule, sound cannot be transmitted or subsequently heard (or in the case of ultrasound, received).

The following is a list of some common propagation velocities of ultrasound in various materials and tissue. Keep in mind that propagation velocity depends on the character of the medium (density and stiffness) and not the frequency of the transducer.

Air: 330 m/sec	Skull: 4,000 m/sec
Lung: 600 m/sec	Liver: 1,555 m/sec
Water: 1,480 m/sec	Muscle: 1,600 m/sec
Fat: 1,565 m/sec	Blood: 1,560 m/sec

(The average for most soft tissue is 1,540 m/sec.)

Sound Waves

Let's look at a few different ways sound waves propagate. Have you ever put your head under water and tapped two rocks together? In this case, you are creating a source from within the medium (water), and sound also propagates through the medium in all directions. For example, consider a small spherical object such as an air bubble in water (Fig. 4-5). Now imagine this air bubble pulsating back and forth around its mean position, causing waves to move spherically outward at a constant speed. This is approximately referred to as a *point source*. Sound waves are moving out in *all* directions.

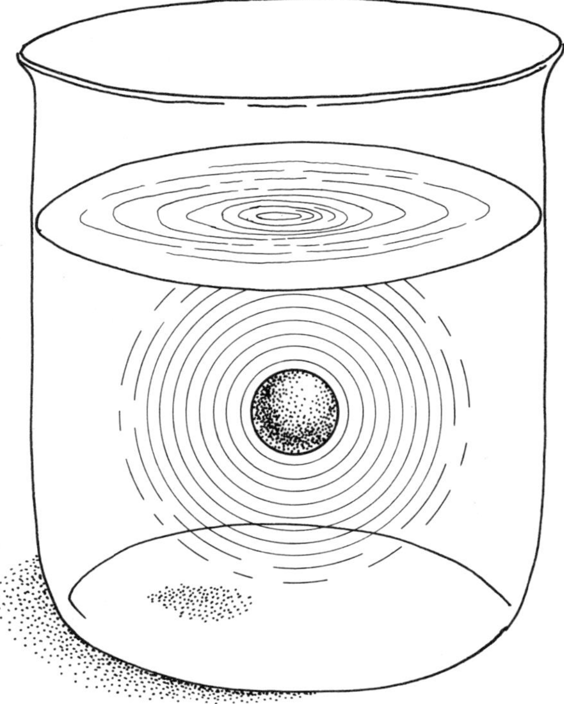

Fig. 4-5. Waves from within the medium move away from the source in all directions like rays from the sun.

Transverse Waves

If we take a periscope to the surface of water to look at waves on the surface, it will appear as if all the water on the surface is moving rapidly toward the shore (Fig. 4-6). If a small boat were sailing on the surface of the water, however, we would see that the boat moves up and down, and the craft is not necessarily propelled toward the shore (unless it rides down the surface of a steep wave). The wave moves across the surface of the water, but the medium itself oscillates up and down (Fig. 4-6). In this case, the particle displacement of the medium moves up and down, but the wave moves perpendicular to this motion. This is referred to as a *transverse wave*.

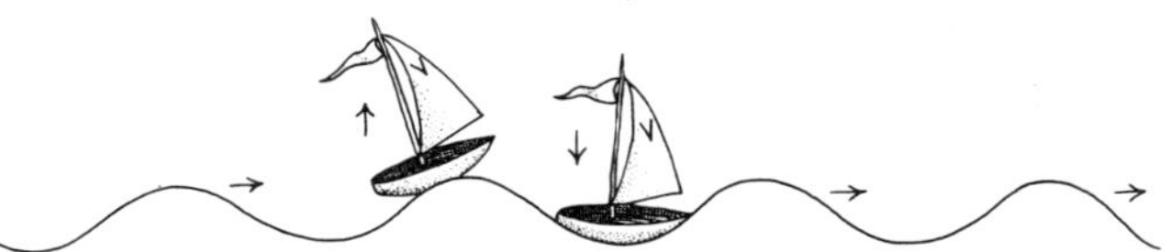

Fig. 4-6. The waves move toward the shore, but the boat rides up and down.

Longitudinal Waves

Remember the Slinky toy? If you hold one end in each hand and alternately move your hands back and forth, you will note that the slinky "wave" moves from one hand to the other. Unlike the wave of the ocean water, each part of the Slinky moves back and forth. All motion is either forward or backward, not up and down.

In the case of sound waves, the particle displacement is in parallel with the wave propagation. This type of wave is referred to as *longitudinal wave*.

Compression and Rarefaction

When we struck the bell with a hammer, we caused a chain reaction of molecules interacting with each other to move a signal from the bell to your ear. Keep in mind that it is not just one molecule that is affected, but millions and millions of molecules all oscillating in a large group.

This large group bunches up as it propagates in longitudinal waves away from the source. This results in a *compression* of molecules in a "wave," and therefore subsequent imbalance in the medium. The imbalance on either side of the compression is an area where the molecules are spread out. This area is called *rarefaction*, the anatomy of an ultrasound wave (Fig. 4-7).

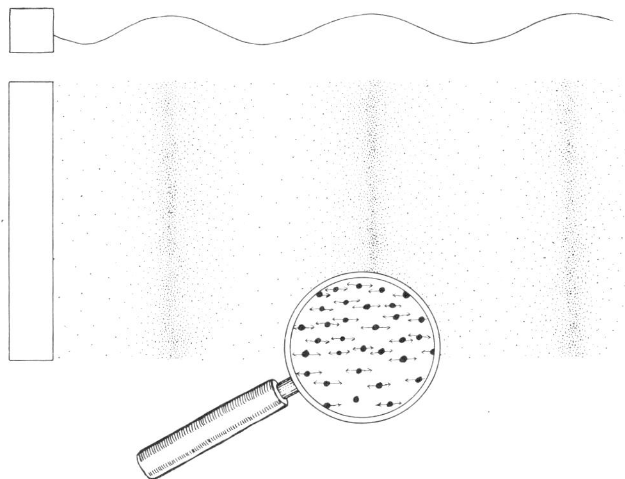

Fig. 4-7. Compression and rarefaction. If we look at the movement of the molecules, we can see they are moving back and forth, but if we look at the movement of the waves, we can see they are moving away from the sound source in a longitudinal plane. Note the wave on the top of the illustration representing compression (increase in the wave above the base line) and rarefaction (decrease in the wave below the base line).

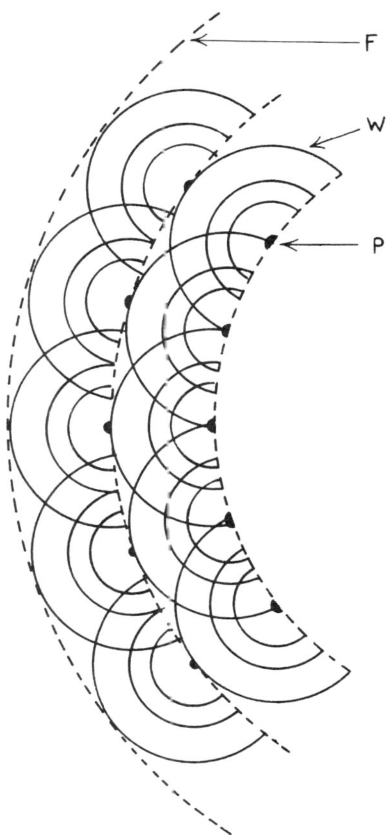

Fig. 4-8. Each point (P) on the waves acts as a new point source for new waves (W). A whole new wavefront (F) is formed by connecting all the wave positions at the same point in time.

Wavefront, Rays, and the Ultrasound Beam

The rapid forward-and-reverse vibration of an ultrasound transducer in a medium results in longitudinal waves being transmitted away from the source. To represent this wave, a line or a surface is drawn through all points of the wave that are in the same phase. This is called a *wavefront* (Fig. 4-8). The lines pointing in the direction of the wave propagation and perpendicular to the wavefront are called *rays*. In ultrasound imaging, wavefronts heading in a particular direction are referred to as an *ultrasound beam*.

Wave Properties

As mentioned earlier, vibrating molecules are like pendulums swinging in a series. Although we can't look at individual molecular motion, we *can* look at the collective compression and rarefaction of groups of molecules. The compression usually corresponds to the positive parts, and the rarefaction corresponds to the negative parts of the acoustic pressure *waveform*. By plotting the course (Fig. 4-9) of this compression and rarefaction on a strip-chart recorder, we can begin to evaluate some characteristics of sound wave properties.

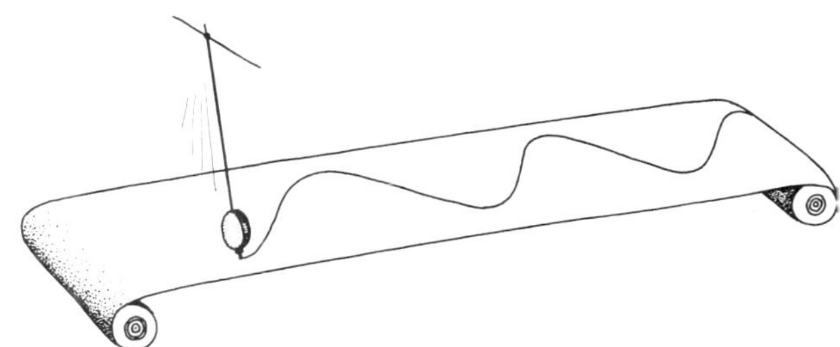

Fig. 4-9. Strip-chart recorder plotting compression and rarefaction of a waveform.

Amplitude

One of the first characteristics we could define would be the *amplitude*, which is the range from the mean to the extreme (Fig. 4-10). There are three types of amplitude in ultrasound:

1. Particle displacement amplitude (distance)
2. Particle velocity amplitude (speed)
3. Acoustic pressure amplitude (pressure)

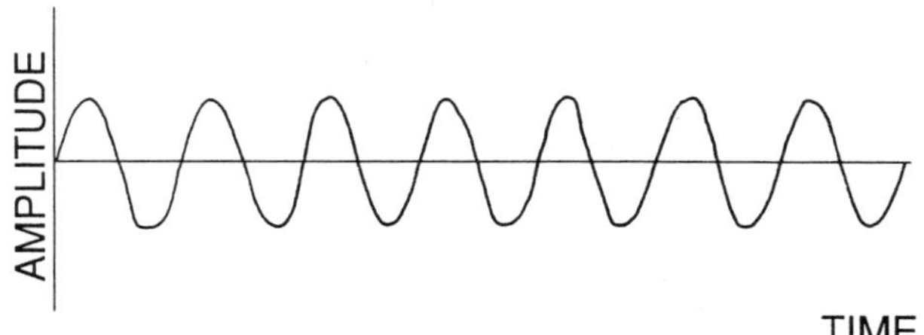

Fig. 4-10. Plotting the amplitude of a waveform over time.

Particle Displacement Amplitude

Once again, the sound wave traveling through a medium isn't an actual object moving from one point to another; it is the mechanical interaction of molecules. An individual particle in the medium oscillates back and forth around its mean position as sound propagates in the medium. In other words, the position of the molecule varies in time. At one point, the particle has moved forward and at the other point, it has moved back.

The maximum displacement (the greatest distance) the particle has moved in relation to the mean position is referred to as the *particle displacement amplitude* of the wave, the basic unit for which is the meter (m). In sum, particle displacement amplitude is a measurement of how far the particle moved when it oscillated.

Particle Velocity Amplitude

When an individual particle in the medium moves back and forth around its mean position, the particle velocity varies in time as well as position. In this case, the particle speed varies. The particle reaches its maximum velocity at the maximum particle displacement. This is referred to as the *maximum particle velocity amplitude* and is measured in meters per second (m/sec).

Note: Don't confuse particle velocity with ultrasound velocity; they are two different things. Particle velocity refers to how fast the particle oscillates around its mean position. The speed of sound is how fast the sound wave propagates through a medium.

Acoustic Pressure Amplitude

When sound wave propagates in a medium, the pressure at any point varies with time, above and below the pressure surrounding the wave. The *acoustic pressure amplitude* is then defined as the difference between the total pressure of the wave and that in the surrounding or ambient medium, the maximum acoustic pressure.

Acoustic Variable

A sound wave propagating through tissue has several biological effects. These effects in the medium are a result of a change or variation from its normal condition. This change is referred to as the *acoustic variable*. There are several changes in the medium that occur as a result of acoustic variables:

1. Pressure
2. Density
3. Temperature
4. Particle motion or distance

Cycle

The completion of a particle's forward-and-reverse movement is referred to as one *cycle*. One complete cycle of a wheel brings you right back to the starting position (Fig. 4-11). And so it is with an oscillation of a molecule; one complete cycle also brings you back to the starting position of that molecule.

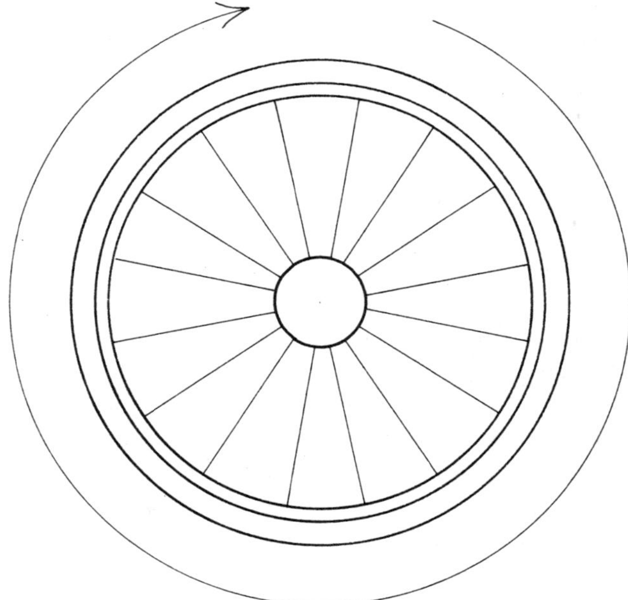

Fig. 4-11. One cycle of a wheel.

Frequency

Other than the distance (particle displacement amplitude), the speed (particle velocity amplitude), and the pressure (acoustic pressure amplitude), it is also important to know how often in a unit of time (the frequency) a particle oscillates around its mean position. Frequency provides us with much specific information about the oscillation of the molecules, specifically, the number of cycles that occurred over a certain period of time (Fig. 4-12).

I DROVE 200 MILES TODAY!
I DROVE 200 MILES IN ONE HOUR!!

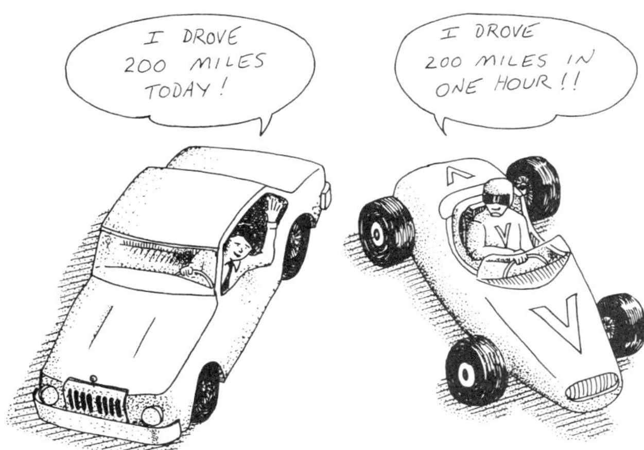

Fig. 4-12. Producing a large number of cycles is not as important as how many cycles were produced in a specific period of time.

In ultrasound, as mentioned earlier, we measure the number of cycles per second (Fig. 4-13). The unit of measure we use for sound is called hertz. One complete cycle of a wave, in one second, equals 1 hertz; five complete cycles equals 5 hertz. One thousand hertz is called 1 kilohertz or 1 kHz, and one million hertz is called 1 megahertz or 1 MHz.

Diagnostic Ultrasound Frequencies

Ultrasound is defined as sound whose frequency is above the range of human hearing, which is 20,000 cycles per second, or 20 kHz. Diagnostic ultrasound is generally between 2,000,000 Hz and 10,000,000 Hz, or 2 MHz and 10 MHz. Although this may seem to be an extremely large number of cycles, it is relatively low when compared with other imaging frequencies, which can go as high as 20 MHz.

Lower frequency indicates that the wavelength is longer and can therefore penetrate deeper. These frequencies are typically used for deep abdominal or transcranial imaging. The higher frequency has more cycles per second and, therefore, poor penetration. The higher frequencies are used for more superficial imaging, such as small parts and carotid artery duplex.

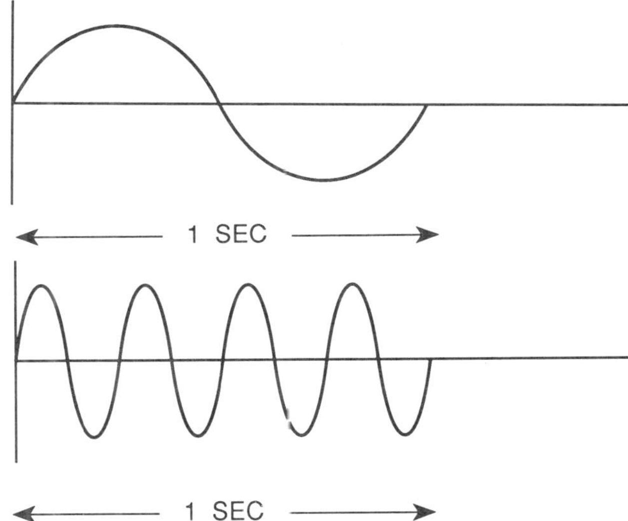

Fig. 4-13. Top: 1 cycle in 1 second = 1 Hertz (1 Hz). Bottom: 5 cycles in 1 second = 5 Hertz (5 Hz).

Wavelength

The ultrasound *wavelength* is important to the vascular specialist. It determines *how far* the ultrasound will penetrate in tissue. If we want to measure the wavelength, we can look at the waveform plotted over a distance (Fig. 4-14). The wavelength is defined as the distance between adjacent peaks and is referred to by the symbol λ (a Greek lambda). There can be only one cycle in a wavelength (Fig. 4-14).

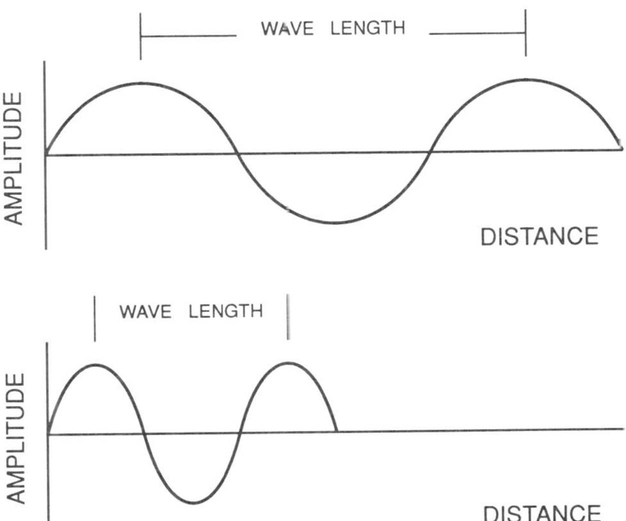

Fig. 4-14. Each cycle contains one wavelength, regardless of the length of the cycle.

Pulse Length

Pulse length is often confused with wavelength; the *difference* between the two, however, is very important. Pulse length is the distance from the start of the pulse to the end of the pulse (Fig. 4-15). A pulse length may contain several complete cycles or less than one complete cycle. The pulse length determines the resolution of an image, which is determined by how long the ultrasound transducer is allowed to "ring."

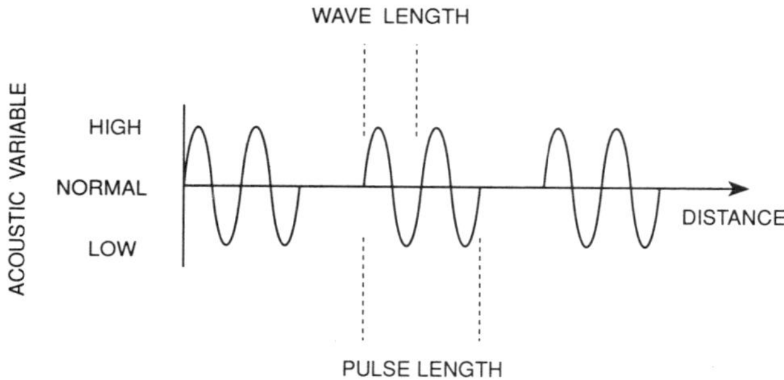

Fig. 4-15. A pulse length may contain several cycles but a wavelength has only one cycle.

For example, a drummer strikes the brass cymbal with the drumstick and then, for effect, damps the cymbal between thumb and forefinger (Fig. 4-16). This, in effect, shortens the length of time the cymbal rings. To shorten the pulse length, the same principal is applied, except that the damping of the ultrasound is constant in time.

The transducer, in conjunction with the backing material used for damping or cutting off the vibrations, determines how long the transducer will ring, thus producing the pulse length. The pulse length determines what is called *axial resolution*, or the ability to distinguish two separate objects along the ultrasound beam's path.

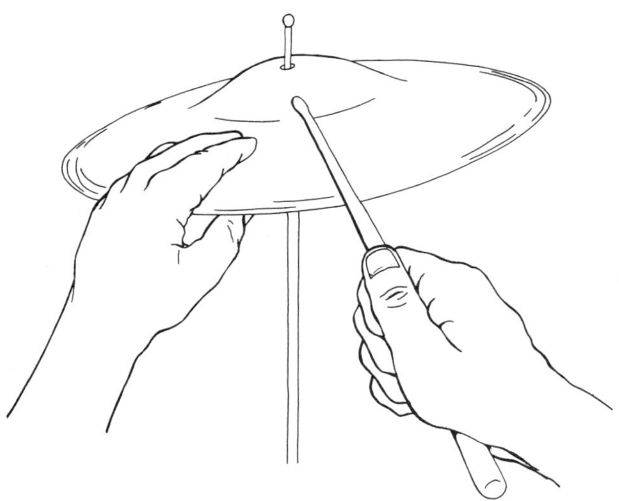

Fig. 4-16. Damping the cymbal's ring to make a short pulse length.

Wavelength Versus Pulse Length

Some students get confused between the terms *pulse length* and *wavelength*. The difference between these two terms is important to understand because they refer to two different characteristics of the waveform and the effects they produce. Wavelength, or lambda, refers to the length of one complete ultrasound cycle. A wavelength contains only one cycle. Pulse length is the distance from the beginning of the pulse to the end of that pulse. A pulse length may contain several cycles, but there can be only one cycle in a wavelength. Be sure to understand this difference.

Let's review what we have learned so far about ultrasound waves. First, if we could freeze an ultrasound wave in time and put it on a graph, we could look at the physical characteristics of the wave. If we want to measure the wavelength, we would measure the distance of the beginning of one complete wave cycle to the beginning of the next. To measure the pressure amplitude of the wave, we would measure the highest pressure point of the wave cycle relative to the surrounding or ambient pressure. If we wanted to look at the pulse length, often referred to as the *spatial pulse length*, we would measure the "wave train" from the beginning of the signal to the end.

Continuous Wave Versus Pulsed Wave

If a sound source oscillates continuously, the sound wave generated by the sound source will continuously propagate in the medium. This is called *continuous wave* (CW). On the other hand, if the sound source operates in an off-on fashion, the sound wave produced in the medium will also consist of a series of pulses. This is referred to as a *pulsed wave* (PW). Pulsed wave ultrasound is typically used in imaging ultrasound. The differences between CW and PW will be covered in depth later in this section.

Pulse Repetition Frequency and Pulse Repetition Period

Each time the bell is struck, a pulse of sound is emitted. The more often we repeat the strikes on the bell, the more pulses are emitted. The number of short pulses generated in a second is called the *pulse repetition frequency* (PRF).

The PRF is, in the case of the ringing bell, the number of times one hits the bell with the hammer during a particular period of time. In ultrasound, it is the number of times the transducer pulses with electricity. The PRF is usually measured in 1-second units. If you hit the bell 5 times 1 second, the PRF is 5. Ultrasound pulse, however, usually occurs in thousands of times per second. Therefore, the PRF in ultrasound is measured in kilohertz (thousands).

The time interval *between* corresponding points on the waveform of two successive pulses is referred to as the *pulse repetition period*. The basic unit for measuring the pulse repetition period is seconds.

Band Width and Center Operating Frequency

Transducers are commonly labeled as 3.5 MHz or 7.5 MHz. This refers to the resonance frequency of that particular transducer or the frequency with which the crystal "likes" to ring. A CW transducer that rings continuously produces only one precise frequency. The *center operating frequency* is the greatest amplitude of the band width.

A PW transducer is allowed to ring only in short bursts. In general, the shorter the burst, the broader the range of frequencies produced. This is just the opposite of CW transducers that ring continuously and produce a very narrow range of frequencies. In sum, the longer the pulse duration (letting the crystal ring), the narrower the band width. Inversely, the shorter the pulse duration (dampening the ring), the broader the band width.

A 7.5-MHz PW transducer produces its greatest amplitude at 7.5 MHz. This is referred to as the *center operating frequency*. The transducer doesn't only transmit signals at exactly 7.5 MHz, however; there are some higher and some lower frequencies at either side of the center frequency as well. The range of these frequencies is referred to as the *band width*. Although these frequencies at either end of the band width do not have the amplitude of the center frequency, they may be beneficial in allowing the transducer to utilize the advantages of higher frequency (resolution) and lower frequency (penetration).

The band width's greatest amplitude is at the center (i.e., 7.5 MHz) and gradually diminishes in a bell-shaped curve. A broad-band transducer will provide a greater range of frequencies but at a lower amplitude all over. This is how some equipment manufacturers can make claims that 7.5-MHz transducers can operate between

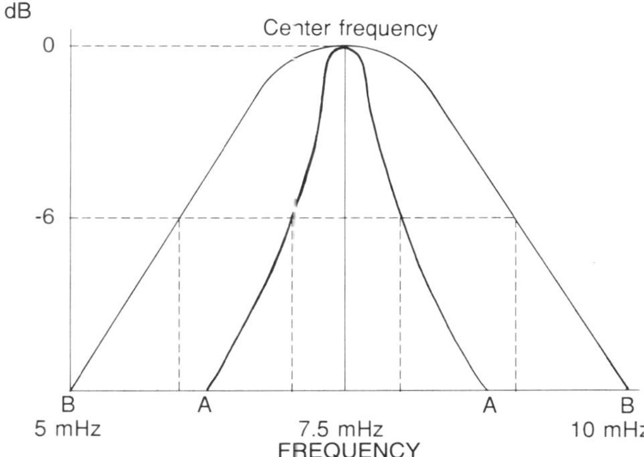

Fig. 4-17. The band width shows the amplitude and range of the signal. A narrow band width transducer (A) shows that the amplitude drops off quickly on either side of the center frequency (7.5 MHz). The broad band width transducer (B) shows that the amplitude remains higher on either side of the center frequency, providing a greater range of usable frequencies.

5.0 and 10.0 MHz. But as you can see from Fig. 4-17, the farther the signal moves from the center frequency, the lower its amplitude or signal strength. If you want a lower frequency imaging transducer to penetrate deeper, it is advisable to choose a transducer with a lower center frequency.

Table 4-1 lists typical frequencies used in ultrasound imaging and examples of applications for which the transducers are used.

Table 4-1. Typical frequencies in ultrasound imaging.

Tranducer	*Application*
2.25 MHz	Deep abdominal, large patients, transcranial Doppler
3.5 MHz	Cardiac, abdominal, iliac arteries
5.0 MHz	Neonates, pediatrics, peripheral arterial, venous
7.5 MHz	Carotid arteries, saphenous vein mapping, small parts

Acoustic Power

The amount of energy that is emitted from a source and transmitted along a beam over 1 second of time is called the *acoustic power*. The instantaneous value of acoustic power varies periodically in time. For example, as mentioned earlier, PW ultrasound is turned on and off between bursts of ultrasound emission. When the transducer is in the off position, the acoustic power is zero. If we were to measure the acoustic power during this particular interval, it would not reflect the true acoustic power being transmitted overall. Therefore, acoustic power is averaged over a period of time to include pulses in both the on and off modes. The basic unit for acoustic power is measured in watts (W).

Intensity

The best term to describe the magnitude of a signal is *intensity*. Intensity is similar to the loudness of sound, and like the loudness of a loud rock and roll band, the intensity of the signal (music) can be dangerous if it is concentrated in a small area. Intensity is the average power of a wave divided by the area normal to the direction of propagation in which it is spread. The intensity of a rock and roll band playing in a small room is very high. It is much better to have the band play in a large auditorium.

Intensity can also be described using sunlight and a magnifying glass. Sunlight can be more intense by focusing the rays with a magnifying glass. All the energy becomes concentrated into one small spot. In fact, the light may be so intense that it can cause a fire! (Fig. 4-18)

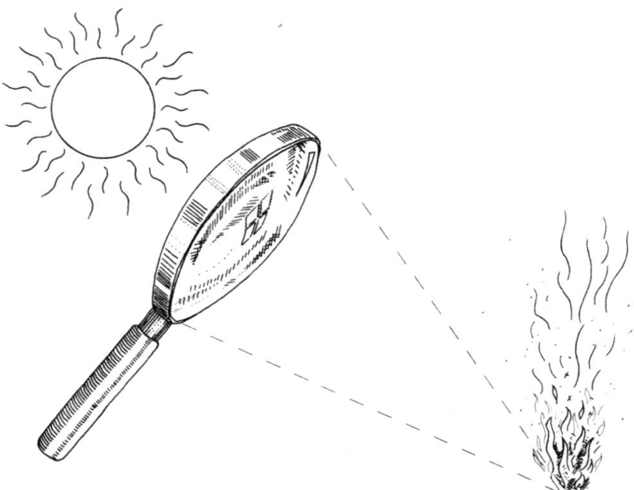

Fig. 4-18. The magnified intensity of sunlight can cause a fire!

Intensity is particularly important when the ultrasound wave enters sensitive areas such as a fetus or the brain. One has to be careful not to concentrate too much ultrasound into too small an area for too long a time. Health providers and the Food and Drug Administration (FDA) are concerned about ultrasound intensity, and specific guidelines on the limits of intensity must be adhered to rigidly.

The units for intensity are expressed as follows:

$$\text{intensity (W/cm}^2\text{)} = \frac{\text{power (W)}}{\text{area (cm}^2\text{)}}$$

Frequency and Ultrasound Imaging

High-frequency ultrasound provides better image resolution, or clarity of the image. However, high-frequency ultrasound is absorbed quickly and does not travel deeply into the tissue. Lower frequency ultrasound travels deeply into tissue but does not provide the quality of image produced by high-frequency ultrasound. In sum, there is always some type of trade-off with ultrasound frequencies. In general, the vascular specialist always should attempt to use the highest frequency possible with the penetration necessary to obtain the proper image.

Characteristic Acoustic Impedance

Characteristic *acoustic impedance* is an important property of a medium. It is defined as

$$\text{acoustic impedance} = \text{density} \times \text{the speed of sound in tissue}$$

Acoustic impedance changes at the tissue interfaces. In the case of the mountain yodeler, the interface is the boundary between the air and the rocky mountain wall. In the body, an interface is the boundary between two different types of tissue. That difference of tissue may be large, as between a calcified vessel and blood, or it may be more subtle, as within soft plaque or the liver. It is important to remember that the propagation velocity of ultrasound is dependent on the medium, and anytime that medium changes, so do the propagation velocity and the acoustic impedance.

Attenuation

Because the propagation of sound through tissue is constant, one might think that the sound waves would just continue on into the depths of the body. We know that doesn't happen. Several conditions affect ultrasound transmission on its journey through the body. Consequently, acoustic pressure, amplitude, particle velocity amplitude, and intensity all decrease exponentially with distance. This reduction in acoustic energy is called *acoustic attenuation*. The basic unit for measuring impedance is the decibel (dB).

The Attenuation Coefficient

As ultrasound travels through tissue, it loses its energy at a fairly steady rate. Consequently, the pressure amplitude decays exponentially with distance. The rule of this decay in soft tissue is one half a decibel per centimeter per megahertz. The loss of signal amplitude through attenuation in soft tissue is approximately 0.5 dB/cm/MHz.

Ultrasound Energy Loss

In ultrasound imaging, acoustic energy is constantly being lost from an ultrasound beam through several kinds of processes:

1. Reflection
2. Refraction
3. Scattering
4. Absorption

All of these interactions, in one way or another, reduce the intensity of (attenuate) the ultrasound beam.

Echo-Reflection

Up to this point, we have been talking only about the pulse in the pulse-echo principle. Now it's time to talk about the echo, or *reflection*, of the ultrasound signal. What exactly causes an echo?

An echo is the sound that returns to you if you make a loud noise in a large room. When you yell, "hello" you might hear "hello . . . hello . . . hello . . ." in decreasing amplitude as the sound bounces back and forth between the walls. The first "hello" you shout is the pulse and the subsequent "hello . . . hello . . . hello . . ." is the echo.

Most people are familiar with the yodeling mountaineer (Fig. 4-19). This mountaineer yodels high on a mountain peak and that signal returns to him over and over if the conditions are right! Those conditions are well known to the yodeler, and his expertise in obtaining the return of his yodeling skill depends on his knowledge of the pulse-echo principle and acoustic impedance.

First, in order to get an authentic mountain echo, you need a large mountain wall. It can't be some dinky little hillside or your yodel will pass right over it onto the wilderness, and little if any sound will be echoed back. Second, you need a hard, flat mountain wall so that the echo will bounce directly off the large rock surface. Finally, you need to sing your echo directly in front of the wall. Otherwise, you will deflect the returning signal to some other mountain.

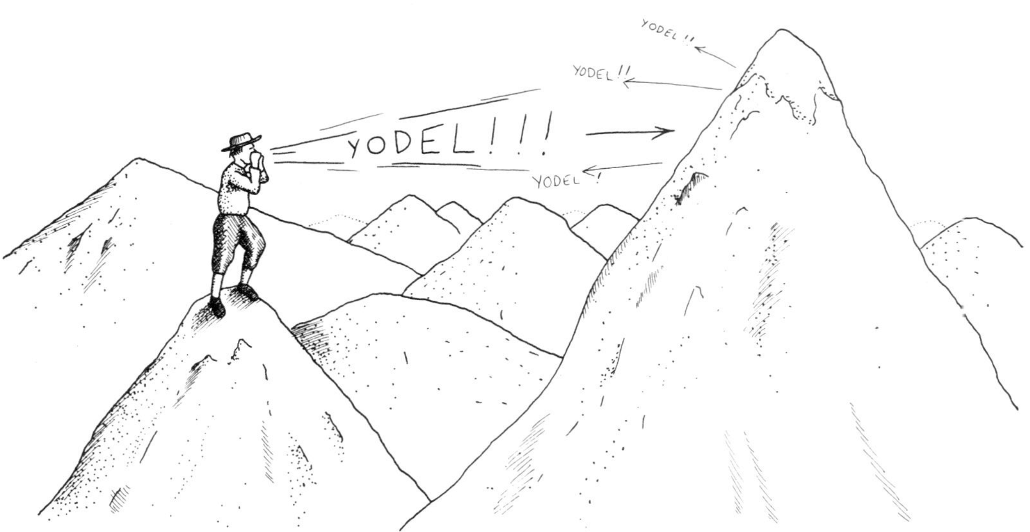

Fig. 4-19. The mountain yodeler demonstrating the pulse-echo principle.

In ultrasound, the yodel is the incident beam and the mountain wall is the boundary of the tissue interface. The echo, or ultrasound signal that is reflected back to the transducer, is called the reflected beam. In general, the greater the difference between characteristic acoustic impedances of the two media, the greater the energy of the incident beam that is reflected back. Conversely, the smaller the interface in relation to the wavelength, the more ultrasound signal will be scattered. In addition, the strength or amplitude of that signal is dependent on the acoustic impedance difference between the two interfaces.

Imaging ultrasound beams provide the strongest returning signal when they strike an interface at 90 degrees to the interface. If a baseball player wants to hit a home run, the batter must strike the ball as close to 90 degrees as possible in order to send the ball out of the park (Fig. 4-20). That is why it is best to aim the ultrasound probe perpendicular, or 90 degrees to the structure you want to image. In this manner, the borders of bodily structures are imaged.

When an ultrasound beam is directed at an interface that is larger than the sound beam, that beam will be partially reflected back at the sound source (Fig. 4-21). The rest of the ultrasound energy continues to propagate through the tissue until it meets the next interface.

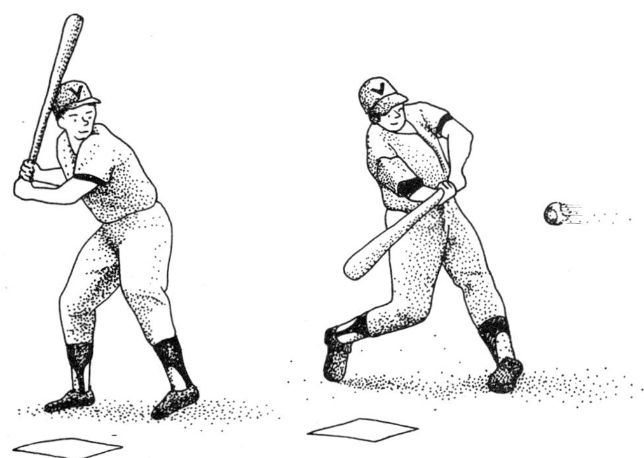

Fig. 4-20. The ball is best knocked out of the park when hit at 90 degrees.

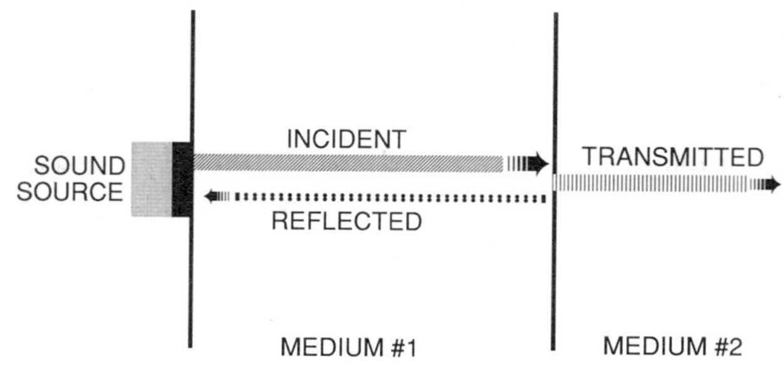

Fig. 4-21. The sound source transmits an ultrasound beam through a medium. Part of the beam is reflected back to the transducer and part of the beam passes through the next interface.

Specular Reflectors

Specular reflectors occur where ultrasound reflects off a smooth surface. This is equivalent to light reflecting off a smooth mirror. Specular reflectors occur at interfaces that are much larger than one wavelength in diameter. In other words, the reflectors are larger than the wavelength that strikes them. The wavelength is pretty small; for example, the wavelength of a 10 MHz transducer is only 0.15 mm. Specular reflectors are responsible for the important details imaged in diagnostic ultrasound.

Refraction

In ultrasound, *refraction* occurs when the incident beam (that which is transmitted from the transducer) strikes an interface (the boundary between different density tissue with different wave velocity propagation) at an angle and the actual beam bends away from the expected line of travel (Fig. 4-22). In sum, this amount of bending from the expected straight-line path of travel changes with two factors:

1. The change in angle of incidence away from 90 degrees
2. The sound velocities associated with the media

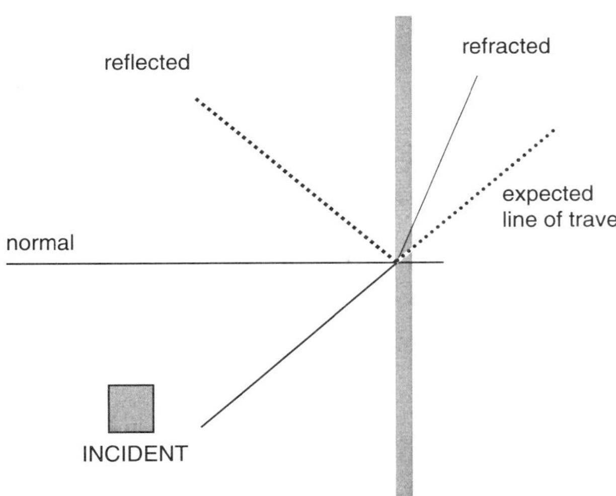

Fig. 4-22. When an ultrasound beam strikes an interface at an angle, part of the beam is reflected back but *away* from the transducer. The transmitted ultrasound beam passes through the interface but is refracted away from the expected line of travel.

Angles

If you are bouncing a ball off a wall and want that ball to return to you, you must keep the angle of incidence (your tossed ball) close to the angle of reflection (the returned ball). With ultrasound, the same principle applies. In order to obtain the maximum reflection, one must aim the ultrasound beam as close to 90 degrees as possible. As an angle of incidence approaches 90 degrees, or perpendicular to the interface, the portion of energy reflected back is almost constant. Once the angle starts to deviate from 90 degrees, the returned signal also returns at a different angle, and most likely away from the transducer.

Propagation Velocities

Propagation velocity is dependent on the medium. Subsequently, as the ultrasound passes through different organs containing different medium characteristics, so will the propagation velocity change. As an example, the average velocity in soft tissue is 1,540 m/sec. However, various soft tissues have different propagation velocities:

Muscle: 1,630 m/sec
Liver: 1,570 m/sec
Kidney: 1,560 m/sec
Brain: 1,520 m/sec

As an ultrasound beam passes from the liver to the kidney in an abnormal way, the change in propagation velocity causes the beam to be partially transmitted, but at an angle away from the incident beam. This is called *refraction* and is described by *Snell's law*.

Scattering

Scattering occurs when the ultrasound wave strikes an interface with irregularities close to the size of, or smaller than the wavelength; sound is reflected in many *different* directions (Fig. 4-23).

Fig. 4-23. Ultrasound scattering from an irregular interface.

Scattering is a valuable interaction of ultrasound that has profound benefits for imaging the internal texture of the image.

Scattering provides the examiner with the ability to detect specific changes in tissue, thus providing a clear understanding of the tissue type or tissue characterization. Scattering occurs in soft tissue as well as blood.

Rayleigh Scattering

Rayleigh scattering occurs when the size of the scatterer is much smaller than the wavelength, and ultrasound is then reflected in *all directions*.

Speckling

When Rayleigh scattering occurs *uniformly in all directions*, speckling occurs (Fig. 4-24). Speckling differentiates types of tissue. It is a result of scattering plus interference. Almost all soft tissue produces scattering because of its cellular structure and small internal detail.

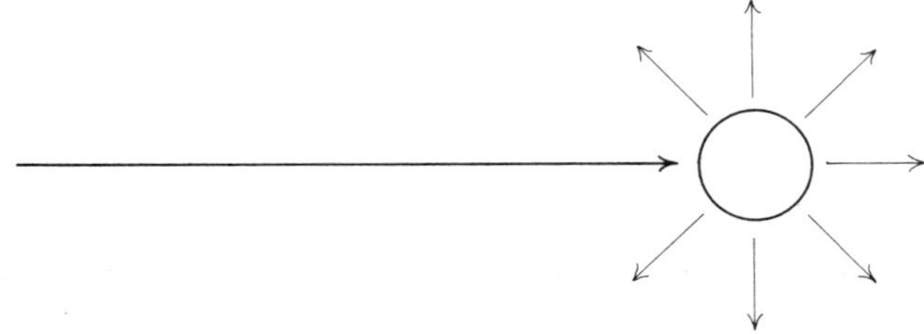

Fig. 4-24. Ultrasound scattering uniformly when the interface is smaller than the wavelength.

Absorption

Absorption is the only process whereby sound energy is dissipated by the medium. In all other modes of ultrasound interactions, the decrease in ultrasound intensity is a result of redirecting the ultrasound beam. Absorption is the process whereby ultrasound energy is transformed into another form of energy, primarily heat. The absorption of the ultrasonic beam is related to the

1. frequency of the beam
2. viscosity of the medium
3. relaxation time of the medium

Although the vascular specialist cannot control the medium of the tissue, she can learn to operate the ultrasound system (gain, power, time-gain compensation) and choose a transducer (higher or lower frequency) that will provide the best image possible. Time-gain compensation allows the operator to increase the gain at various depths in order to provide a balanced image.

Image Artifacts

Artifacts can be defined as any interference of the normal ultrasound display that decreases the operator's ability to acquire imaging or Doppler data. Artifacts can occur due to normal anatomic variations within the tissue. They can also exist secondary to the structure or the mechanics of the transducer. Understanding the nature of the artifact, therefore, can lead the vascular specialist to the source and, many times, the solution of the problem.

Origin: Air

One of the most common artifacts confronted in imaging ultrasound occurs in the presence of air in or near tissue. This air can result from poor contact between the transducer and the skin, attempting to image in the chest, or imaging the abdomen of a patient who has excessive bowel gas. Ultrasound, for the most part, is incapable of penetrating these areas.

You will recall from your lessons on ultrasound physics that sound waves need to propagate through a medium, preferably tissue that contains molecules in close proximity to each other. This interaction of molecules allows the transmission of the ultrasound wave. Air molecules have very low stiffness; subsequently, ultrasound energy is absorbed and the transmission of ultrasound ceases.

In abdominal vascular imaging, the presence of air in the bowel is a constant problem. Because ultrasound cannot penetrate under these conditions, you will see a "shadow" just beyond the area containing air. As with a shadow created by any blocking of light, your ability to view is blocked by the absence of the proper "illumination" behind the object. The condition of air in the bowel can be limited by asking the patient not to have anything to eat or drink after midnight on the night before the examination. In this way, digestive activity, and the subsequent production of air, is limited.

Origin: Poor Skin Contact

Another condition in which air causes artifacts is due to poor transducer-to-skin contact. This seems especially true on patients with thin necks or legs where contact is difficult to make. Sometimes there will be just a tiny bubble of air in the gel, which prevents the ultrasound from traveling through that single spot. If you are not paying attention, you will not necessarily notice an air bubble in the gel; you will just know that, for some reason, the image isn't very clear. By de-emphasizing your sight from the area of interest and looking at the whole image, you will pick up these types of artifacts a little easier. Two simple measures that should relieve contact problems are first, using more gel and, second, trying a different scan plane. Often, you can obtain better surface contact on a more lateral approach.

Origin: Calcium

Calcium also interferes with obtaining ultrasound images. The nature of that interference is just the opposite of that of air. Calcified plaque contains molecules that are so densely packed, they have very little room to move around. The ultrasound waves strike the hard interface of calcified tissue, but like a tennis ball hitting a solid wall, they simply deflect all the ultrasound waves back. The result is no ultrasound penetration beyond the plaque and, subsequently, no image beyond the interface.

One possible solution to this type of artifact is to scan the vessel or structure you are imaging from a different plane. For example, if you are imaging a vessel from an anterior approach and encounter a great deal of calcium on the anterior aspect of the vessel, bring your probe around to take a more lateral or posterior lateral view. If the plaque does not involve the entire vessel, you may be able to "sneak" a look behind the plaque to identify tissue you would otherwise be unable to see. In sum, don't confine yourself to regimented approaches; use various scan planes freely in order to obtain the images you require.

Origin: Vessel Walls

Vessels need not be calcified to cause a shadowing artifact. Often times, thick vessel walls, especially on a transverse view, may cause shadowing due to the way the vessel is aligned with the ultrasound transducer. Because the ultrasound waves need to penetrate a good portion of the vessel walls, much of the energy gets absorbed. The result is shadowing distal the vessel you are attempting to image.

Origin: Reverberation

The construction of the transducer includes a facing, or matching material at the point where the transducer comes into contact with the skin. The importance of the matching material is to limit the amount of acoustic impedance between the transducer and tissue. Without this matching material, a large reflection would occur between the skin and transducer because of the large acoustic impedance between them. This large reflection is then transmitted out toward the tissue where it reverberates once again.

Another term used for reverberation is *re-echo*. If an echo is a signal being sent and bounced back to the sender, then the re-echo, or reverberation, is the re-bouncing back of that signal.

In ultrasound imaging, a reverberation artifact may appear as a series of interfaces that are inconsistent with the tissue you are imaging. This is particularly true in mechanical sector scanners that require a fluid path and, subsequently, a thick housing to prevent the fluid from leaking. The result is that some of the ultrasound waves bounce off the housing back to the transducer where they are once again bounced into the tissue. This will appear as a series of lines in the image that are aligned parallel to the transducer face.

Review Exercise

1. The principle that refers to sending and receiving an ultrasound signal is called the ______________-______________ principle.

2. The auditory nerve translates ______________________________ into volume and tone.

3. Sound most commonly originates from a

   a. medium
   b. source
   c. horizontal wave
   d. oscillation

4. Sound begins as ______________________________ of molecules.

5. The pace at which molecules "like" to vibrate is called the ____ frequency.

6. For sound to propagate, it must be transmitted through a ______________.

7. The transmission of sound requires the substance in which the signal is moving through to be

   a. expandable and contractible
   b. solid, liquid, or gas
   c. soft tissue
   d. elastic and deformable

8. Propagation velocity is dependent on the

   a. transmitted frequency
   b. power
   c. PRF
   d. mechanical properties of the medium

9. Sound is ______________________________ by nature.

10. To propagate means to

    a. multiply
    b. speed up
    c. diminish
    d. reproduce

11. The propagation velocity depends on what two mechanical properties of the medium?

    a. ____

    b. ____

12. The average velocity of sound through soft tissue is

    a. 1,540 cm/sec
    b. 1,560 m/sec
    c. 1,555 m/sec
    d. 1,540 m/sec

13. List four acoustic variables.

a. ______________________________

b. ______________________________

c. ______________________________

d. ______________________________

14. Sound cannot be transmitted in

a. air
b. water
c. solids
d. a vacuum

15. Sound moves in specific patterns called ______________.

16. The number of times a transducer pulses during a specific time is called the ______________ ______________ ______________________________.

17. A large group of molecules propagating in a group is referred to as (compression/rarefaction).

18. The area on either side of a large group of propagating molecules is referred to as (compression/rarefaction).

19. A number of different waves oscillating to form a common wave is called the ______________________________.

20. Ultrasound moves in

a. transverse waves
b. longitudinal waves
c. spherical waves
d. helical waves

21. A CW Doppler transducer rings ______________________________, as opposed to a PW Doppler transducer, which rings in ______________________________.

22. List three types of particle amplitude in relation to ultrasound.

a. ______________________________

b. ______________________________

c. ______________________________

23. Identify the wavelength and pulse length:

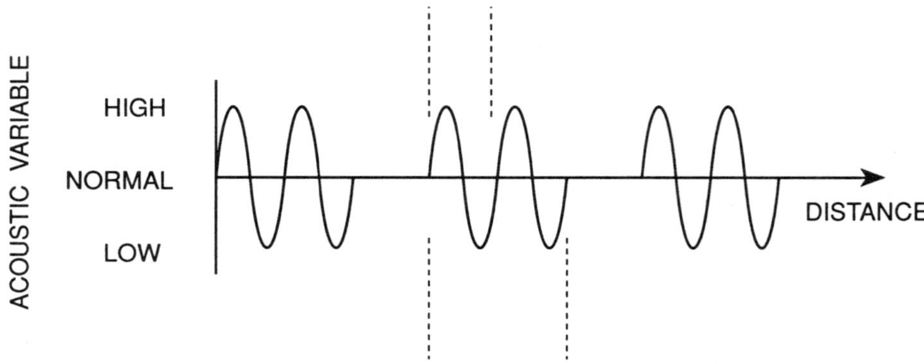

24. The best term to define the magnitude of a signal is

a. amplitude
b. intensity
c. power
d. strength

25. The completion of a particle's forward-and-reverse movement is referred to as a ____________

26. The number of cycles occurring over a period of time is referred to as ultrasound ________________________.

27. Ultrasound tends to be in a range of about

a. 1 MHz to 15 MHz
b. 5 MHz to 15 MHz
c. 15 MHz to 20 MHz
d. 20 kHz and above

28. Medical imaging uses frequencies between

a. 2 MHz and 10 MHz
b. 5 MHz and 15 MHz
c. 15 MHz and 20 MHz
d. 20 MHz and above

29. A wavelength is measured over

a. time
b. distance
c. both time and distance
d. none of the above

30. Pulse length is determined by how long the transducer is allowed to ____________.

31. Match the following frequencies:

a. 100,000 cycles/sec ___ 15 MHz
b. 10 cycles/sec ___ 100 kHz
c. 15,000,000 cycles/sec ___ 13.5 kHz
d. 13,500 cycles/sec ___ 10 Hz

32. The range of frequencies a transducer may display is referred to as the

a. wave train
b. pulse length
c. wavelength
d. band width

33. The highest frequency amplitude a transducer displays is referred to as the

a. center operating fequency
b. pulse length
c. wavelength
d. band width

34. The length of a sound wave is the _____________ from one event in the wavelength to the beginning of that event in the next cycle.

35. Amplitude is the amount of ___________________________ from a central point, which is usually the baseline.

36. Match the probe frequencies with the general applications for the following:

a. 2.25 MHz
b. 3.5 MHz
c. 5.0 MHz
d. 7.5 MHz

___ carotids superficial vessels
___ transcranial Doppler, deep abdominal
___ normal abdominal
___ deep veins in the legs

37. The higher the frequency, the greater the amplitude. True or False?

38. The amount of energy that is emitted from a source and transmitted along a beam over 1 second is called

a. acoustic power
b. intensity
c. amplitude
d. acoustic variable

39. The formula for expressing intensity is

Intensity (W/cm^2) =

40. The formula for expressing acoustic impedance is

Acoustic impedance = ____

41. One complete cycle of a wave, in one second, equals

a. 1 kHz
b. 1 MHz
c. 1 MHz
d. 1 Hz

42. Five thousand complete cycles a second equal

a. 5 MHz
b. 5 kHz
c. 5 MHz
d. 5 Hz

43. Which ultrasound has a higher frequency?

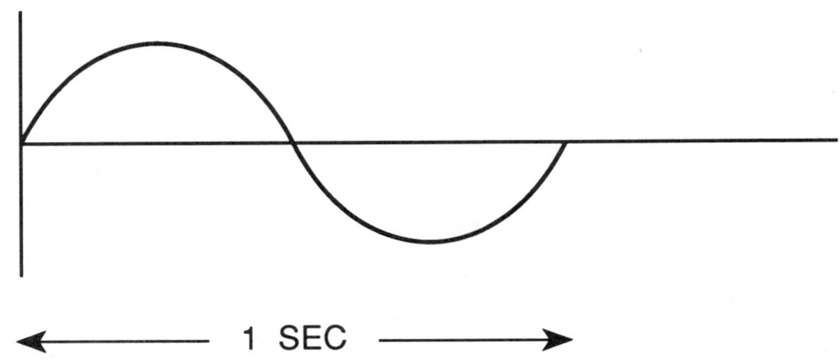

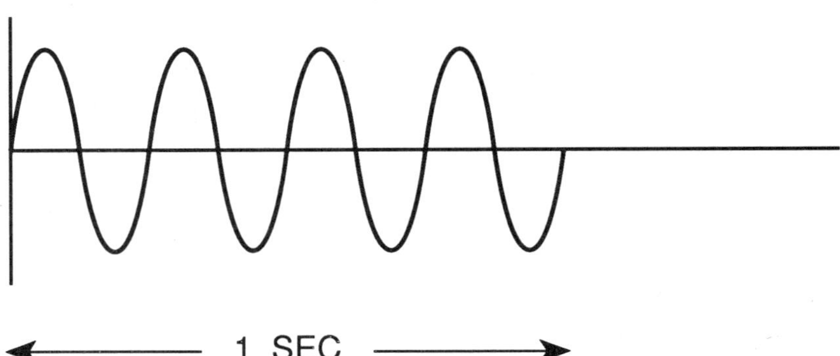

44. All of the following are mechanics of the medium that affect the reflected wave *except*

   a. angle of the incident beam
   b. transducer frequency
   c. size of the interface
   d. difference in acoustic impedance

45. In ultrasound, penetration is dependent on the

   a. amplitude of the wave
   b. wavelength
   c. pulse length
   d. shape of the wave

46. An ultrasound wave moving away from a source and through a medium is called ____________________________.

47. The speed at which a wave moves through a medium is called

   a. ultrasound velocity
   b. propagation velocity
   c. wave propagation
   d. medium propagation

48. The formula expressing the attenuation coefficient is

   a. 10 MHz/dB/0.5
   b. 1 Hz/dB/cm
   c. 0.5dB/mm/kHz
   d. 0.5dB/cm/MHz

49. Propagation velocity is faster in air than in bone. True or False?

50. The velocity of sound is directly proportional to the density of the medium. True or False?

51. The denser the medium, the (greater/lesser) the velocity of sound.

52. Acoustic energy is constantly lost by what four common factors?

a. ____________________

b. ____________________

c. ____________________

d. ____________________

53. Ultrasound intensity is measured in

a. frequency
b. watts/cm
c. decibels
d. cm/sec

54. Attenuation is defined as a decrease of ____________________ strength.

55. The operator can, to some extent, overcome the limits of attenuation. True or False?

56. When an ultrasound is directed at an interface that is larger than the sound beam, much of the beam will

a. be partially reflected back through the medium
b. scatter in many directions
c. scatter in all directions
d. not be affected

57. When an ultrasound is directed at an interface that is smaller than the sound beam, much of the beam will

a. be partially reflected back through the medium
b. scatter in many directions
c. scatter in all directions
d. not be affected

58. When an ultrasound is directed at an interface with surface irregularities close to the size of the wavelength, much of the ultrasound beam will

a. be partially reflected back through the medium
b. scatter in many directions
c. scatter in all directions
d. not be affected

59. Ultrasound scattered in all directions is called

a. specular reflection
b. speckling
c. Rayleigh scattering
d. absorption

60. Ultrasound *uniformly* scattered in all directions is called

a. specular reflection
b. speckling
c. Rayleigh scattering
d. absorption

61. The only process whereby ultrasound energy is dissipated by the medium is called

a. reflection
b. absorption
c. scattering
d. refraction

62. The best angle to transmit an ultrasound signal at an interface is

a. 0 degrees
b. 45 degrees
c. 60 degrees
d. 90 degrees

63. If the ultrasound strikes an interface at a different angle than 90 degrees, the beam is ______________________________ from its expected course.

64. Specular reflection occurs at interfaces that are larger than the _______________ diameter.

65. In refraction, the amount of bending from the expected straight-line path of travel changes with two factors:

a. The change angles away from _______________ degrees.
b. The velocities associated with the _______________.

66. The greater the deviation from the angle of ______________________________, and the greater the difference in tissue ______________________________, the greater the refraction that will occur.

67. Scattering is not a beneficial interaction of ultrasound. True or False?

68. In scattering, because each irregular interface is seen as a separate sound source, sound scattering is reflected

a. toward the transducer
b. away from the transducer
c. in many different directions
d. in one direction only

69. Scattering provides the examiner with the ability to detect specific changes in tissue. True or False?

70. Ultrasound energy is _______________ by converting this high-frequency molecular interaction into heat.

71. Artifacts can be defined as any ____________________ of normal ultrasound display that decreases the operator's ability to acquire imaging or Doppler data.

72. List four common artifacts confronted in ultrasound imaging

a. ____________________

b. ____________________

c. ____________________

d. ____________________

IMAGING ULTRASOUND PRINCIPLES

In this section, we will review the principles of imaging ultrasound. We will also learn how images are converted from sound to images on the ultrasound screen and include the technical capabilities available to manipulate ultrasound signals for better images.

Key Terms

A-mode
Analog scan converter
B-mode
Cathode ray tube
Compound B-mode imaging
Digital scan converter
Dynamic range
Frames per second
Gain
Gray scale
M-mode
Real time
Reflectors
Scan converter
Time-gain compensation

A-Mode

A-mode can be thought of as referring to "amplitude-mode" scanning. The term *amplitude* refers to the strength of the reflected ultrasound signal. The greater the signal that is reflected back, the greater the amplitude "spike"

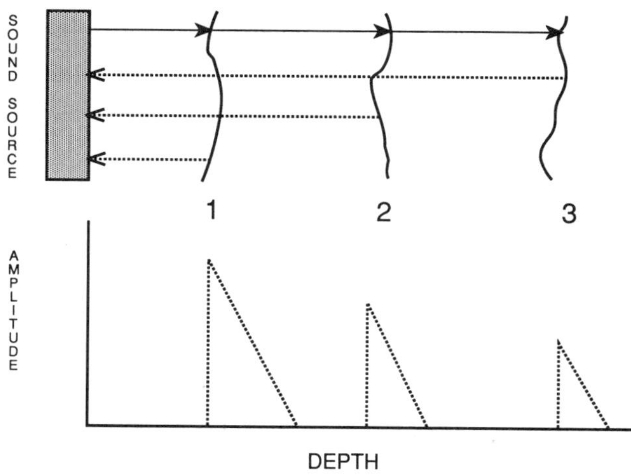

Fig. 4-25. A-mode produces a "spike" providing very specific information about distance and depth.

that will occur on the monitor or graph (Fig. 4-25). A-mode scanning is rarely, if ever, used in traditional noninvasive vascular testing. It is primarily used in ophthalmic (eye) ultrasound and echoencephalography (brain).

B-Mode

B-mode ultrasound refers to the "brightness mode." It can be best understood by looking back at the A-mode illustration. When you look at an A-mode graph, it appears as a series of mountains; the larger the mountain, the greater the amplitude. If we were to fly over these mountains, we would see a quite different pattern (Fig. 4-26). Assuming the bigger mountains had bigger bases, we would be able to "see" them better from our airplane; the image would appear brighter.

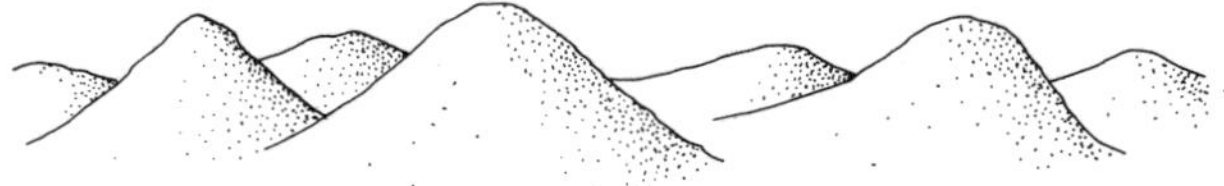

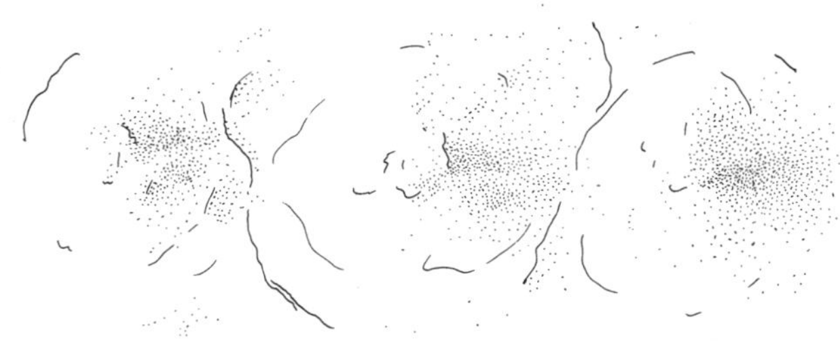

Fig. 4-26. (Top) Looking at the mountains from the side of the road is like A-mode ultrasound. (Bottom) Getting a bird's eye view of the mountains is like B-mode ultrasound.

Because the brightness of the dot corresponds to the amplitude of the signal, we can interpret that brighter reflections occur when signals reflect from stronger interfaces, such as hard calcified plaque, which would cause a high-amplitude signal (Fig. 4-27).

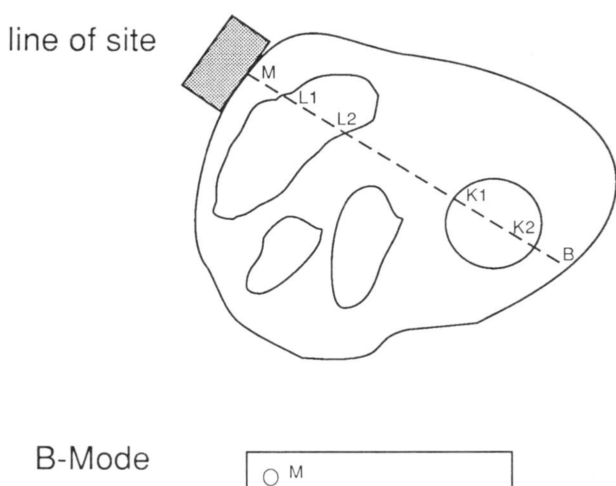

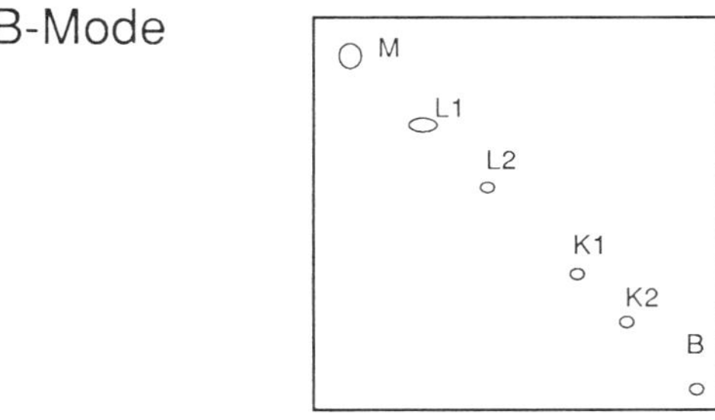

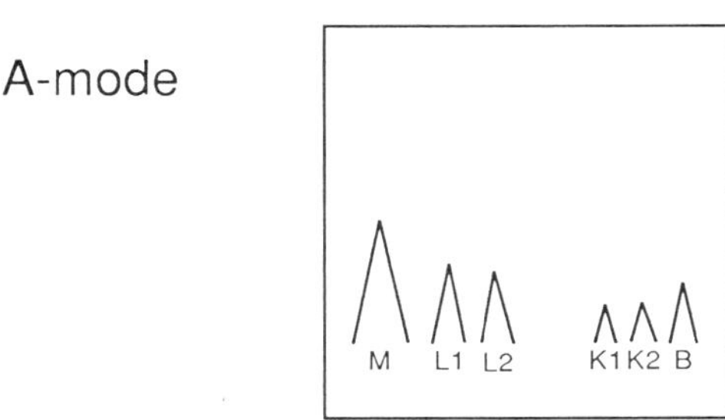

Fig. 4-27. The transducer interprets brighter dots (B-mode) relating to the higher spikes (A-mode) corresponding to the structures reflected from the line of sight.

Clearly, just a few spikes of A-mode or the bright dots of B-mode will provide little benefit in interpreting complex tissue structure of the abdomen or vascular structures. B-mode scanning needs millions and millions of dots compiled together to form an image. The more dots accumulated, the more likely one can compile the different information and make interpretations, such as fresh clot versus normal vein, or mixed plaque composition (Fig. 4-28).

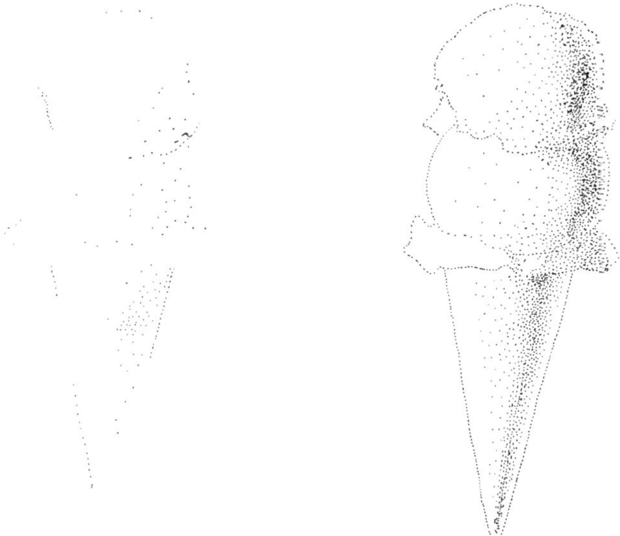

Fig. 4-28. The image on the left has too few dots to complete the picture. The image on the right has enough dots to show accurate detail of this double-scoop ice-cream cone.

Compound B-Mode Imaging

Compound B-mode scanning allows the sonographer to "look" at structures in several different directions. We can move the transducer around obstacles such as gas, bone, or calcified plaque. For example, the best way to describe an object is to describe its height and width (Fig. 4-29). By limiting your observation to only one perspective, you can be fooled by *lack* of information.

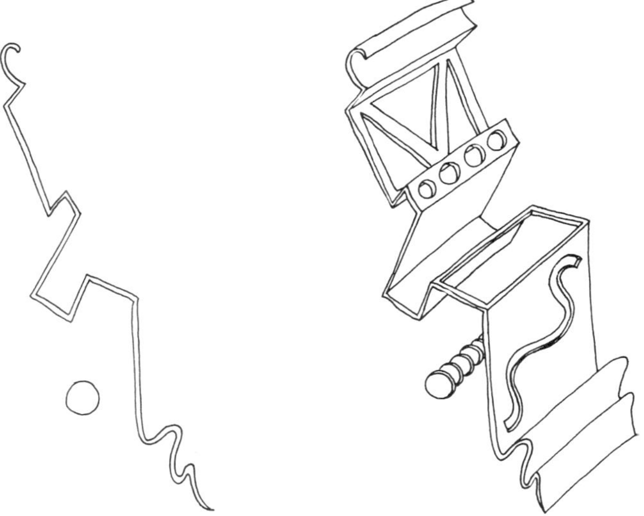

Fig. 4-29. The figure on the left doesn't give us much information about this structure, but by moving the transducer and employing compound B-mode imaging at several different lines of sight, the description of this structure becomes clear.

Compound B-mode imaging uses multiple dots in two dimensions to form static images of internal structures in the body. In addition, scanning from various directions allows for some perspective of the different echos in relation to each other. In order to have these dots form a pattern that is consistent with the anatomical structures, a special "arm" is connected to the ultrasound system (Fig. 4-30). This arm tells the computer that you have moved 10 cm across the abdomen to the left or the right, and the dots that are stored and processed form the picture of what they see.

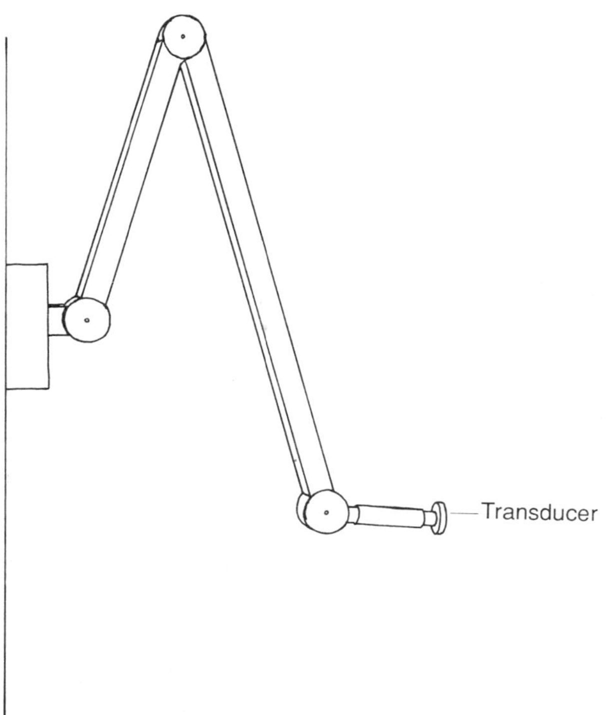

Fig. 4-30. This mechanical arm "knows" when the examiner moves right or left, up or down. It displays the ultrasound dots on a screen in relation to the position of the arm.

Motion Artifact

If you are taking a photograph of a group of friends, one of the first things you may ask the group to do is, "Hold still!" The reason for this is to avoid getting blurry pictures. If somebody is moving during the snapshot, the camera will see the person in two different places and you will end up with an unclear picture.

One of the problems with B-mode imaging is that you cannot always get the patient's organs to hold still during your sweep of the scan. You may attempt to limit that motion by having the patient hold her breath, but inevitably there is some motion that the ultrasound "sees" in two different places. This is especially true with children, very ill, or otherwise uncooperative patients.

M-Mode

M-mode addresses the motion artifact caused by the movement of internal structures. M-mode refers to "motion mode," or time-motion mode, and is specifically designed to look at the motion of the heart and its valves. Using a strip chart recorder, the reflected B-mode dot is traced over a period of time (Fig. 4-31). If the dot is being reflected from the left ventricle of the heart, we will see a trace of the distance the dot moved first in systole and then in diastole.

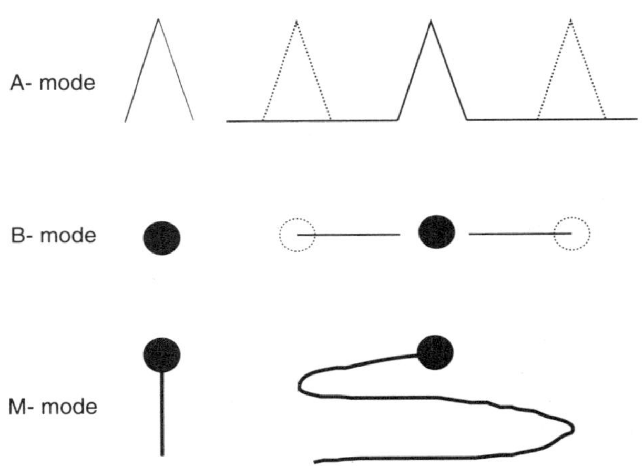

Fig. 4-31. This illustration shows the schematic difference of A-mode, B-mode, and M-mode. M-mode is valuable when objective measurements of motion are necessary.

Scan Converter

So far, we have discussed a few of the different methods of obtaining sound waves. There still remains a problem, however; you not only cannot hear sound waves, you cannot see them either! The sound waves that are reflected back to your transducer must be converted (changed into another form) in order to be seen. Subsequently, one needs a *scan converter* to change ultrasound waves into images that can be seen.

There are two principle types of scan converters: analog and digital. Both have advantages and disadvantages. A simple comparison of analog verses digital technology can be made by comparing a analog wrist watch having a "sweep" second hand with a digital watch that displays numbers only (Fig. 4-32). The analog watch, as you have observed, provides a continuous flow of movement, providing you with an everpresent update of the correct time. The digital watch, on the other hand, gives *exact* numbers of time as it blinks through the seconds, minutes, and hours. There is never a half step with the digital watch; you will have either 32 seconds or 33 seconds, never 32.5.

If you ask an analog watch person the time, she may answer, "About ten minutes to nine," even though the time may be nine minutes to nine. But if you ask the person with a digital watch, she most likely will reply, "Eight fifty-one," because that is precisely what the watch reads.

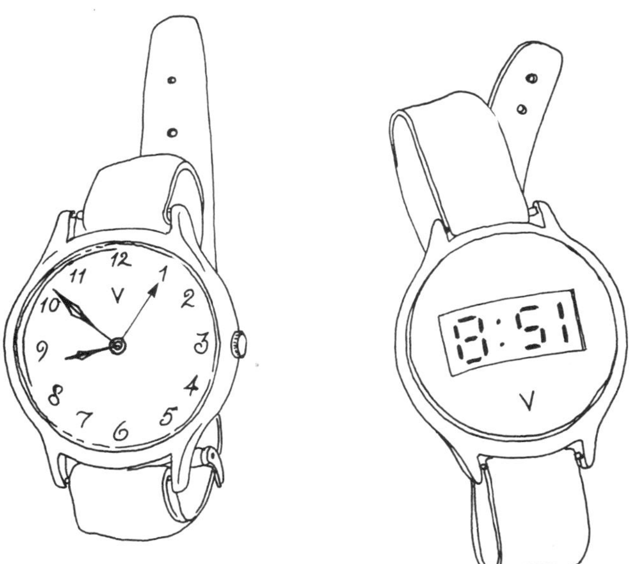

Fig. 4-32. The digital watch always displays very precise numbers. The analog watch shows the ongoing actual time.

Analog Scan Converter

An analog scan converter is very much like a cathode ray tube (discussed in next section) except the phosphorus screen is replaced by a dielectric matrix. A dielectric matrix is a nonconductor of electricity which causes the electrons that hit the matrix to "stick" to the screen, leaving a positive charge on the material. The positive charge left on the matrix is proportional to the number of electrons that strike the matrix, which in turn is proportional to the amplitude of the processed signal. The greater the ultrasound amplitude, the greater the positive charge on the matrix. The electrons are then distributed on the matrix at a very rapid rate through a process called *raster scanning*.

There are, however, a few drawbacks with analog scan converters. One of the major problems is that the image tends to drift, that is, the images created are not consistent from day to day. Because of these problems, most systems now utilize digital scan conversion.

Cathode Ray Tube

A cathode ray tube (CRT) is a device that allows you, in a sense, to "see" electricity or electromagnetic waves. Your television is a cathode ray tube and so is your computer monitor, as is the monitor on the ultrasound system.

The *cathode ray tube* (CRT) consists of a tube in which some air has been extracted, thus creating a moderate vacuum. On one end of the tube is a negatively charged cathode filament. This filament is similar to the filament on a light bulb, but instead of creating light, the cathode filament creates heat. The electrons emitted from the cathode in the form of heat are then focused into a beam and sent through the evacuated tube, like a mini laser. This beam is accelerated by a positively charged anode. After passing through deflector plates that channel the beam either in a lateral or horizontal direction, they strike the phosphorus-covered screen at the other end (Fig. 4-33).

Phosphorus is an element that lights up when struck by electrons. You have seen phosphorus on the Fourth of July in the fireworks display. It is also used in matches to ignite the chemicals on the stick. But, we are talking about heat that brightens up just enough to see how the electrons "perform" on the screen. Electricians and electrical engineers use CRT, such as oscilloscopes, on a regular basis to look at how electricity is performing in various electronics.

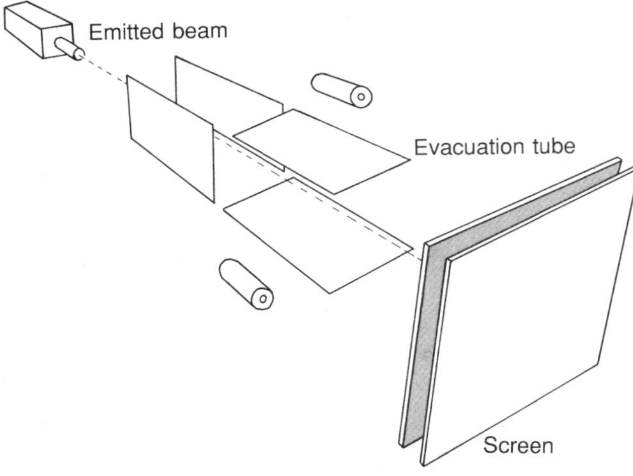

Fig. 4-33. The cathode ray tube.

Digital Scan Converter

Digital scan converters are solid state computer memories that do not use vacuum tubes. In order for a digital scan converter to work, it must first convert the analog signal into a digital signal. This is referred to as analog-to-digital or A-to-D conversion. The digital scan converter scans an area, then divides that area into pixels; small, square picture elements. If you take a number of these elements and put them together, you will get a whole picture, pretty much like a jigsaw puzzle (Fig. 4-34).

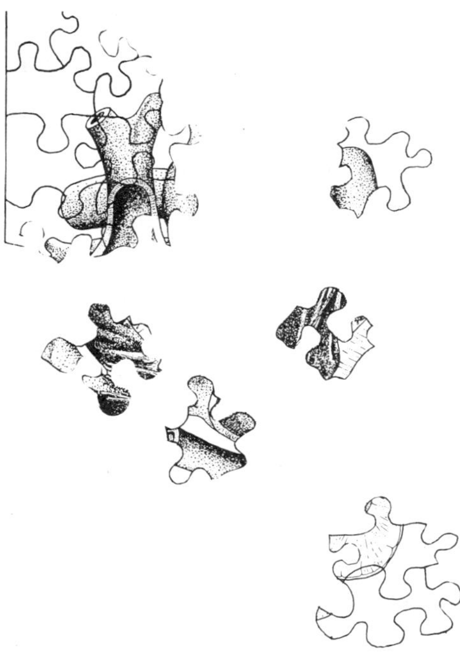

Fig. 4-34. The digital scan converter changes analog information into bits of digital information to form pieces of the puzzle.

The pixels are assigned a position on the X-Y axis and are associated with the amplitude of the signal at that point. Each pixel amplitude is assigned a number by the computer. This assignment of numbers on a screen is very much like putting all the pieces together to form a picture (Fig. 4-35).

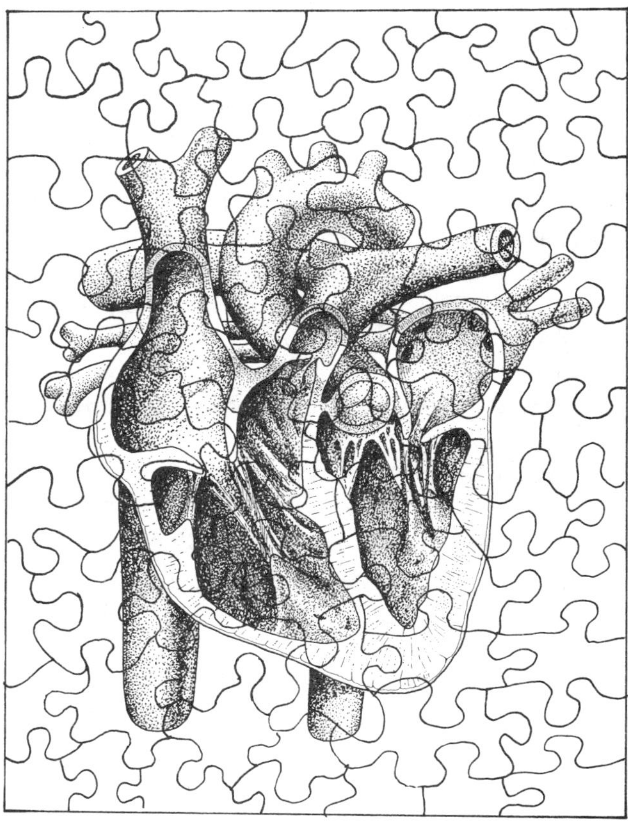

Fig. 4-35. Once all these pieces are collected, an image can be formed.

Gray-Scale Display

B-mode images are acquired by displaying the A-mode "tip" as a dot; the higher the A-mode amplitude, the brighter the B-Mode dot. If the amplitude of the B-mode image is strong enough, it is displayed. If it is not strong enough, you will not see it at all. This "on or off" situation gives rise to so-called bi-stable images. It would be like trying to paint clouds by using only black and white paint, not being allowed to mix them together to make different tones of gray.

In bi-stable images, only strong reflectors of tissue are picked up, and subtle and often important tissue changes are unfortunately missed. The lack of *gray scale* would be equivalent to trying to make physical assumptions about people by looking only at their shadows, not being able to see their skin, clothes, features, smiles, or eyes (Fig. 4-36).

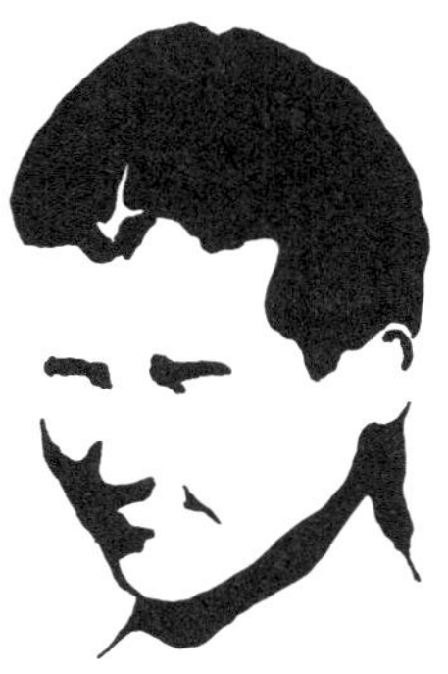
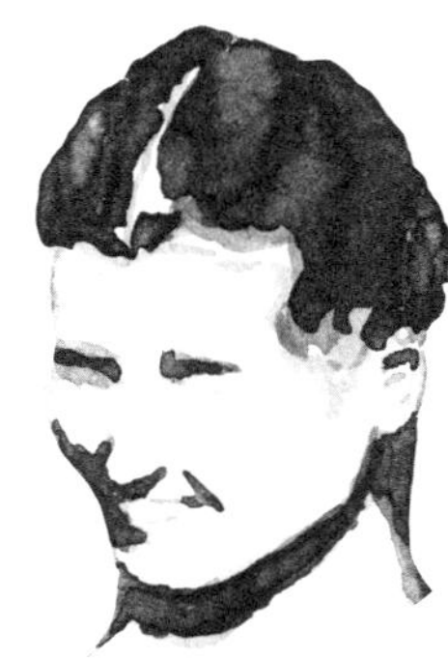

Fig. 4-36. Gray scale provides even more specific information in an image. The more gray scale in the image, the more diagnostic information.

In the early '70s, an improvement was developed to allow the display of gray-scale shades. The scan converter provided images of various levels of black and white that related to the tissue being examined. Soft plaque has a lower amplitude reflector than hard calcified plaque. Complex plaque has various tissue densities, suggesting a mixture of new hemorrhages, calcium, and new plaque formation (Fig. 4-37). All of this is important to the examiner in order to determine not only the extent of the narrowing of the artery, but the composition of the plaque itself.

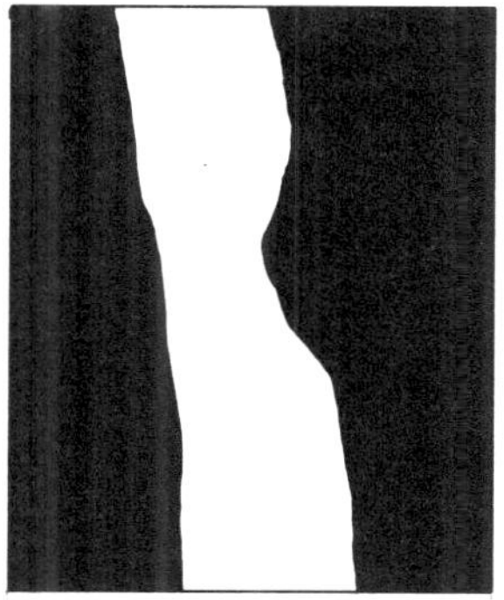
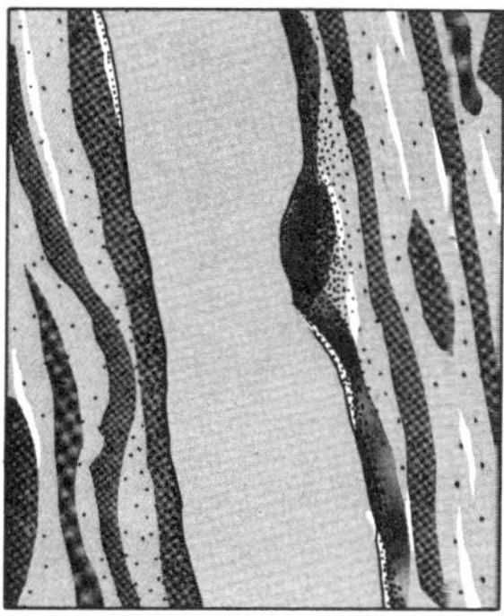

Fig. 4-37. The image on the left lacks gray scale, and diagnostic information is lost. The image on the right shows valuable information of plaque surface characteristics and morphology.

Static B-Mode Image

So far we have discussed how ultrasound systems process and store collective reflections to form a picture. The special arm connected to the system tells the computer where the transducer has moved to give relationship to the picture that is obtained. That image, in turn, is stored and a picture is taken on x-ray film.

What we have seen at this point with A-mode and B-mode is purely a snapshot. The sonographer essentially "sweeps" the transducer across the abdomen one time, and a picture is formed. One repeats that procedure in a different plane to obtain a different perspective of the structure being examined. After a while, the collection of different images helps form an overall pattern of the structure(s) being examined and hopefully allows for an interpretation. Obviously, this is not the most efficient way to ultrasound tissue.

Real Time

Real time is to motion picture as static B-mode is to the snapshot (Fig. 4-38). Most of us have seen the movie picture film close up. It is basically a series of still photographs that are shown in rapid succession to give the visual impression of instantaneous motion.

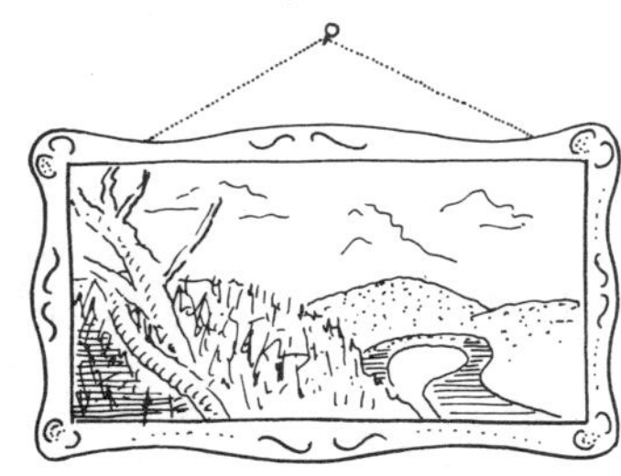

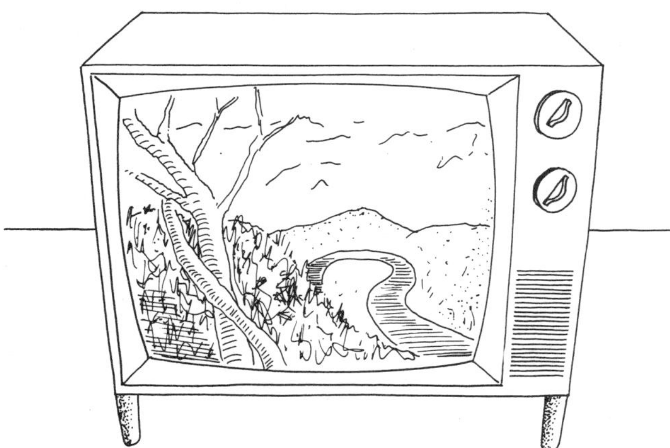

Fig. 4-38. (Top) Static B-mode imaging versus (bottom) real-time B-mode imaging.

Cartoons work the same way. By putting together a series of still pictures and showing them in rapid succession, one gets the image of moving characters. The more images that can be shown in the shorter span of time, the better the sense of quality. Real time allows us to see information as it arrives, unlike static B-scan information which must be retrieved over a period of time and stored for display.

Frame Rate

Due to the integration of computers into ultrasound systems, the rapid process of acquiring, processing, and displaying real-time images is possible. Depending on the type of real-time scanners, anywhere from 5 to 120 *frames per second* (fps) can be produced. Later, when we discuss color flow imaging, we will see the sacrifices in fps that occur when trying to make the ultrasound system perform many functions (image, color, and Doppler). The goal of real-time ultrasound imaging is to obtain a smooth continuous movement of images without the "windshield wiper effect"; that is, the visual perception of images being updated at such a slow pace.

Dynamic Range

Earlier, we described the benefits of gray-scale ultrasound over bi-stable ultrasound. By means of scan conversion, gray scale can display much more information about the tissue we are examining. Instead of seeing just a dot or a blob, we are seeing a whole range of grays—from bright white to almost as black as the background on the CRT.

The significance of this ability to see a large range of grays is that subtle changes of tissue can be detected where they were previously missed. Abnormal and potentially dangerous changes in tissue, such as soft plaque or fresh clot in a vein, can be distinguished from normal anatomy. Good gray scale is perhaps the most important benefit your system can provide in ultrasound imaging.

Dynamic range, the difference between the brightest and weakest received signal, is a measure of the range of signal magnitudes that can be detected by an ultrasound system. The greater the dynamic range, the greater the ability of the system to detect and display different signals. The more different signals one can detect, the easier it is to distinguish between normal and abnormal tissue.

In human tissue, received echos can vary between 100 and 150 dB. That represents a wide dynamic range, depending on the depth and the frequency of the transducer. A wide dynamic range is good, just as your stereo's ability to provide a wide dynamic range of tones is preferable.

However, the wide dynamic range that is detected via the received signal goes through significant degradation in the processing. Because of attenuation, the transmitted signal may drop to 40 dB (Fig. 4-39). Further reduction in the dynamic range occurs when the signal is displayed on the CRT. Finally, video recording of the ultrasound signal may drop the dynamic range to as low as 10 to 20 dB. That is a significant drop from the 150 dB we started out with!

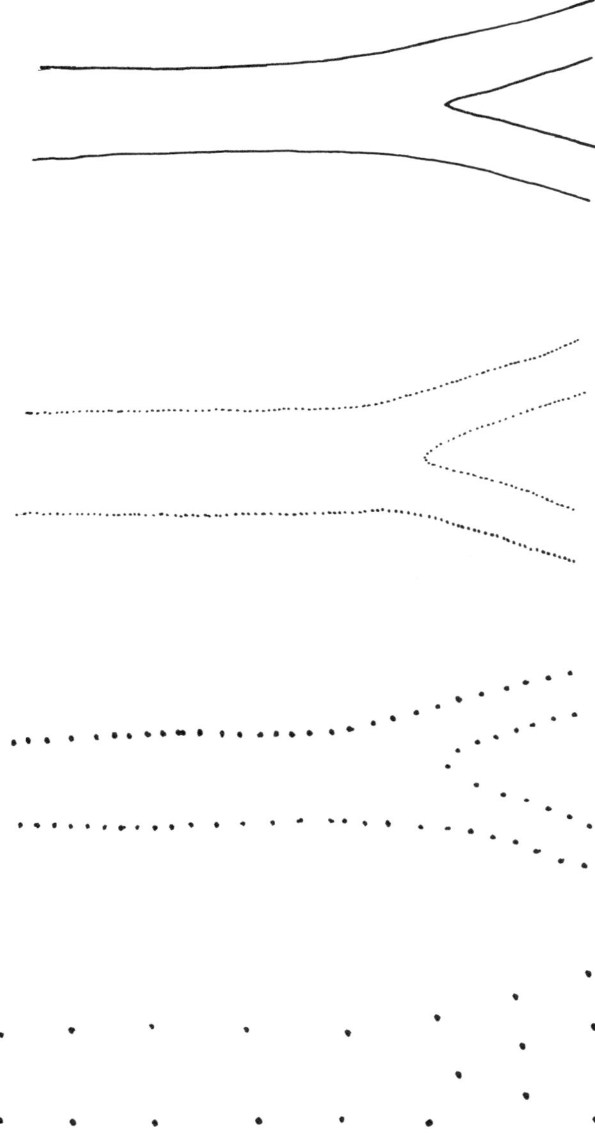

Fig. 4-39. Dynamic range diminishes (from top to bottom) through attenuation, analog-to-digital conversion, and recording devices.

Gain

Gain is the ratio of output power to input power; in other words, how much the input signal is amplified. It is similar to the volume control on your radio. Increasing the volume does not necessarily increase the quality of the music coming out, but it does allow you to hear audio signals that you could not otherwise hear. In ultrasound, the concept is the same, except that gain allows one to "see" sound that has been "turned up" by increasing the gain.

Time-Gain Compensation (TGC)

There exists the natural tendency for signals to attenuate as the ultrasound penetrates deeper into tissue. To compensate for this attenuation, a *time-gain compensation* (TGC) or depth-gain compensation (DGC) is used to adjust for the signals with time or depth. In other words, the farther a signal penetrates the body, and the weaker the signal becomes, the more it needs to be amplified. The purpose of TGC is to provide a signal that is "balanced," and to do so, signals in the far field require amplification. The deeper the signal passes, the greater the need for amplification (Fig. 4-40).

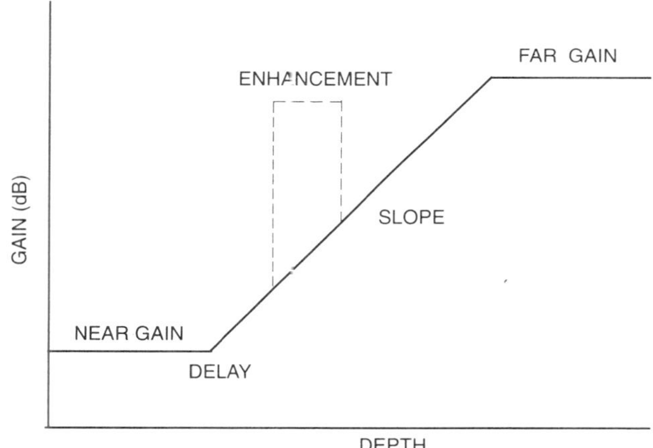

Fig. 4-40. This illustration shows gain being increased at the slope in order to balance the ultrasound image of the near field to the ultrasound image of the far field.

Review Exercise

1. Sound waves that are reflected back to your transducer must be ______________________ in order to be seen.

2. A ______________________ changes ultrasound waves into images that can be seen on a screen.

3. There are two principle types of scan converters:

   a. ____

   b. ____

4. An analog scan converter is very similar to

   a. a digital scan converter **b.** an ultrasound system
   c. a transducer **d.** a CRT

5. An analog scan converter produces very clear images. True or False?

6. One drawback to an analog scan converter is that the image tends to

   a. be pixely **b.** fade
   c. be fuzzy **d.** drift

7. Digital scan converters are solid state computer memories that do not use

   a. vacuum tubes **b.** CRTs
   c. ultrasound waves **d.** analog signals

8. Digital scan converters scan an area, then divide that area into

   a. parameters **b.** pixels
   c. shades of gray **d.** colors

9. A pixel is a small, square picture element. True or False?

10. Pixels are assigned a position on an X-Y axis and are relative to the ______________________ of the signal at that point.

11. In order for a digital scan converter to work, it must convert the ____________ signal into a ____________ signal.

12. An A-to-D converter converts a digital signal to an analog signal. True or False?

13. The term *amplitude* refers to the ____________ of the reflected signal.

14. A-mode is most often used in

    a. cardiac
    b. ophthalmic
    c. encephalography
    d. b and c

15. B-mode ultrasound refers to the "______________ mode".

16. The brightness of the dot corresponds to the ______________________________ of the signal.

17. ______________ B-mode scanning allows the sonographer to "look" at structures in several different directions.

18. A-mode refers to the "______________ mode."

19. M-mode refers to "______________ mode" or time-motion mode.

20. B-mode images are acquired by displaying the ______________ "tip" as a dot.

21. The higher the A-mode amplitude, the brighter the ______________ dot.

22. If the amplitude of the B-mode image is strong enough, it is ______________.

23. The "on or off" condition of early B-mode images gives rise to so-called ______________ images.

24. Bi-stable images display excellent gray scale. True or False?

25. The ability to see ultrasound images constantly updated is called ______________.

26. The ______________________________ provides images of various levels of black and white that relate to the tissue being examined.

27. Real time is to motion picture as static B-mode is to the ______________.

28. Real time allows us to see information as it actually happens. True or False?

29. Due to the integration of ______________ into ultrasound systems, the rapid process of acquiring, processing, and displaying real-time images is possible.

30. Depending on the type of real-time scanners, anywhere from ______________ to ______________ frames per second (fps) can be produced.

31. Dynamic range is a measure of the ____ that can be detected by an ultrasound system.

32. The greater the dynamic range, the greater the ability of the system to detect and display

    a. bright signals
    b. low level signals
    c. deep signals
    d. different signals

33. The more different signals one can detect, the easier it is to distinguish between normal and ______________ tissue.

34. In human tissue, received echos can vary between

    a. 5 and 10 dB
    b. 10 and 50 dB
    c. 50 and 100 dB
    d. 100 and 150 dB

35. A wide dynamic range is not always good. True or False?

36. The wide dynamic range that is detected via the received signal goes through significant ______________________ in the signal processing.

37. Through various attempts at "improving" the signal, such as time-gain compensation and amplification, dynamic range may

    a. improve to 20 dB
    b. improve to 40 dB
    c. drop to 40 dB
    d. not be likely to change at all

38. Reduction in the dynamic range occurs when the signal is displayed on the CRT. True or False?

39. Conventional VCR recording does not affect dynamic range. True or False?

40. Gain is the ratio of ______________power to ______________ power.

41. Gain is similar to the ______________________ on your radio.

42. There exists the natural tendency for signals to ______________________ as the ultrasound penetrates deeper into tissue.

43. To compensate for attenuation, a time-gain compensation (TGC) or depth-gain compensation (DGC) is used to adjust for the signals with

    a. time
    b. frequency strength
    c. depth
    d. time or depth

44. The purpose of TGC is to provide a signal that is "balanced," and to do so, signals in the far field require

    a. gain
    b. lower frequencies
    c. amplification
    d. all of the above

TRANSDUCER AND SYSTEM TECHNOLOGY

Now that we have developed an understanding of how different ultrasound waves are acquired and displayed, we can start to look at some of the specifics of the ultrasound system and transducer technology. In this session, we will learn about what makes a good image and how different transducers benefit various applications.

Key Terms

Axial resolution
Backing material
Dipole
Far field
Focusing
Lambda
Lateral resolution
Linear array transducer
Matching material
Mechanical sector transducer
Mirror transducer
Near field
Near-field boundary
Phased array
Piezoelectric effect
Pressure-electric effect
Resolution
Rotating mechanical transducer
Sector scanning

Mechanical Transducers

The first ultrasound scanners consisted of a transducer that, when physically dragged across the skin, provided a single bi-stable image of the tissue below the surface. Relative to equipment these days, this procedure was time consuming and primitive.

In the early '70s, equipment manufacturers constructed imaging transducers connected to a small electric motor within the probe housing that would mechanically "sweep" the transducer back and forth at a very fast rate and update the image at each sweep. The imaging crystals are contained in a watertight compartment filled with a fluid. The ultrasound waves are transmitted through this liquid and membrane onto the skin surface and into the tissue beyond and back again. The pictures are then displayed and updated with each sweep in order to provide an image in real time. *Focusing*, which will be discussed later in this section, is accomplished by using acoustic lenses.

One of the important characteristics of the imaging field of mechanical sector scanners is that the field of view is much narrower in the *near field* (that field closest to the transducer) as opposed to the *far field* (that field farthest from the transducer). This divergence, or spreading out, of the ultrasound beam means that the image line density is much higher closer to the transducer and gradually becomes less at larger depths. Subsequently, the clarity, or *resolution*, becomes worse in deep tissue.

The value of real time versus the older B-scan is the constant image update, occurring every 5 to 120 times per second. This difference is analogous to seeing a snapshot versus a motion picture; with real time, one can appreciate movements within the body that were previously unavailable.

The three primary types of mechanical scanners are

1. mechanical sector
2. rotating head
3. mirror

Mechanical Sector

The *mechanical sector transducer* is still very popular and used widely in vascular and general ultrasound examinations. The transducer mechanically sweeps back and forth in a pie-shaped arc, thus providing its name "sector scanner" (section of a circle like a piece of the pie).

Although mechanical sector transducers are still respected for their image quality and value, they are prone to the problem of any device that has rapidly moving parts: they break down. Imagine the small transducer sweeping rapidly from one side to the other, constantly changing direction (Fig. 4-41), and this happening as many as 3,000 times a minute! In addition, the movement of the crystal interferes with the reception of imaging and Doppler signals, especially if one is performing color Doppler.

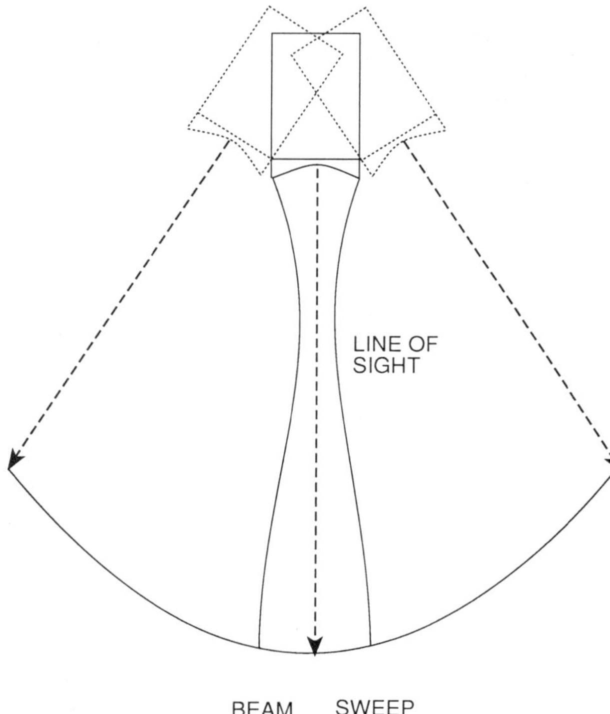

Fig. 4-41. The mechanical sector transducer.

Rotating Mechanical Transducer

The rotating scanner uses several transducers attached to a rotating axis (Fig. 4-42). As the active transducer faces the scan plane, it takes an image. These images are updated as fast as the system can rotate the axis and display the images. This rotation somewhat reduces the problems associated with the crystal's sweeping back and forth.

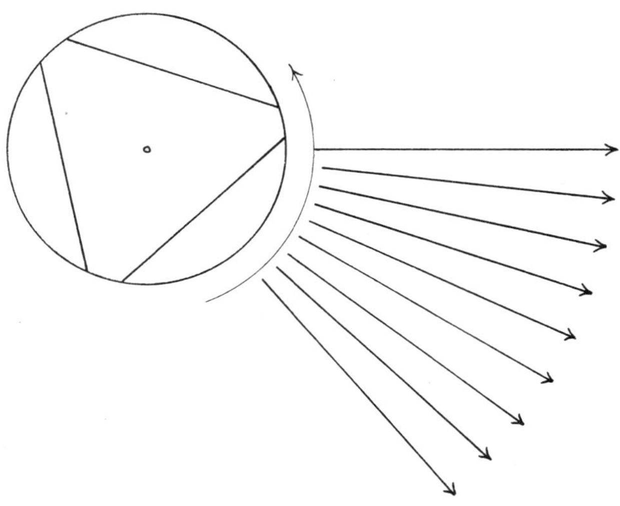

Fig. 4-42. The rotating mechanical transducer.

Mirror Mechanical Transducer

The mirror scanner uses a reflecting device that "flips" a reflected ultrasound beam back and forth (Fig. 4-43). In this fashion, the mirror makes all the movement instead of the imaging crystal. Both the rotating- and mirror-type transducers are not often used for vascular ultrasound, however. Mechanical movements cause interference of transmitted and received Doppler ultrasound signals, which is disadvantageous to the vascular examination.

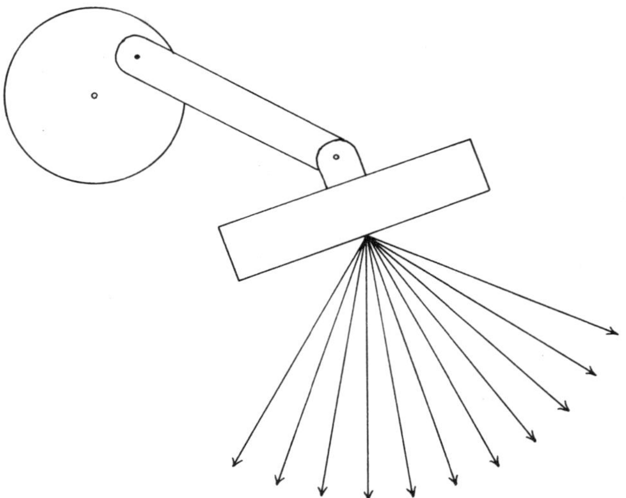

Fig. 4-43. The mirror mechanical transducer.

Electronic Transducers

Electronic transducers are subclassified into linear array and phased array.

Linear Array System

A *linear array* system has a sequential row of crystals, each of which acts individually to first produce and then receive echoes. For example, 130 crystals may be lined up in a row to produce different "lines of sight."

Linear array is a single slab of *piezoelectric material* cut into a collection of separate pieces called *elements*. Each element is connected to its own electronic circuitry. Elements are fired in groups along the transducer (Fig. 4-44). In a system with 64 individual crystals, a microprocessor coordinates the firing sequence of the transducer. For example, crystals 1–4 will fire and then wait about 200 milliseconds. Then crystals 2–5 will fire and wait for the same period. Then crystals 3–6, and so on down the line until the process reaches the end and the sequence repeats.

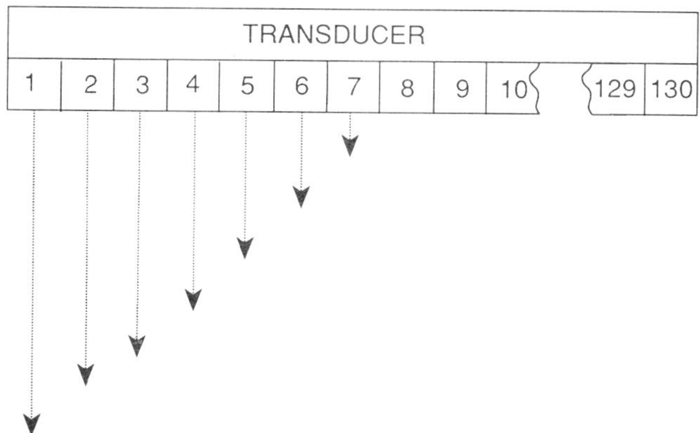

Fig. 4-44. The linear array transducer fires crystals in groups. For example, first elements 1–4 transmit and then receive, then elements 2–5 transmit and then receive, then elements 3–6 transmit and then receive. These elements continue to fire sequentially in "groups" at a rapid rate along the transducer.

It is not uncommon to have as many as 256 elements in a transducer and produce large fields of view. By controlling the aperture of the transducer, the beam width can be made narrower or larger. A narrow beam width results in good *lateral resolution* (ability to distinguish two separate objects side by side). However, it also results in a short *near field* and a rapidly diverging *far field* (discussed later). A larger aperture improves the far field, but produces poor lateral resolution.

Phased Array

Phased array transducers fire all the crystals at nearly the same time. Phased array transducers produce only one line of sight over the entire array each time the crystal is pulsed. By using delays in the crystals, the imager can be "steered" to create a sector image (Fig. 4-45).

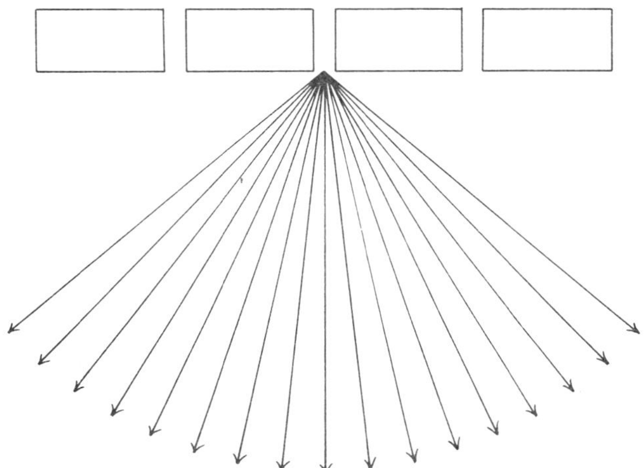

Fig. 4-45. The phased array transducer.

Annular Array

The annular array transducers represent a mix of both the mechanical and phased array scanners. In the annular array transducer, the elements are constructed in concentric rings, one inside the other. This allows for symmetry of focusing by controlling the excitation phase of each ring. The rings must be "wobbled" like the mechanical sector scanner in order to produce an image, however. Annular array transducers are still highly respected for image quality, particularly in cardiac ultrasound. In addition, the "footprint," or size, of the transducer head is small, enabling the user to scan in difficult areas, such as between the ribs.

Transducer Construction

The construction of the transducer consists of a single or series of piezoelectric crystals connected by a positive and negative charge (Fig. 4-46). In back of the crystal is *backing material*, which buffers the ultrasound signal in order to keep the "ringing" as brief as possible. Finally, the transducer is housed in an insulated material with a facing, or matching, material to reduce the difference between the acoustic impedance of the transducer and the tissue being scanned. The importance of this feature is that it will reduce the reverberation artifact (discussed previously).

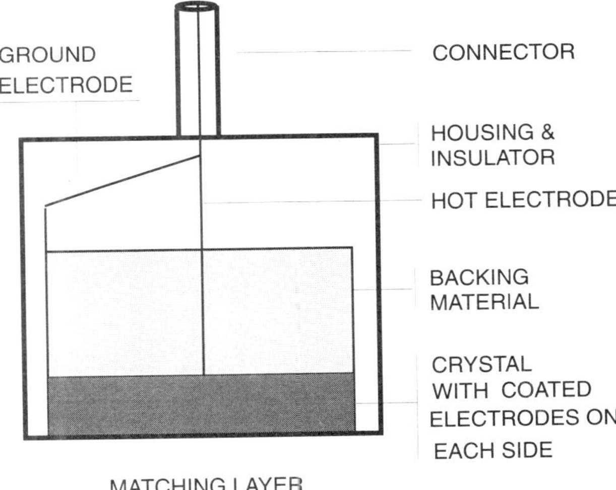

Fig. 4-46. Ultrasound transducer construction.

Piezoelectric Effect

A transducer is a device that transforms one form of energy into another. An ultrasound transducer converts electrical energy into mechanical energy (Fig. 4-47) and then back to electrical energy. This process is obtained due to the specific properties of the piezoelectric (sounds like "piece of electric") material.

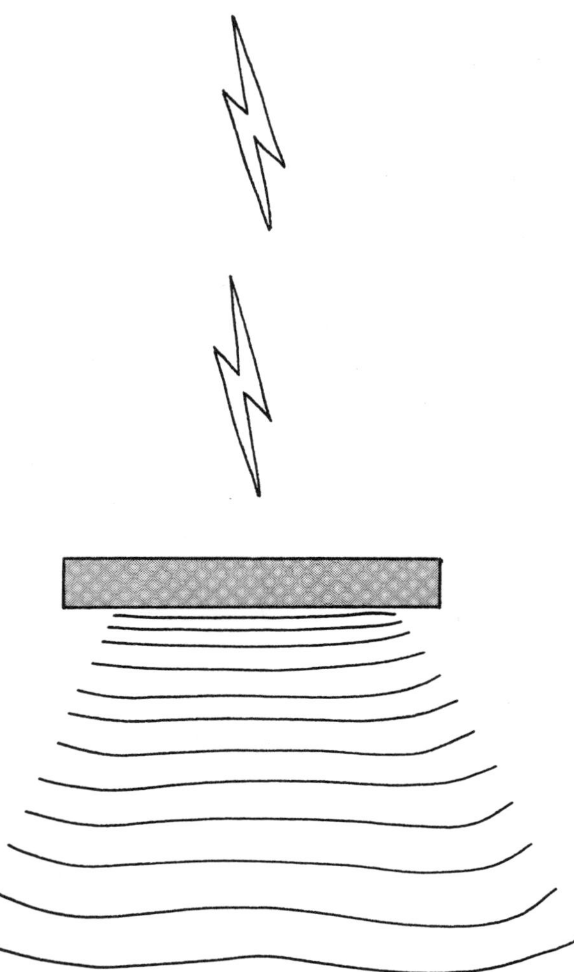

Fig. 4-47. The piezoelectric crystal converts electrical energy into mechanical energy to transmit an ultrasound signal. It then converts received mechanical energy into electrical energy to form a picture.

The piezoelectric effect is also known as the *pressure-electric effect*, in that we are transferring the electric energy to pressure energy in order to manufacture ultrasound waves. When a rhythmic pattern of electricity is applied to the piezoelectric material, it responds by producing rhythmic vibrations, therefore providing rhythmic ultrasound waves.

Piezoelectric Properties

The piezoelectric device is constructed of crystalline (crystal-like) material that is made of *dipoles* on each molecule. Dipoles are molecules that are electrically positive on one end and negative on the other (Fig. 4-48).

In normal crystalline material, dipole molecules are arranged randomly and do not normally move around. When the material is *heated up to a certain temperature*, however, the molecules can move freely. When a positive and negative charge is placed on either end of this material, it causes the dipole molecules to line up: the negative end of the dipole molecule toward the positive charge and the positive end of the dipole molecule toward the negative charge. (Keep in mind that like charges repel and opposite charges attract.) Then the material is cooled again so that the dipole molecules maintain their alignment in the crystal.

Now you have piezoelectric material. By placing conducting plates on either side of the material and on the top and bottom of the material, one can control the direction of the dipole molecules and, subsequently, the thickness of the material. By placing a charge on the walls of the material, the molecules line up in that direction, causing the crystal to contract. By reversing the charge to the surfaces of the crystal, the molecules flip in that direction and, because they are longer, the material expands (Fig. 4-49).

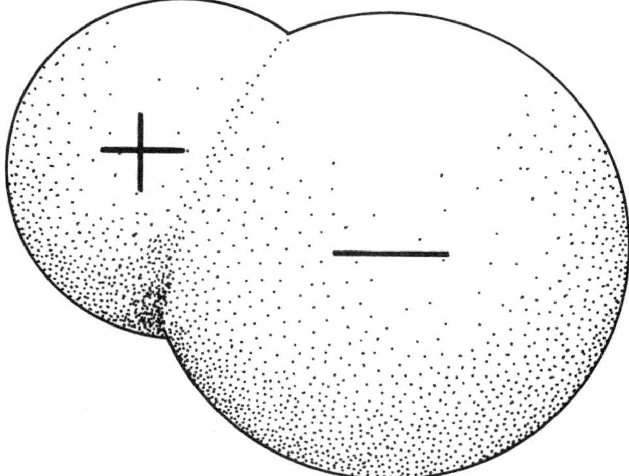

Fig. 4-48. Dipole molecule of crystalline material.

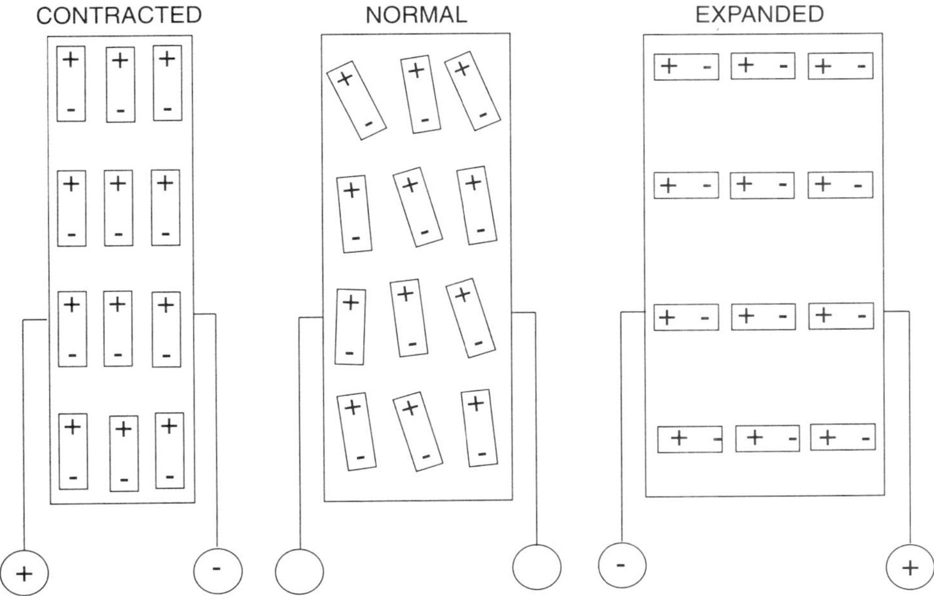

Fig. 4-49. Changing the shape of the piezoelectric crystal by reversing the electrical charge of the material.

Piezoelectric material can not only send ultrasound waves but also receive them. The piezoelectric material can "listen" for signals being bounced off interfaces in the body. Those returning sound waves are similar to the effect that sound has on the human ear. The pressure from the sound moves the eardrum, which, in turn, sends a signal through a series of small bones to the auditory receptors. That signal is then transmitted to the brain where it becomes interpreted as tone and volume.

In ultrasound, the returning signals strike the crystal, causing it to expand and contract. That change in shape produces an electrical signal. This electric signal is then converted and displayed as an image or Doppler signal on your monitor.

Ringing

When you strike a bell with a hammer, the bell doesn't just send off one contraction and one expansion for each blow of the hammer. The bell itself may vibrate at the note C, for example, which is 256 vibrations per second. But that doesn't mean you have to hit the bell 256 times per second. Rather, the bell vibrates, or "rings," at its own resonance frequency for a while.

Piezoelectric crystals also ring on their own for a while, too. The crystal has a natural vibration frequency as sound bounces back and forth between the two surfaces of the material. Now, we are not talking about a whole lot of room between surfaces. In order for a sound wave to move back and forth within the crystal, the material must be the size of at least one half of the wavelength. That's pretty thin! Therefore, the higher the frequency, the shorter the wavelength, the thinner the piezoelectric material.

Backing Material

In some cases, specifically for therapeutic ultrasound, we want the crystal to ring continuously in order to obtain maximum output of energy in the form of heat. For diagnostic ultrasound, however, we usually want just a short burst of ultrasound. This has the benefits (discussed shortly) of shortening the pulse length and therefore increasing axial resolution.

To ensure a crystal doesn't keep on ringing (due to its own resonant qualities), damping material is placed on the back of the transducer, away from the direction we want ultrasound to travel. This is a highly energy-absorbing substance that functions like the shocks on an automobile. The result of this damping is a very short burst of ultrasound transmission.

Resolution

When looking at an ultrasound system, you may have heard people viewing the monitor say, "Nice resolution!" or "I don't think the resolution is good in the far field!" But, what does resolution mean beyond just a pretty picture?

To resolve is to break something up into separate parts in order to analyze it. *Resolution*, then, is the act of resolving. Put in ultrasound terms, resolution is the ability to identify separate parts in an image in order to obtain information regarding its various properties; the more information you have, the better chance you have of analyzing the separate parts.

Image resolution is the ability to resolve or distinguish between two closely located echo-producing tissue reflectors. A high-resolution system means that it can identify two reflectors that are close together. In B-mode imaging, we are concerned with two-dimensional imaging:

1. Axial resolution
2. Lateral resolution

In addition to axial and lateral resolution, line density affects image quality. Each line in the image represents a transmission pulse and the reception of echoes from reflectors located along the line of sight. The closer together the image lines, the finer the detail and spacial resolution (Fig. 4-50).

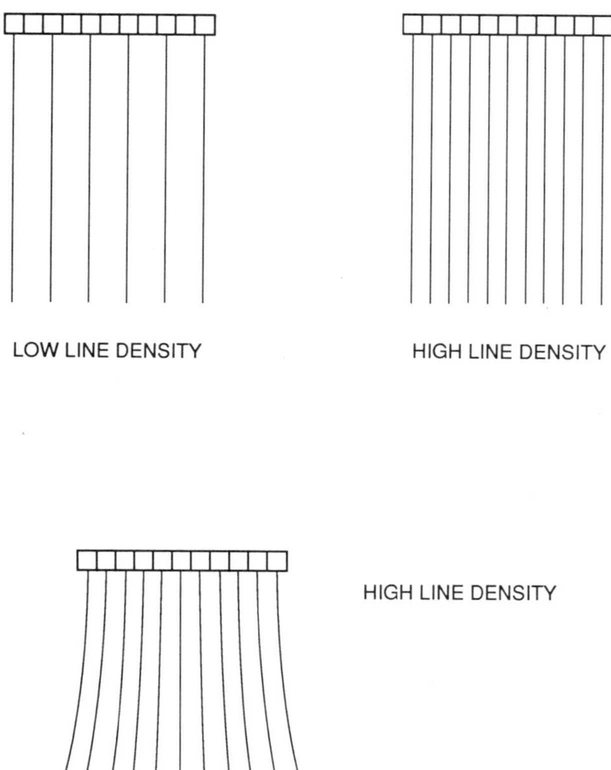

Fig. 4-50. The tighter the line density, the better the image resolution. Note that as ultrasound lines of sight move away from the transducer, they diverge or spread apart.

The transducer must wait for the echoes to be received from the farthest depth in the image, however, before the next transmission pulse. Therefore, the repetition of the pulse depends on the depth of the image field of view and the propagation velocity of the tissue. In sum, the deeper the image field, the lower the pulse repetition.

The resolution of an ultrasound transducer is directly related to the wavelength (*lambda*) and the beam width it produces. The shorter the wavelength, the better the axial resolution. The narrower the beam width, the better the lateral resolution. So, how can we determine the expected resolution of a transducer, given the information we have learned so far?

Axial Resolution

As previously mentioned, a piezoelectric crystal is first excited by an electrical impulse and then damped almost immediately after. The purpose of the damping is to send out the shortest ultrasound cycle possible. In fact, the ideal situation would be to stimulate the piezoelectric crystal to produce one cycle only.

Axial resolution is the ability to distinguish two reflectors close together along the same line of sight. In order to achieve high axial resolution, the time the transducer is allowed to ring, or the pulse duration, must be short. The value of the short pulse lengths is in the ultrasound beam's ability to distinguish different reflectors as it travels into the depths of a tissue (Fig. 4-51).

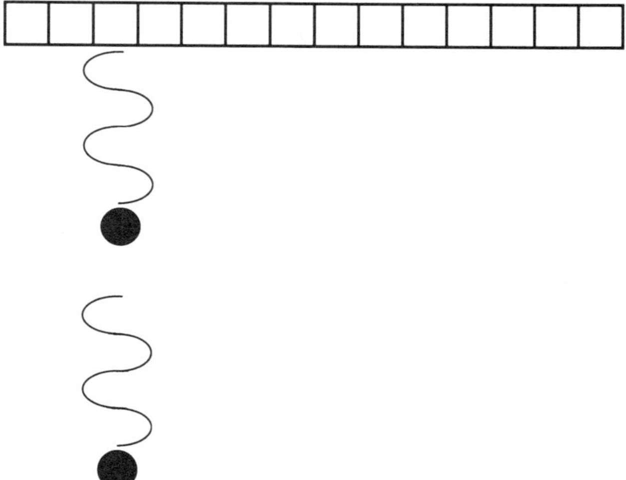

Fig. 4-51. Short pulse lengths provide the ability to "see" two separate reflectors on an axial plane individually. This results in improved resolution.

If a pulse length is too long, it will have difficulty distinguishing between two different objects that are very close to each other, and two objects would tend to be seen as one. In other words, the axial resolution would be poor (Fig. 4-52).

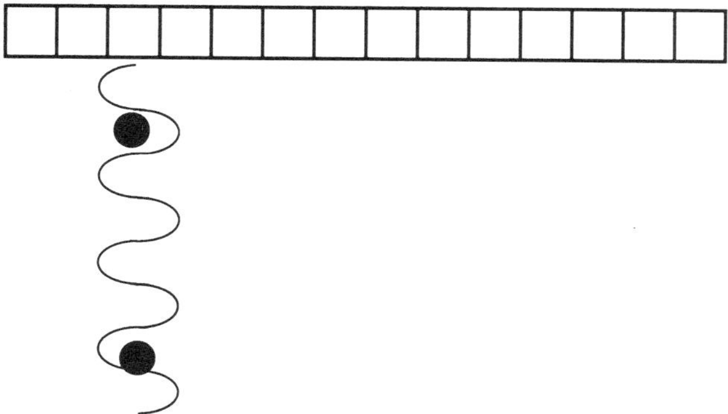

Fig. 4-52. Long pulse lengths will "see" two separate reflectors as one. This results as one blurry dot instead of two sharp separate dots, or poor axial resolution.

Lateral Resolution

Lateral resolution is the ability to distinguish between two reflectors closely spaced along a direction perpendicular to the line of sight (Fig. 4-53). The lateral resolution is determined by the width of the beam, or the beam width, at the depth of the reflectors. If the two-point reflectors are so close that the separation between them is smaller than the beam width at that depth, their respective images will overlap and they will be seen as one reflector (Fig. 4-54).

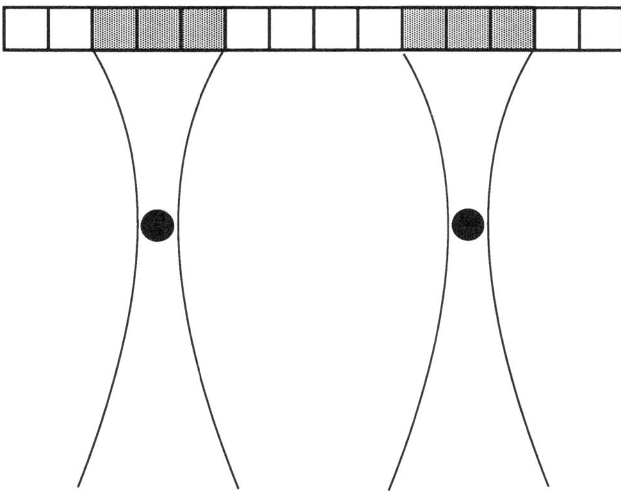

Fig. 4-53. A narrow beam width will see two reflectors lateral to each other individually. This results in good lateral resolution.

In general, lateral resolution is worse than axial resolution. That is, the smallest distance the ultrasound system can identify is two to three times greater in lateral resolution than in axial resolution. Therefore, lateral resolution is a big concern in ultrasound imaging.

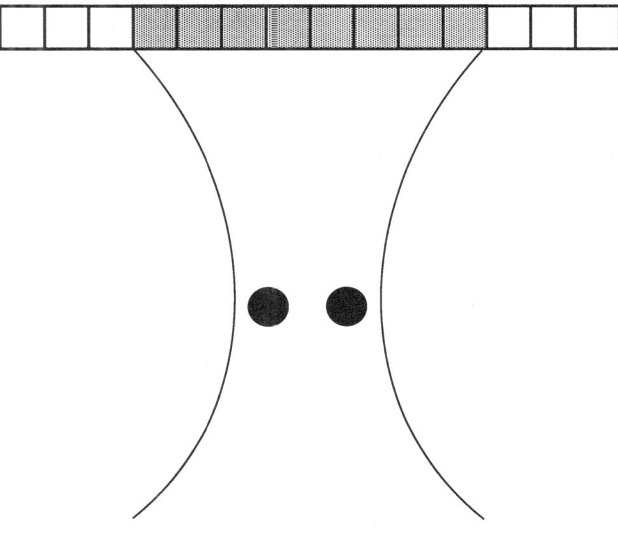

Fig. 4-54. A wide beam width will see two reflectors as one. This results as one blurry dot instead of two sharp separate dots, or poor lateral resolution.

Near Field/Far Field

Ultrasound waves leaving a transducer move in a field relatively close to that of the transducer; there is very little divergence in the beam at this point. As we begin to move a little farther from the field, however, the width of the field begins to change a little; the waves begin to diverge at a steady rate. The portion of the beam where the ultrasound waves stay in a close field is called the *near field.* The zone before the point where the ultrasound beam begins to diverge is called the *focal zone*. Finally, beyond the *near-field boundary* is the *far field* (Fig. 4-55).

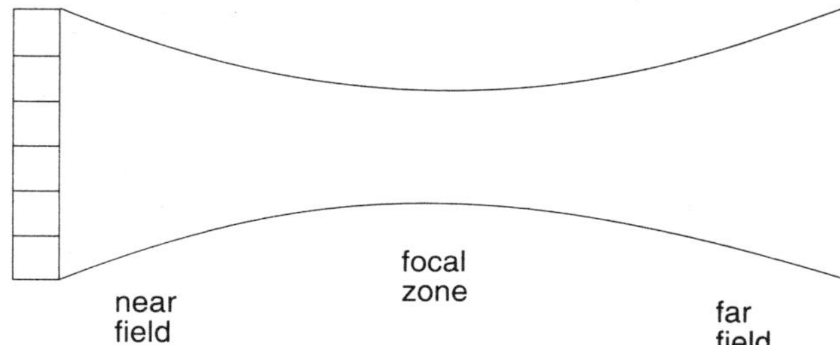

Fig. 4-55. Ultrasound beam narrows in the near field to the focal zone and then diverges in the far field. The image is generally clearest in the focal zone.

The near field is also called the *Fresnel zone*, and the far field is called the *Fraunhofer zone*. Both Fresnel and Fraunhofer were nineteenth-century mathematicians and physicists who first described these various zones in relation to light diffraction.

More on Beam Width

One might think that by having a very small front-face dimension, or aperture, of a transducer, a very narrow beam width would be produced. Well, this is true to an extent. In fact, the beam width actually starts getting narrower as it leaves the transducer. The problem is that it starts spreading out, or diverging, rapidly after that. So, although we may have a narrow beam width close to the transducer or the near field, the beam width gets very wide shortly thereafter in the far field (Fig. 4-56). The result is good lateral resolution close to the transducer and poor lateral resolution as the diverging beam moves away from the transducer.

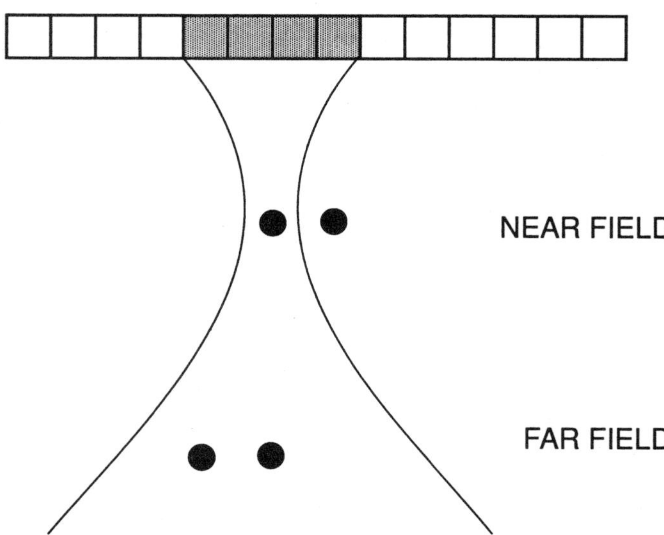

Fig. 4-56. Good near-field resolution but poor far-field resolution.

What if we develop a transducer with a large face-front dimension or large aperture? In this case, the beam will begin to narrow farther away from the transducer or in the far field (Fig. 4-57). Therefore, lateral resolution will be quite good in a zone farther away from the transducer. The problem here lies in the poor lateral resolution close to the transducer or the near field.

So how do we design a transducer that can provide good lateral resolution in both the near and far fields? One solution is ultrasound *focusing*.

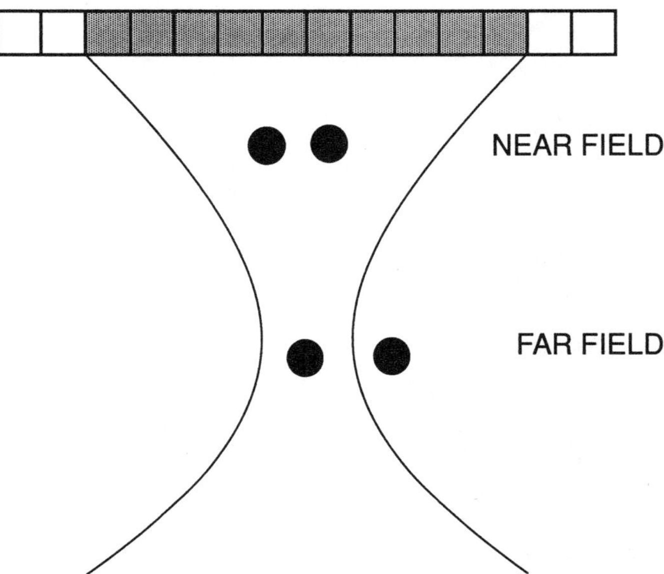

Fig. 4-57. Good far-field resolution but poor near-field resolution.

Focusing

One of the most important objectives of an ultrasound transducer is to direct ultrasound waves in one direction. We want ultrasound waves to be transmitted in the way light is emitted from a flashlight, not a light bulb. In order to obtain this, a number of focusing techniques must be used. As ultrasound waves are initially generated, they are emitted in all directions. By focusing the ultrasound beam, however, we can concentrate the ultrasound beam into a narrow column.

Do you remember when, as a child, you would play with a magnifying glass in the sun? If you held the glass just right, you could focus the rays of sun into a point of light. By doing so, you could make a concentration of heat so strong, that you would be able to burn a hole through a leaf or even light it on fire!

Camera lenses work in somewhat the same way. By focusing the lens, you are able to get a clear picture of the subject you are photographing, although by doing so you make the background more blurry. Ultrasound carries the same properties as any mechanical wave, including light waves, and, as with the camera, ultrasound uses focusing in order to concentrate on a specific area of interest. The uneven bend of an ultrasound lens causes the waves to advance toward a common point. In this way, the intensity of a sound beam can be increased without increasing the power.

The transducer itself can be curved in order to bend the waves into a concentric point, or the unfocused transducer can reflect waves off of a mirror, which is bent in order to focus the ultrasound beam. There are so many nonmechanical means of focusing ultrasound waves; linear array transducers focus waves by forming a curved wave front electronically. In sum, focusing is either externally focused (mirrors or lenses) or internally focused.

Unlike the magnifying glass, the ultrasound transducer will not focus a beam into a tight dot. Rather, the beam forms a narrow beam region. As mentioned earlier, this is referred to as the focal zone. After this region of narrowness, the beam begins to diverge again, becoming wider and wider. It is in the region where the beam is the most narrow that we have the best lateral resolution.

The ideal ultrasound system would provide us with an absolutely clear image with great axial and lateral resolution at all depths. As yet, that ideal system does not exist. The ultrasound scientists, engineers, and vascular specialists, however, are striving to reach this goal.

Review Exercise

1. The three primary types of mechanical scanners are

   a. ______________________________

   b. ______________________________

   c. ______________________________

2. With the introduction of linear array transducers, the mechanical sector is no longer a practical transducer. True or False?

3. Mechanical sector transducers are still respected for their

   a. dependability
   b. color imaging
   c. resolution and value
   d. duplex

4. One drawback that mechanical transducers are prone to is that they ______________________.

5. The rotating scanner uses several transducers attached to a ______________________.

6. The ______________________ uses a reflecting device that "flips" a reflected ultrasound beam back and forth.

7. Mechanical sector transducers

   a. are expensive
   b. cannot be used for duplex
   c. cannot focus
   d. cannot be electronically steered

8. Name that transducer!

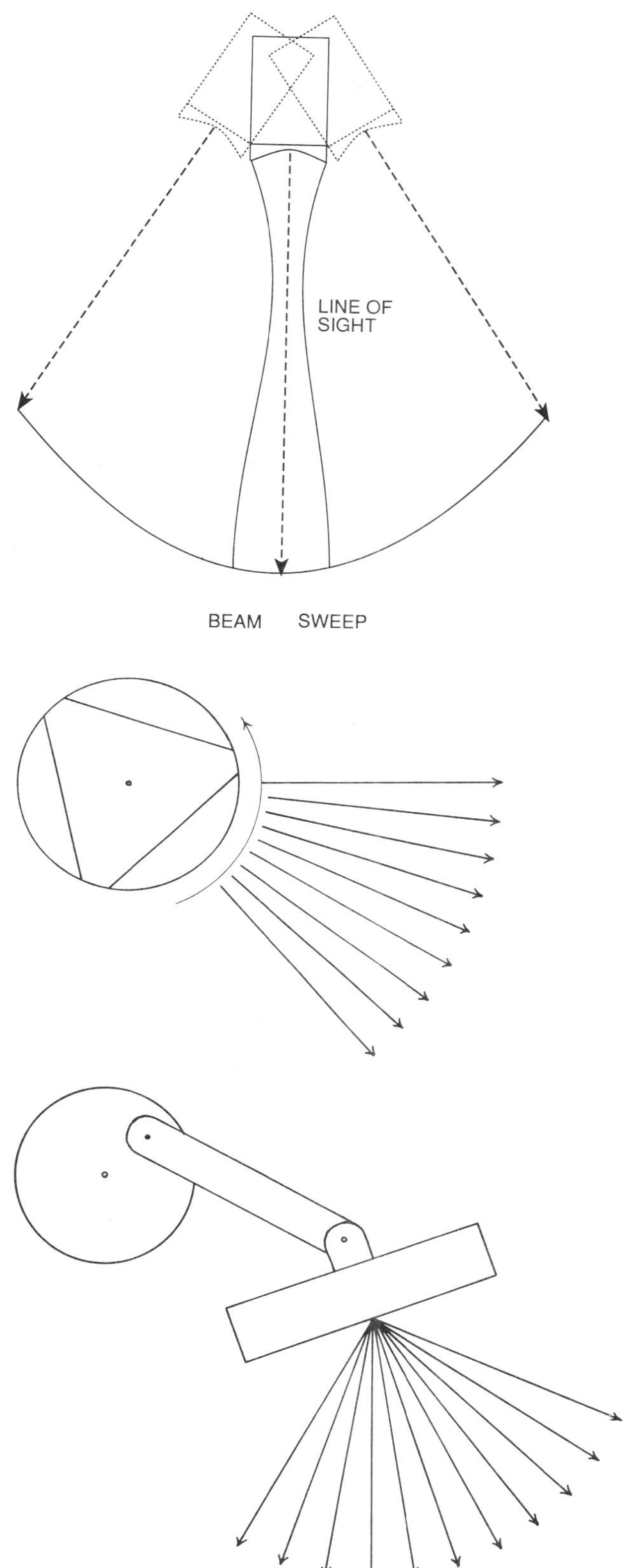

9. Electronic transducers are subclassified into

   a. ______________________________

   b. ______________________________

10. A linear array system has a sequential row of crystals, each of which acts individually to first ______________ and then ______________ returning echoes.

11. Each crystal of a linear array transducer is activated sequentially, producing (at shallow depths) images at up to ______________ frames per second.

12. The multiple small crystals used in linear array ultrasound systems produce a ______________ beam.

13. Linear array transducers can produce good ______________ resolution.

14. Larger crystals improve the (near/far) field, but produce poor (medial/lateral) resolution.

15. Smaller crystals improve the (near/far) field, but produce poor (medial/lateral) resolution.

16. Linear array transducers fire crystals

    a. nearly all at the same time
    b. one at a time
    c. every other one
    d. in groups

17. Phased array systems fire all the crystals

    a. at nearly the same time
    b. every other one
    c. one at a time
    d. in a group

18. By using ______________ in the crystals, the linear array image can be steered in one direction or another.

19. In vascular imaging, ______________________________ allows the operator to "aim" the ultrasound waves in order to strike an interface at 90 degrees.

20. The construction of the transducer consists of a single or series of ______________________________ connected by a positive and negative charge.

21. In back of the crystal is ____, which damps the ultrasound signal in order to keep the "ringing" as brief as possible.

22. The transducer is housed in an insulated material with a ____ to reduce the difference between the acoustic impedance of the transducer and the tissue being scanned.

23. The importance of backing material is to

a. increase ringing
b. decrease ringing
c. increase reverberation
d. decrease reverberation

24. An ultrasound transducer converts __________________________ energy into __________________________ energy.

25. When a rhythmic pattern of __________________________ is applied to the piezoelectric material, it responds by producing vibrations.

26. The piezoelectric device is constructed of __________________________ that is made of dipoles on each molecule.

27. Dipoles are molecules that are electrically ____________ at one end and ____________ at the other.

28. When a positive and negative charge is placed on either end of crystalline material, it causes the dipole molecules to

a. line up
b. expand
c. contract
d. oscillate

29. The negative end of the dipole molecule moves toward the ____________ end, and the positive end of the dipole molecule moves toward the ____________ end.

30. By placing a charge on the walls of the material, the molecules line up in that direction, causing the crystal to ____________.

31. By reversing the charge to the surfaces of the crystal, the molecules flip in that direction and, because they are longer, the material will

a. expand
b. contract
c. vibrate
d. oscillate

32. Piezoelectric material can not only ____________ ultrasound waves but also ____________ them.

33. In ultrasound, the returning signals strike the crystal, causing it to

a. expand
b. contract
c. both expand and contract
d. heat up

34. Changing the piezoelectric shape produces

a. heat
b. ultrasound
c. an electrical signal
d. either c or b

35. For improved axial resolution, we usually want a ______________ burst of ultrasound.

36. Short "bursts" equal a short

a. wavelength
b. cycle
c. frequency
d. PRF

37. The result of damping is a very short burst of ultrasound transmission, which is beneficial for

a. all resolution
b. lateral resolution
c. axial resolution
d. penetration

38. A narrow beam width provides better ____.

39. The more information you have in an ultrasound image, the better ability you have in analyzing the separate parts. True or False?

40. The resolution of an ultrasound system is directly related to the ______________________________ it produces.

41. The ______________ the wavelength, the better the axial resolution.

42. As ultrasound leaves the transducer, it diverges as it moves away from the scan head. True or False?

43. Divergence only affects the ultrasound waves as they move away from the reflector. True or False?

44. Ultrasound beams can be ______________ to control a narrow beam to limit the effects of divergence.

45. The purpose of the damping is to send out the ______________ ultrasound wavelength possible.

46. The value of the short wavelength is in its ability to

a. not travel far
b. increase propagation speed
c. penetrate deeper
d. improve axial resolution

47. For the best *axial* and *lateral* resolution, your transducer should provide

a. ______________________________

b. ______________________________

48. With long pulse lengths, the ______________resolution is poor.

49. If the damping is constant, the pulse length is ______________.

50. The ability to distinguish two distinct objects in the same axis as the beam is called

a. penetration
b. axial resolution
c. lateral resolution
d. sensitivity

51. Axial resolution is determined by the

a. dampening material
b. piezoelectric material
c. beam width
d. pulse length

52. The ______________ the beam width, the better the lateral resolution.

53. One of the most important objectives of an ultrasound transducer is to direct ultrasound waves

a. as quickly as possible
b. as far as possible
c. in as many different directions as possible
d. in one direction

54. In order to assist ultrasound waves in traveling in one direction only, a number of ______________ techniques must be used.

a. firing
b. guiding
c. steering
d. focusing

55. If the diameter of the transducer is wide, it has difficulty in distinguishing two reflectors

a. one on top of the other
b. side by side
c. of the same tissue
d. of different tissue

56. A trade-off of a narrow beam width is

a. reverberation
b. poor axial resolution
c. poor lateral resolution
d. rapidly diverging far field

57. Ultrasound waves leaving a transducer move in a field relatively close to that of the transducer; there is very little ____________________________ in the beam at this point.

58. The portion of the beam where the ultrasound waves stay in a close field is called the ______________________________.

59. The point at which the near field *begins* to diverge is called the

a. near field
b. far field
c. focal zone
d. near-field boundary

60. Beyond the near-field boundary is the

a. near field
b. far field
c. focal zone
d. near-field boundary

61. The near field is also called the ______________________________ zone, and the far field is called the ______________________________ zone.

62. Ultrasound uses ______________ in order to concentrate on a specific area of interest.

63. The uneven bend of an ultrasound lens causes the waves to advance toward

a. specular reflectors
b. near-field boundary
c. the far field
d. a specific area of interest

64. The transducer itself can be curved in order to bend the waves into a concentric point. True or False?

65. Linear array transducers focus waves by forming a curved wavefront

a. mechanically
b. electronically
c. a or b
d. neither a nor b

5

Electronics and Doppler Physics

BASIC ELECTRONICS

So much of what we do in vascular technology requires the use and understanding of electrical instruments. To better comprehend how these instruments work, it is important to learn the fundamentals and physical principles of electronics. So let's begin with the basics, including the metric system (Table 5-1).

Key Terms

Ampere
Atoms
Charge
Compound
Conductor
Current
Electrons
Energy
Ions
Kinetic energy
Load
Megawatts
Microamperes
Milliamperes
Milliwatts
Negatively charged ions
Nucleus
Ohm's law
Positively charged ions
Potential energy
Power
Protons
Resistance
Resting energy
Static electricity
Voltage
Watts

Table 5-1. The Metric System

Powers of 10	*Prefix*	*Symbol*	*Meaning*
10^9	Giga	G	Billion
10^6	Mega	M	Million
10^3	Kilo	k	Thousand
10^2	Hecto	H	Hundred
10^1	Deci	d	Ten
10^{-1}	Deca	da	Tenth
10^{-2}	Centi	c	Hundredth
10^{-3}	Milli	m	Thousandth
10^{-6}	Micro	μ	Millionth
10^{-9}	Nano	n	Billionth

Atoms and Electrons

As you may recall from basic studies, *atoms* are the building blocks of life. All matter, whether it is solid, liquid, or gas, is made up of atoms. Atoms of the same kind, formed together, produce elements. There are 104 basic elements, including oxygen, hydrogen, sodium, and carbon. When two or more different elements are combined, a *compound* is formed. A familiar compound is water (H_2O)—a combination of two elements containing two parts hydrogen to one part oxygen.

If you were to look at an atom under a sufficiently powerful microscope, you would notice that the atom is made up of further components: neutrons, protons, and electrons. The core of the atom, the *nucleus*, is composed of tightly packed protons and neutrons. The *protons* are positively charged; neutrons have no charge (discussed later) and are neutral electrically. Rotating around the nucleus, like planets around the sun, are the negatively charged electrons (Fig. 5-1).

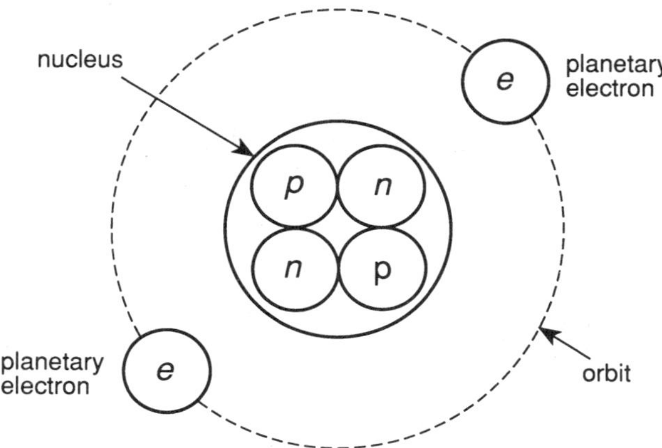

Fig. 5-1. Negatively charged electrons (e) rotating around the nucleus, which contains protons (p) and neutrons (n).

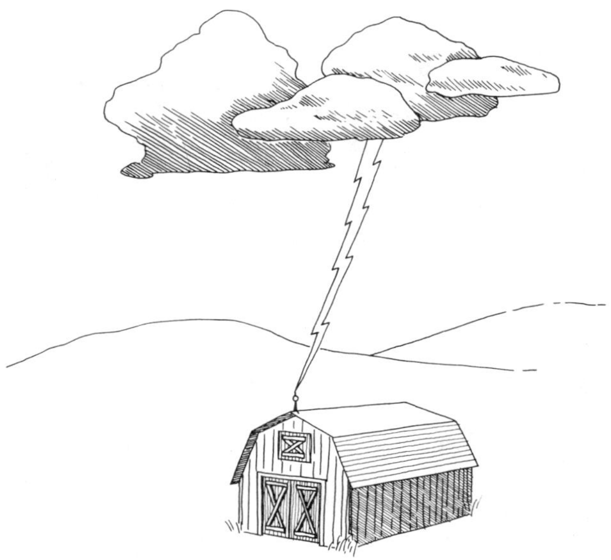

Fig. 5-2. An example of static electricity.

Ions

Atoms attempt to maintain an equal number of electrons and protons in order to balance the electrical charge. It is a law of physics: Things want to be in balance. If there are six electrons rotating around the nucleus, then the atom wants six protons in the center—no more, no less. It is possible, however, for an atom to pick up or lose electrons, or even store the electrons. Such an atom, which has an imbalance of electrons to protons, is called an *ion*. If you upset this balance by moving some electrons out of the atom, the atom becomes agitated; it seeks its missing electrons. This atom is positively charged and therefore called a *positively charged ion*. If, on the other hand, the atom picks up a few extra electrons, it is negatively charged. This atom is called a *negatively charged ion*.

Static Electricity

We have all experienced the sensation of getting "zapped" after shuffling across a thick carpet and touching a doorknob. That zap is the result of electrons from negatively charged ions jumping through the air trying to neutralize their charge (*static electricity*). Another example of static electricity is lightning. The clouds become negatively charged and the earth positively charged; the result is an enormous zap (lightning) as the electrons stream through the air to neutralize the positively charged ions (Fig. 5-2).

Static electricity is referred to as a *stationary charge*; electrons are built up in one object and reduced in another. As the two objects become closer, that charge leaps out as a spark, or lightning, to neutralize the condition. Static electricity isn't always helpful for doing work (unless it's a spark plug), however, because we have little or no control of the power.

Dynamic Electricity

If we can control the flow of electrons from one point to another, we can put electricity to practical use. Electricity flowing in a tungsten filament produces light. Electricity flowing in a heating coil on the stove produces heat. Electricity flowing to a piezoelectric crystal produces ultrasound. This flow of electrons is called *dynamic electricity*.

Potential Electricity

If we have an object with negatively charged ions at one end and positively charged ions on the other end, we have an electrical potential between them. This potential, which has the ability to perform work, is called *voltage*, or stored energy. Voltage can cause a static electricity discharge if the objects get too close to each other, as in the example of thunder clouds and the earth.

The basic law of electrical *charge* states that opposite charges attract and like charges repel. The simplest example of this can be demonstrated with two horseshoe magnets. If you put the two positive ends or two negative ends together, you will notice that the magnets push away (or repel) from each other. By flipping one magnet around so that the positive pole is close to the negative pole, you'll feel the two magnets pull toward each other. This is the effect of the electrons on the negatively charged ion attempting to jump over to the positively charged ions. The pull you feel in between is called the *electromagnetic field.*

Voltage

So far, we have learned that electricity is produced when electrons are either added or subtracted from an atom. These negatively or positively charged ions have stored potential for work. The greater the charge, the greater the potential or voltage to perform work. Voltage provides the pressure necessary to make electrons flow.

Stored charges often dissipate in one way or another. Rapid dissipation through the air is called *static discharge* and is often referred to as a spark, whereas flow of electrons is called dynamic energy. Because dynamic energy is more controllable, it is felt to be more practical for work. Electricity as we know it in electrical applications is dynamic energy.

There are many sources of voltage; the most commonly known is the cell battery, such as that in your car or a flashlight. Through a process of chemical reaction inside the battery, positively charged ions are produced at one end and negatively charged ions are moved to the other end (Fig. 5-3). As long as this chemical reaction is sustained, the oppositely charged ions remain at either end.

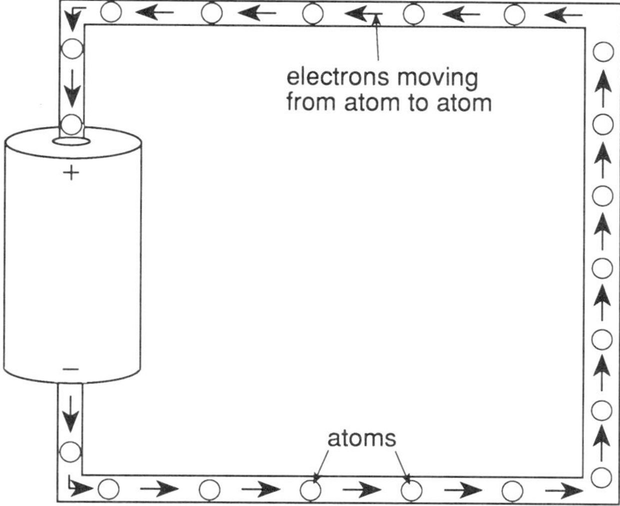

Fig. 5-3. Electrons flow from negative to positive charge in the cell battery.

Current

A good conductor is material that offers little *resistance* to the electrons passing through it. (Other types of conductors make it difficult for electrons to pass.) Copper is a good conductor, so in this example we use a copper wire to connect one end of the battery to the other. The negatively charged electrons, finding a "path" to the positively charged pole, can flow through the wire. This flow, just like a river's flow, is called *current.*

Direct Current/Alternating Current

There are two types of electrical current: direct (DC) or alternating (AC). Direct current is electron flow in one direction only. The flow of current may be fixed and steady or switch on and off periodically. In all cases, the electrons flow in one direction: from negative to positive. A battery operating a flashlight is a common example of direct current.

An alternating current, as its name implies, is current that alternatingly flows in each direction in a conductor. The electrons move in one direction for a short period, or cycle, and then reverse direction for a short period. An AC voltage is one that reverses polarity (positive or negative) periodically. During one cycle, one pole may be positive and the other negative. Then, the poles switch—the positive one becomes negative and the negative one becomes positive. This is why you can insert the plug of a light into house current, which is AC, in reverse position without a problem. However, if you were to hook the cables up backward to the DC battery of your car, you would be in for a big shock!

Ampere

Current is measured by counting the number of electrons that passes a point in a conductor during a specific period of time. The more electrons that pass in the conductor, the greater the current. The unit of measure for those electrons is the *coulomb.* It takes 6.2×10^{18} electrons to make one coulomb. If one coulomb moves through a conductor in one second, we call this an *ampere* (A). In sum, current is the flow of electrons in a conductor and is measured in amperes.

Charge

As discussed earlier, although nothing is really "happening" when there is an excess of electrons in an atom, there is a potential for static or dynamic electricity to occur. As explained, this potential is referred to as a charge, and it is measured in voltage.

When you charge your car battery, you provide the potential for it to do work (start your car). Your battery has a 12-volt pressure to move electrons. If you don't secure the cables to the battery post properly, you may get a spark of static electricity. When you do turn the key, electrons flow though the wires (current) in a controlled fashion, and that current is measured by the number of electrons that flow through the wire during a particular period of time (amperes).

Ohm's Law

Now that we have a basic understanding of voltage, current, and charge, let's examine some practical aspects of electricity. When we connect a wire from one pole of the battery to another, we allow the flow of electrons to pass through the conductor, which helps neutralize ions at either end. This, however, is not a practical application of electricity. What we're interested in is how we can make this electricity work for us. The term *load* is used to describe a device operated by electricity. The load could be a light bulb, heating coil, or Doppler instrument. The load is the instrument or device that performs useful work.

An example of a simple electric circuit (Fig. 5-3) describes this process schematically. The battery is the voltage source, and the rectangle is the load. The lines connecting the battery to the load are conductors (e.g., copper wires). The electrons travel from the negative terminal and pass through the copper wires to the load, where some type of useful work is performed. The current continues though the copper wires to connect with the positive terminal, thus completing its round-trip, or circuit. If at any point this circuit is disconnected, all flow of electricity will stop; current is dependent on a continuous loop in order to move.

It should be noted that even though the flow of the electrons is from the negative to the positive, it is a convention when showing schematic electrical circuits to diagram the current from the positive to the negative. Engineers adopted this convention many years ago, before electricity was really understood, and it remains the standard, however confusing, today.

As stated earlier, copper wires are good conductors because they allow electrons to flow easily through the material, but if wires were made of heating elements, which resist the flow of electrons, they would get too hot to be of use. If they were made out of a material such as tungsten filament, they would glow (Fig. 5-4). We do not want electrons to perform work in the wire; we want them to get to the load.

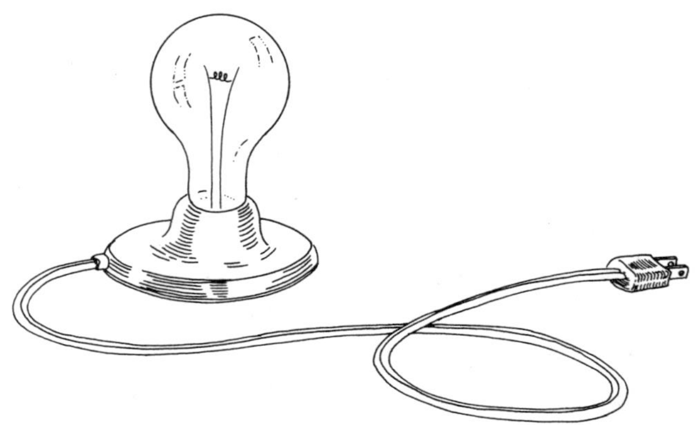

Fig. 5-4. Resistance to the flow of electricity in this electric bulb causes light.

The main characteristic of a load is that it offers some opposition, if work is to be done, to the current. This opposition to current is called *resistance* and it is measured by a term called *ohm* (sounds like "home" without the "h"). The letter symbol for ohm is **Ω**. If the resistance to current is high, the ohm value is high. Conversely, when there is little resistance to current, the ohm value is low.

The amount of resistance in a current directly affects the amount of current flow. In addition, the amount of voltage applied to the resistance will affect the current. (Does this sound a little familiar in regard to vascular flow and resistance?) The entire relationship between flow, resistance, and current is known as *Ohm's law*. In electrical law, Ohm's law is the most important of them all. Ohm's law states

> The current in a circuit is directly proportional to the applied voltage and inversely proportional to the resistance.

Ohm's Law is expressed

$$I = V/R$$

where I is the current (measured in amperes), V is the voltage (measured in volts), and R is the resistance (measured in ohms).

We can look at this law in several different ways. If we increase the voltage by two, we increase the current by two, but if we double the resistance, we cut the current by one half. If we lower the voltage by ten, we reduce the resistance by ten. In sum, current depends on how much voltage is applied and how much resistance electricity meets; to increase the current, you need high voltage and low resistance.

It will help to give some examples here. If voltage is 5 volts and current is 0.1 ampere, the resistance is

$$R = V/I = 5/0.1 = 50 \text{ ohms}$$

If we know what the resistance is and what the current is, we can solve for voltage. Let's say the resistance is 10 ohms and the current is 5 amperes. Then,

$$V = R \times I = 10 \times 5 = 50 \text{ volts}$$

What you need to know here is Ohm's law (I = V/R). Then you must be able to solve not only for resistance, but also for current and voltage. *Note*: Don't memorize the other formulas; learn how to solve for each.

Algebra Review

1. If I = V/R, in order to solve for R we get rid of the V from V/R by dividing both sides by V.

$$I/V = V/R/V$$

Because V divided by V = 1, it cancels each other out.

$$I/V = R, \text{ or } R = I/V$$

2. If I = V/R and we want to solve for V, then get rid of the R by multiplying both sides by R.

$$R \times I = V/R \times R$$

Because 1/R × R = 1, it cancels each other out.

$$R \times I = V, \text{ or } V = R \times I$$

Milliamperes and Microamperes

When we discuss current in electrical systems, especially in noninvasive vascular instruments, we are often dealing with very low figures. Because of this, different terminology is applied to express these otherwise very long decimal fractions. For example, a *milliampere* (mA) is 1/1,000 of an ampere, and a *microamperes* (μA) is 1/1,000,000 of an ampere. To avoid a long decimal series of .0000005 amperes, we write 0.5 microamperes, or 0.5 μA.

Energy

The term *energy* was first expressed by Aristotle and is defined as *power* in the form of action, vigor, or performance. Energy in physics is defined as the work that a physical system is capable of doing in changing from its actual state to a specific reference state. For example, the sun's energy (heat and light) can be converted into a different energy (dynamic electrical energy) to perform work.

There are three forms of energy:

1. Potential
2. Kinetic
3. Resting

For purposes of this section, we will concern ourselves only with potential and kinetic energy.

Potential Energy

Potential energy refers to the ability to do work that is derived from position rather than motion. The build-up of a massive amount of water in a dam has the potential for producing electricity. Blood in the left ventricle has the potential to do the work of moving blood cells to the periphery of the vascular system. The potential energy in a freshly charged battery has the ability to do work (or play) by running appliances or portable Dopplers.

Kinetic Energy

Kinetic energy refers to the ability to do work on the basis of the energy's motion. Although a dam has the capability of performing work, it does not actually do so. It is the water escaping through a culvert that turns the turbine and creates the electricity. It is the kinetic energy of moving blood that carries the red cells to their destinations.

Power

We have discussed a number of ways for calculating different measurements of what is put into a system—voltages, current, charge, and resistance—but how do we measure the output? Once the work is done and the energy is consumed, we can measure those results in terms of power. *Power* is defined as the rate at which work is done. Electrical power is expressed in units called *watts* (W).

The most common result of the consumption of energy while performing work is *heat*. Heat is a form of power. At times, the heat is desirable, particularly when we want to toast some bread in a toaster or warm up a room with a portable heater. At other times, however, power in the form of heat is not desirable. For example, light bulbs produce light and some heat. The heat is not necessarily beneficial, but it is difficult to get light without heat. A particular problem with the complex circuitry in ultrasound systems is the heat produced by the circuits. This is caused by the enormous amount of energy dissipated in the form of heat as the electrons pass though wires, circuits, and resisters.

We use our understanding of Ohm's law to determine the power in an electrical circuit. Because power is a result of the work performed, there is a relationship between power, voltage, current, and resistance. The basic power formula is as follows:

$$P = V \times I$$

Because I (current) represents the charge moving through the circuit and V (volts) represents the driving voltage, we can understand how the more voltage that is introduced and the greater the current moving around, the greater is the power (P) that results. For example, if the voltage in your home is 120 V (normal voltage in American houses) and the amperes in a light bulb are measured at 0.5 A, that light would produce 60 watts (W) of power.

Other methods of computing power can be utilized by combining the power formula with Ohm's law. Assume we know the voltage and resistance, but not the current. Because $I = V/R$, then $P = V \times V/R$. If $V = 100$ volts and resistance = 10 ohms, then

$$P = 100 \times 100/10, \text{ or}$$

$$P = 10{,}000/10, \text{ or}$$

$$P = 1{,}000 \text{ watts}$$

If we know values for current and resistance but not for voltage, and because $V = I \times R$, we can use the formula

$$P = I \times I \times R$$

If current (I) equals 0.05 amperes and resistance (R) equals 50 ohms, then

$$P = 0.05 \times 0.05 \times 50, \text{ or}$$

$$P = 0.0025 \times 50, \text{ or}$$

$$P = 0.125 \text{ watts}$$

Milliwatts

Again, because vascular technology utilizes equipment with many low-power settings, it is convenient to use terms appropriate for the exceedingly small numbers. Because 100 milliamperes equal 0.1 ampere, it would be more useful to express the figure in the previous formula as 125 *milliwatts* (mW).

Megawatts

On the other hand, if we are dealing with very large power values, then we use the terms *kilowatt* or *megawatt*. Simply stated, a kilowatt is a thousand watts, and a megawatt (like megabucks) is a million watts.

Review Exercise

1. All matter, whether it is solid, liquid, or gas, is made up of

   a. protons
   b. electrons
   c. neutrons
   d. atoms

2. Similar atoms, formed together, produce

   a. elements
   b. matter
   c. compounds
   d. solids, liquids, gases

3. There are ______________ basic elements.

4. When two or more elements are formed together, a ____________________________ is formed.

5. Atoms are made up of

   a. ____

   b. ____

   c. ____

6. The core of the atom is called the ______________.

7. The protons are (positively/negatively) charged.

8. Rotating around the nucleus are negatively charged

   a. atoms
   b. protons
   c. electrons
   d. neutrons

9. Atoms try to keep an ____________________________ of electrons and protons.

10. It is possible for an atom to pick up or lose electrons. True or False?

11. An atom that has an imbalance of electrons to protons is called a

    a. compound
    b. ion
    c. positively charged ion
    d. either b or c

12. An atom that is minus electrons is called a

    a. compound
    b. negatively charged ion
    c. positively charged ion
    d. either b or c

13. When an atom picks up a few extra electrons, it is called a

a. compound
b. negatively charged ion
c. positively charged ion
d. either b or c

14. Lightning is an example of ______________ electricity.

15. If we can ______________ the flow of electrons from one point to another, we can put electricity to practical use.

16. Electricity flowing in a tungsten filament mainly produces ______________.

17. Electricity flowing to a piezoelectric crystal mainly produces ______________________________.

18. The controlled flow of electrons is called ______________ electricity.

19. An object with negatively charged ions at one end and positively charged ions on the other end has an electrical ______________________________ across it.

20. The electricity that has the ability to perform work is called ______________________________ electricity.

21. Voltage also is referred to as ______________ energy.

22. Electricity is produced only when electrons are removed from an atom. True or False?

23. Voltage provides the necessary ______________ to make electrons flow.

24. Rapid uncontrolled discharge through the air is called ______________ discharge.

25. Controlled flow of electrons is called ______________________________ energy.

26. Dynamic energy is less stable than static electricity. True or False?

27. Electricity as we know it in electrical applications is ______________ energy.

28. The cell battery is a common source of

a. voltage
b. amperes
c. current
d. all of the above

29. The flow of electrons through a conductor is called

a. voltage
b. amperes and current
c. current
d. pressure

30. The more electrons that pass in the conductor, the greater the

a. voltage
b. amperes
c. current
d. pressure

31. The unit of measure for the electrons in question 30 is

a. voltage
b. coulomb
c. current
d. Ohm's

32. Current is the ______________ of electrons in a conductor.

33. The unit for measurement of the electrical potential to do work is called

a. voltage
b. amperes
c. current
d. pressure

34. Current is measured by the ______________ of electrons that flow through the wire during a particular period of time.

35. The term used to describe a device operated by electricity is

a. power
b. load
c. charge
d. unit

36. The load is what does the useful work. True or False?

37. In a schematic drawing, a battery is the ______________ source, and the rectangle is the load.

38. The ______________ continues through the copper wires to connect with the positive terminal, thus completing its round-trip, or circuit.

39. If at any point this circuit is ______________________________, all flow of electricity will stop.

40. Current is not dependent on a continuous loop in order to move. True or False?

41. The main characteristic of a load is that it offers some ______________________________, if work is to be done, to the current.

42. Opposition to current is called ______________________________ and it is measured in a term called

a. voltage
b. amperes
c. current
c. ohm

43. The Greek letter symbol for ohm is ______________.

44. If the resistance to current is high, the ohm value is

a. low
b. balanced out
c. high
d. none of the above

45. The amount of ____________________________ applied to the resistance will affect the current.

46. The relationship between flow, resistance, and current is known as ____________________________.

47. Ohm's law is expressed as I = V/R, where

a. I = ____________________________

b. V = ____________________________

c. R = ____________________________

48. If we increase the voltage in question 47 by two, we increase the current by ______________.

49. If we double the resistance in question 47, we ______________ the current by ______________.

50. If the current stays constant, and we lower the voltage by ten, we ______________ the resistance by ______________.

51. Current is dependent on how much ______________ is applied and how much resistance the current is meeting.

52. To increase the current, one needs

a. high voltage/high resistance
b. low voltage/low resistance
c. low voltage/high resistance
d. high voltage/low resistance

53. If voltage is 5 volts and current is 0.1 amperes, the resistance is R = V/I.

R = ____________________________

54. If the resistance is 10 ohms and the current is 5 amperes, then V = R × I.

V = ____________________________

55. If I = V/R, then the expression for resistance is R = ______________.

56. If I = V/R, then the expression for voltage is V = ___________.

57. When we discuss current in electrical systems, especially in noninvasive vascular instruments, we are often dealing with very ______________ figures.

58. A ______________________________ is 1/1,000 of an ampere.

59. 0.000005 amperes equals ______________ microamperes.

60. There are three forms of energy:

a. ____

b. ____

c. ____

61. ______________________________ energy refers to the ability to do work derived from stored energy rather than motion.

62. ______________ energy refers to the ability to do work on the basis of the energy's motion.

63. Once the work is done and the energy is consumed, we can measure those results in terms of

a. load
b. energy
c. voltage
d. power

64. Electrical power is expressed in units called

a. voltage
b. watts
c. amperes
d. Hertz

65. The most common result of the consumption of energy while performing work is

a. heat
b. light
c. voltage
d. power

66. We use our understanding of ______________ law to determine the power in an electrical circuit.

67. Power is a result of the ______________ performed.

68. There is a relationship between power, voltage, current, and resistance. True or False?

69. The basic power formula is P = V × I, where

a. P = ______________________________

b. V = ______________________________

c. I = ______________________________

70. The greater the load, the greater the ______________________.

71. If V = 1,000 volts and resistance = 500 ohms, then P = V × I.

P = ______________watts

72. If we know the values for current and resistance but not for voltage, we use the formula P = I × I × R. If current (I) equals 0.10 amperes and resistance (R) equals 100 ohms, then

P = _________ watts

73. In conventional terminology, it would be more useful to express the figure 0.125 watts as ______________.

NON-ULTRASONIC VASCULAR INSTRUMENTATION: PLETHYSMOGRAPHY

During the past ten years, there have been numerous changes in the type of noninvasive vascular instruments used in the laboratory. In general, both Doppler and imaging ultrasound now dominate as the equipment preferred by most vascular diagnosis for a majority of the testing performed. It is important, however, to understand other systems that are still used in testing procedures, such as plethysmography.

Key Terms

AC/DC coupling
Calibration
Four-wire resistance
Graphic recording
Impedance plethysmography
Oculoplethysmography
Plethysmography
Resistance
Skin temperature
Strain-gauge plethysmography
Two-wire resistance measurement

Plethysmography refers to the volume changes of tissue. The term stems from the Greek work *plethysmos*, which means "to increase." Because transient changes in the limbs or other tissue are related to volumetric alterations of blood flow in the tissue, plethysmography can be used to measure those changes. (The specific procedures will be covered in detail in chapter 6.) The primary instruments used for plethysmographic testing include

1. air plethysmography
2. oculoplethysmography
3. photoplethysmography
4. strain-gauge plethysmography
5. impedance plethysmography

Air Plethysmography

When a vascular specialist initially evaluates a patient with suspected vascular disease, one of the first steps in the clinical assessment is to feel for palpable pulses. One not only feels for the presence or absence of pulses, but also attempts to assess the quality of them: Pulses might be rated as weak, strong, or bounding. Feeling for arterial pulses is limited, however, to the pulse of one particular artery at one particular anatomic position. Indirect assumptions are made about the surrounding tissue based on the quality of that specific pulse.

Imagine that the vascular specialist's fingers were so sensitive that he or she could feel the changes in volume of the entire segment of a limb or small digit. That is essentially what *air plethysmography* does. Blood pressure cuffs with an inflatable rubber bladder are placed around the limb at several different positions. Then, a small amount of air (about 65 mmHg) is injected into each cuff to form a snug fit for the cuff without interfering with normal blood inflow or outflow.

When arterial flow in systole enters the leg or finger, the very subtle increase in volume is sensed by the cuff, just as sensitive fingertips sense the change in volume of the pulse. The increase in segmental limb volume causes a corresponding increase in the pressure in the bladder contained within the cuff. This pressure change is transmitted through the connecting tubing to a sensitive pressure transducer and recorded on a graph. As the heart relaxes in diastole, the subsequent decrease in volume flow also is sensed and recorded.

Air plethysmography can also be used to measure alterations in venous flow. By using two cuffs, one to occlude venous outflow in the thigh and the other to "sense" corresponding volume changes in the calf, an assessment of venous capacitance and outflow can be made.

First, a large cuff is placed on the thigh and inflated to a level just below diastolic pressure. This degree of occlusion will essentially allow arterial blood in without letting venous flow out. As the arterial flow continues to flow into the limb, the sensing cuff on the calf begins to reflect these changes by showing an increase in volume in the calf. This is similar to damming up a stream: as you continue to prevent the water from flowing out, more and more water builds up behind the dam (Fig. 5-5).

If there is no extensive venous obstructive disease already present, the recording of this increase in volume will rise to a significant height over baseline height within

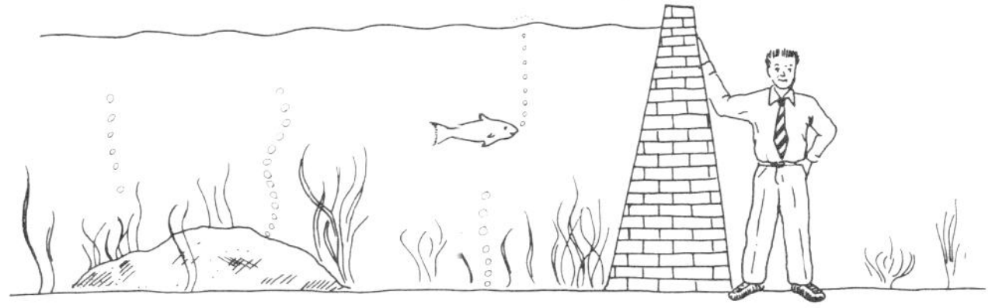

Fig. 5-5. Damming up!

a designated period of time. At this point, the thigh cuff is rapidly deflated, allowing the blood to flow back to the heart, which it does rather quickly due to the built-up pressure. If there is no obstruction in the deep venous system, the venous blood will rush out of the limb, and the cuff on the calf will reflect that immediate change by a drop in the signal. If there is an obstruction of the deep venous system, however, the blood will be unable to rush out because it will have to find its way through smaller collateral vessels and superficial veins. The drop in the recording will be much slower.

It must be noted that while many laboratories feel that plethysmography is helpful in determining arterial or venous blood flows in the limbs, others use plethysmography on a limited basis. It is up to individual departments to determine the worth of the data provided by plethysmographic studies in the specific clinical setting.

Air Oculoplethysmography

The *pneumo* (air) *oculoplethysmography* (OPG) system is still in wide use despite advances in duplex ultrasound technology. The OPG uses eye cups that resemble large contact lenses attached to a small plastic tube. The eye cups are applied to the sclera of both eyes, and a vacuum is applied. By using this vacuum, the actual shape of the eye is temporarily distorted to the point that blood supply to the eyes from the ophthalmic artery is cut off. (Although this may seem somewhat brutal for a noninvasive test, the effect is little more than that caused when rubbing one's eyes.)

Have you ever noticed that while rubbing your eyes you may have caused a little black spot to appear in your vision? That black spot occurs when pressure applied to the eye momentarily cuts off blood supply from the ophthalmic artery. Clear vision returns when the pressure is stopped. This is the same effect that air OPG has, but it is obviously more controlled than an eye massage. By slowly reducing the vacuum through the tubing to the eye cups, we can measure at what pressure the ophthalmic artery occludes and then compare it with the brachial artery pressure. (The ophthalmic artery is normally about two thirds that of the brachial artery).

Photoplethysmography

Photoplethysmography (PPG) is an instrument that measures changes of blood content in the skin and is used in both venous and arterial studies. The PPG has two elements: an element that emits an infrared light into tissue and a receiver to note changes in the reflected light signal. As blood volume increases in systole, more light is absorbed and less is reflected back to the receiver. In diastole, with less blood in the tissue, more light is reflected back to the receiver. The sensor translates this ebb and flow of blood in the tissue into an electrical signal. This signal can be displayed on a monitor and/or can be recorded on a strip chart recorder. This device is particularly valuable for evaluating venous insufficiency and digital arterial flow.

Strain-Gauge Plethysmography

Strain-gauge plethysmography is a device that is similar in physiologic principle to air plethysmography. The electromechanical mechanism for obtaining data, however, is much different. As with air plethysmography, the instrument measures volume changes in a segment of a limb. The strain-gauge, however, uses a small mercury-filled elastic tube that encircles the limb. It is connected on either end by electrodes.

Rather than sensing the pressure changes in a mildly inflated cuff, the strain gauge measures changes in the length of the tube, which is stretched ever so slightly, each time the limb is filled with blood during systole. As the mercury column in the tube (which is an electrical conductor) stretches, its electrical resistance changes dramatically, allowing recording to be made related to limb volume. Unlike air plethysmography, this is a system that can be calibrated to give quantitative flow data. These changes occur with fluctuations of arterial pulses or effects of venous outflow studies.

Impedance Plethysmography

The reason for reviewing electrical principles will become obvious as the subject of two-wire/four-wire *impedance plethysmography* (IPG) is discussed. If you do not feel comfortable with your current understanding of the electrical principles, particularly the subject of Ohm's law, please review that section again before proceeding.

Two-Wire Impedance Plethysmography

As vascular specialists, we have learned about Ohm's law and electrical impedance, but we are not really interested in the resistance of electrons in wires; we are interested in blood flow. Fortunately, flowing blood is a good conductor of electricity. By thinking of the blood as the "wire" or the "load," we can utilize Ohm's law to determine *resistance* in the same way.

You will recall from Ohm's law the basic formula

$$I = V/R$$

Current is equal to voltage divided by resistance. The greater the resistance, the lower the current. We can determine the resistance of a conductor or a load by implementing Ohm's law; that is, if we know the voltage and can measure the current, we can solve for resistance.

$$R = V/I$$

Resistance is equal to voltage divided by current. For example

Resistance = 12 volts divided by 0.240 amperes

Resistance = 0.6 ohms

A further important property of a conductor such as blood is the way in which its resistance changes. Blood within a vessel causes resistance to increase as the vessel gets longer. However, as the vessel's *diameter increases*, the *resistance decreases* inversely proportional to the cross-sectional area. For example, if vessel 1 and vessel 2 have the same cross-sectional area, but vessel 1 is twice as long as vessel 2, it has twice the resistance. If two vessels are the same length, but the first has twice the cross-sectional area as the second, it will have only one half the resistance.

By placing electrodes a fixed length apart and measuring the resistance of electrical flow in a limb, we can determine that if the resistance is low then there is an ample volume of blood and that vessels are dilated. Conversely, if the resistance is high, we can assume that there is lower volume in the limb and that the blood vessels have a small (nondilated) cross-section.

Two-wire impedance plethysmography has a problem, however. The electrodes connected to the skin have an inherently unpredictable impedance. It is not easy to determine whether resistance is from the electrode contacts on the skin or from the blood in the vessel. Therefore, two-wire impedance plethysmography is seldom used clinically.

Four-Wire Impedance Plethysmography

The *four-wire impedance plethysmography* system overcomes the limitations of the two-wire system. The two conducting wires, one to send and the other to receive, are wrapped around the limb in a customary fashion. Then, two additional wires are wrapped around the limb in between the first two; these are the resistance measuring wires. The technique and interpretation for this procedure will be discussed in detail in chapter 6.

Graphical Recording/Calibration

Much of the plethysmography testing is recorded on graphs, which makes it possible to obtain data representing successive changes over a period of time. The graph most commonly used in vascular technology is the strip-chart recorder. This type of graph employs an electric motor to move a long strip of paper under a pen. The pen, either ink filled or heat sensitive, moves in response to electrical signals related to physiologic changes and records those variations on charted graph paper.

Vascular equipment is like a fine musical instrument. A piano player will often tune the instrument by using a tuning fork, for example, in the key of C. The tuning fork gives off a consistent tone in that key because it is designed to vibrate at exactly 256 cycles per second. The key-of-C tuning fork will not vary. A tuned piano, therefore, will provide a consistent tone with every other piano that is also properly tuned.

Medical instruments need to be "tuned" on a regular basis as well. By calibrating instruments, we can be certain that the information obtained is reproducible not only by the same instrument day after day but also between other similar instruments. In this way, data that is shared between laboratories can be trusted and reproduced with only physiologic changes causing variations.

AC/DC Coupling

In recording equipment, the alternating current (AC) mode is used to measure such rapid changes as pulsatile blood flow. Slowly changing physiologic signals, such as occur with venous blood flow, are measured by the direct current (DC) mode. By coupling the two modes into one system, the vascular specialist has both modes available for a variety of vascular testing.

Skin Temperature

All measurements of blood flow impedance should be done in a standard room temperature of approximately 22° to 25° C, to avoid vasoconstriction (cold) or flushing (hot) responses from skin temperature and to provide a stable baseline skin blood flow (Fig. 5-6).

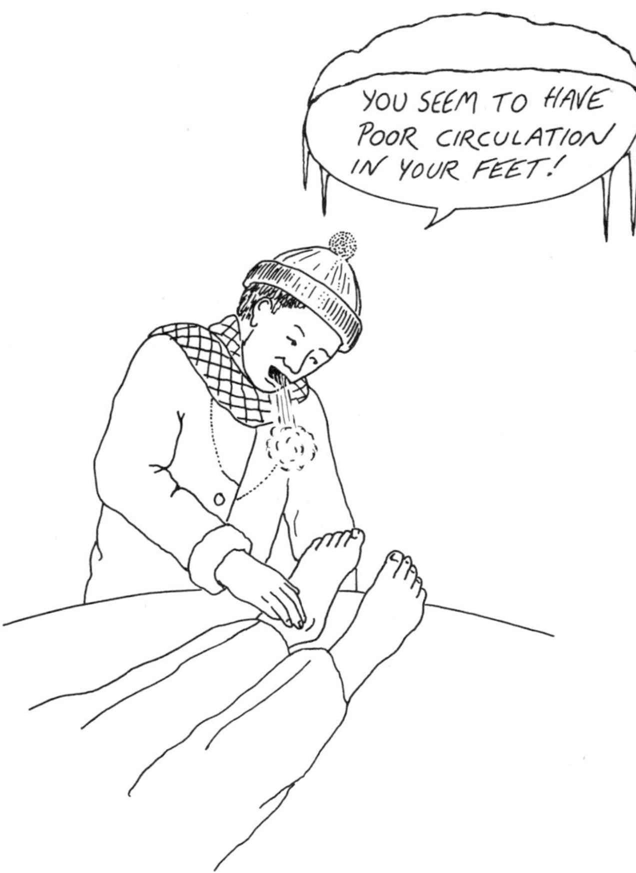

Fig. 5-6. A cold room will affect the circulation in the feet.

Review Exercise

1. Plethysmography measures ______________ changes in tissue.

2. Plethysmography is used only for arterial studies. True or False?

3. When the occluding cuff of a venous outflow plethysmography study is released, the blood flow moves out of the limb ______________ in a normal leg.

4. Oculoplethysmography refers to
   ____.

5. Air-filled OPGs evaluate carotid artery disease by identifying

   a. decrease in ophthalmic artery pressure
   b. delay in ear tracings
   c. delay in eye tracings
   d. both a and b

6. Ophthalmic artery pressure is ______________ that of brachial artery pressure. (Refers to comparative amount.)

7. Photoplethysmography uses ______________ to measure blood volume changes in the skin.

8. Strain-gauge plethysmography uses ______________ in a fine elastic tube.

9. Strain-gauge plethysmography measures changes in ______________ of the tube.

10. Moving blood is a relatively good conductor of electricity. True or False?

11. One can utilize ______________ law to determine resistance in the deep venous system.

12. If we can measure the ______________ to electrical flow in a limb segment, we can determine if there is an ample volume of flowing blood.

13. Two-wire impedance plethysmography is equally as good as four-wire impedance plethysmography. True or False?

14. The graph most commonly used in vascular technology is the
    ____________________________ recorder.

15. In plethysmographic equipment, the alternating current (AC) mode is used to measure

    a. venous pressure
    b. venous incompetency
    c. slow physiologic changes
    d. rapid physiologic changes

16. Slower changes in blood volume, such as occur with venous blood flow, are measured by (AC mode/DC mode).

17. AC/DC coupling in a vascular system provides the vascular specialist with

    a. a dangerous electrical situation
    b. no benefit
    c. minimal benefit
    d. significant benefits

18. All measurements of blood flow impedance should be done in a room temperature of approximately

    a. 20° C
    b. 22° to 25° C
    c. 25° to 28° C
    d. 30° C

19. When one measures physiologic changes in the body and records them on a strip-chart recorder, it is essential to ensure that the data obtained is

    a. calibrated
    b. accurate
    c. reproducible
    d. all of the above

DOPPLER SIGNAL PROCESSING

In this section, the principles of *Doppler signal processing and spectral analysis* will be reviewed. Because duplex ultrasound combines imaging and Doppler ultrasound, it is essential for the student to be familiar with principles of both noninvasive technologies.

Key Terms

Aliasing
Amplitude
Continuous-wave Doppler
Cosine theta
Doppler
Doppler effect
Doppler equation
Doppler shift
Frequency shift
Nyquist limit
Phase
Pulsed-wave Doppler
Pulse repetition frequency
Range ambiguity
Sample volume size
Single-gate pulsed Doppler

Doppler Effect

For vascular specialists, the Doppler flow meter remains one of the single most important instruments available in the laboratory. Where imaging is valuable in "looking" at blood vessels, Doppler is extremely important in "listening" to blood flow. If we use the analogy of traffic in the road once again, we can begin to appreciate the significant contribution of Doppler ultrasound.

If you are traveling through a city in the early morning and you are unclear of the route you will take, you will obviously want a road map. The map will tell you where the roads lead and whether they are major highways or secondary roads. The map allows you to see what your path is likely to be and how wide or narrow the roads are.

You are unlikely to be the only car on the road, however. Clearly, at 8 A.M. you will have to deal with rush-hour traffic. What roads carry the biggest load of traffic? Have there been any accidents? Is traffic particularly heavy due to an event that a lot of people are attending? Is there any ongoing construction? Your map will be of little assistance with these conditions. On the other hand, you do have another source of information —the traffic report on the radio:

> Good morning! This is the traffic helicopter reporting from the skies. There appears to be heavy traffic on route 91 this morning, heading into town. Traffic is slowed down to 25 mph due to an accident. If you try route 5, watch out for construction. Traffic has been reduced to a single lane for 2 miles. Route 30 is wide open with traffic moving freely.

Now your information is far more complete. You can not only see what the roads are like with a map, but you can know what the traffic is like on those roads.

If we think of ultrasound imaging as providing the vascular specialist with a road map, we can think of Doppler as providing a traffic report. In other words, we are interested not only in what the vessels look like but also in how they are affecting blood flow. With this additional information, one can assess vascular disease with far more accuracy.

The term *Doppler* originates from Christian Doppler, an Austrian physicist who first described frequency shifts in 1842. It is reported that Doppler was interested in the light shifts of stars in order to determine whether they were moving away from or toward each other. His explanation of this effect soon focused on *sound* shifts and the analogy we are all most familiar with—his description of sound shifts using the train whistle. Although many of us rarely travel by train any longer, we are all familiar with the effects of a train's whistle as it approaches and leaves the train station without stopping (Fig. 5-7).

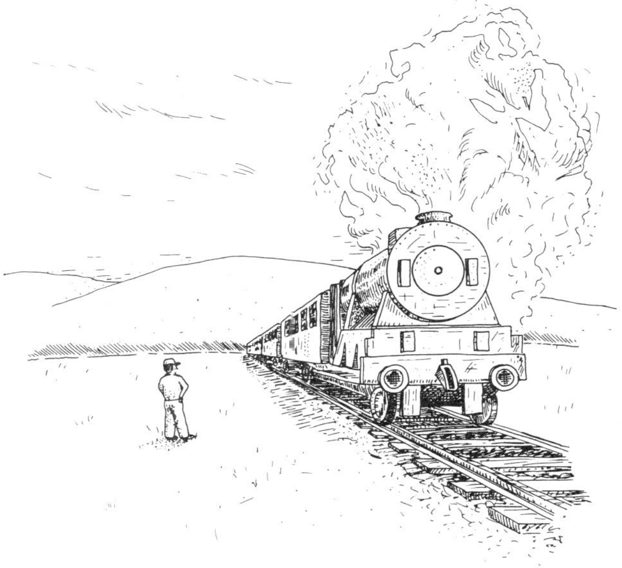

Fig. 5-7. To the stationary observer, the train whistle's pitch appears to increase as the train approaches and then to decrease as it passes. This is the Doppler effect.

The engineer riding the train will hear no change in the sound of the whistle as he blows it, but the observer on the platform will hear the change distinctly as the train passes by. How does this occur? Once again, let's return to the basic concepts of ultrasound physics in order to understand how this change takes place.

You will recall that sound waves are generated from a source and move out in a constant velocity (which is dependent on the medium) in concentric circles. These waves are like the waves made by someone fishing in a clear pond where the bobber creates tiny little waves on the surface of the water (Fig. 5-8).

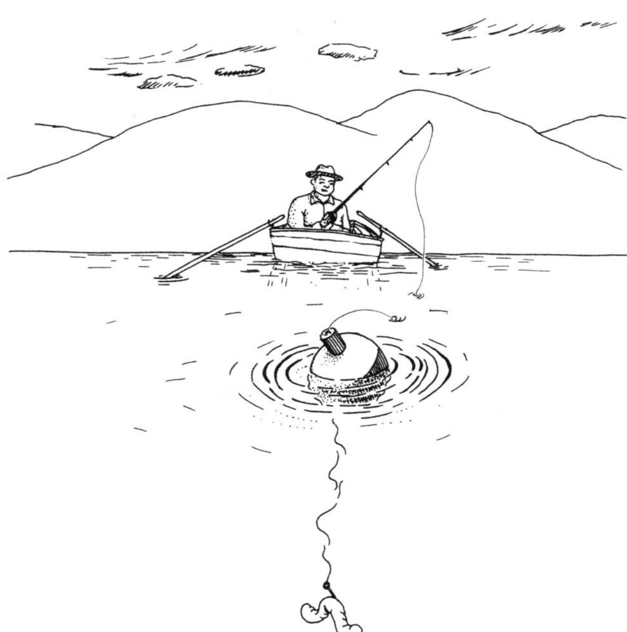

Fig. 5-8. Waves from the stationary bobber move away from it in concentric circles.

If the boat starts moving, there is a change in the pattern of the waves. The waves moving in the same direction as the boat start getting closer together, whereas the waves on the other side start getting pulled apart in the opposite direction. In terms of ultrasound, the observer on the dock would note that the waves coming toward her would have more waves per second (an increase in frequency), whereas the waves on the other side of the bobber would have fewer waves per second (lower frequency) (Fig. 5-9).

If you were a frog hiding behind a rock to avoid being seen by the boat, and all you could see was the waves in the water, you could tell if the boat is moving toward you by the increase in the frequency of waves, or away from you by the decrease in the frequency of waves, or stationary by the fact that the waves did not change in frequency (Fig. 5-10). Being an intelligent frog, you might think, "There is an apparent shift in the frequency of waves I am observing. Clearly, with the increase in this *frequency shift*, the boat is coming toward me. Time to leave!"

The principles of Doppler ultrasound are very much the same as the waves in the water. A Doppler emits a signal and then observes the response of that signal to the target at which it is aimed. The system compares the difference of what was sent and what was received. Are the blood cells moving toward you or away from the Doppler? Is it moving fast, or is it moving slowly? Is it moving at all? In blood flow, the *Doppler effect* helps us answer these questions and more.

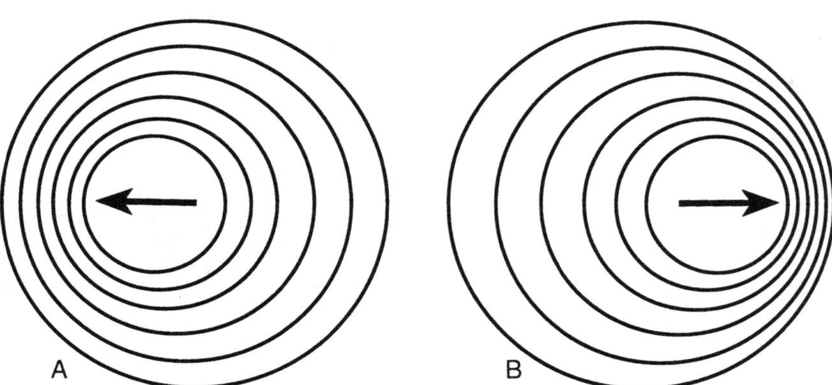

Fig. 5-9. (A) Increased frequency within the left of the sphere as the sphere moves to the left. (B) Increased frequencies to the right of the sphere as the sphere moves to the right.

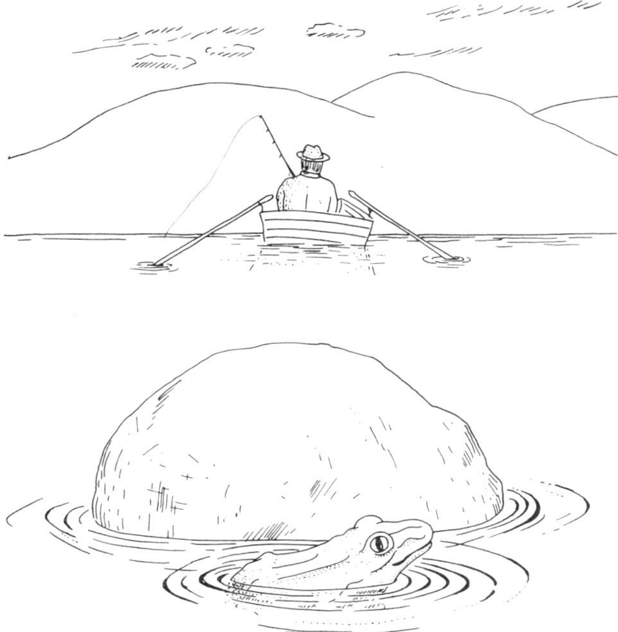

Fig. 5-10. By observing the wave patterns, this frog can tell whether the boat is moving toward or away from him.

Doppler Equation

The *Doppler equation* usually strikes fear in the hearts of many new (and sometimes experienced) vascular specialists. This equation includes letters and symbols that are literally "Greek to me."

Because we *are* vascular specialists, we cannot always go on in our careers describing the Doppler principle by talking about frogs hiding behind rocks and looking at waves made by a boat! We must be familiar with the language that is commonly used by vascular specialists. More importantly, the principles of the Doppler equation will help us to perform our examinations better and understand the results more clearly. Before we actually get into the equation itself, however, let's get a better understanding of why the equation is so important.

If someone were to boast that they drove from the East Coast to the West Coast in three days, you would want to know more information about the trip before you could make a judgment on such a statement. For example, at what speed did she travel? Did she drive a Corvette or a camper? Did she go on the highway or secondary routes? Were the roads dry or did she run into snow in Denver? Did she stop to rest or did she have another driver? The answers to these questions help you better determine the value of a cross-country trip in three days. For example, a solo motorcycle trip may be far more impressive than an airline flight.

With Doppler information, the principle is the same. If someone tells you, "Wow! This artery has a 3-kHz frequency shift," you need to know more about the situation before you can make a judgment about the results. In some cases, a 3-kHz shift may be completely normal, and in others, a 3-kHz frequency shift could indicate significant disease. The minimum information you need to know, other than what vessel you are examining, is the following:

1. What is the frequency of the Doppler transducer?
2. How fast does the ultrasound travel through tissue?
3. What is the angle of the Doppler ultrasound beam to the blood vessel?

The Doppler formula looks like this:

$$Df = \frac{2FV(\text{Cos } \theta)}{C}$$

where Df = Change in frequency (the difference of what was sent and what was received)

2FV = Twice the fundamental frequency of the Doppler transducer, because the ultrasound beam must make the round trip (in and out).

Cos θ = Cosine theta the angle at which the Doppler ultrasound beam strikes the vessel

C = The velocity of ultrasound through tissue

So, as an astute vascular specialist, you react to the 3-kHz Doppler shift by stating

> I noticed that the angle of your Doppler beam was 60 degrees and that the Doppler transducer you were using has a fundamental frequency of 5 MHz. Given the fact that ultrasound travels through soft tissue at approximately 1,540 meters per second, I have calculated, by utilizing the Doppler equation, that a 3-kHz shift is within normal limits!

Doppler Frequency Shift

The Doppler instrument provides three important pieces of information regarding blood flow. From a technical perspective, these are

1. phase
2. amplitude
3. frequency shift

From a practical prospective, they define the following questions:

1. What is the direction the blood cells are traveling?
2. How strong or weak is the signal?
3. How fast are the blood cells traveling?

How does the Doppler provide these data?

As an analogy, imagine you are sitting at the baseball stadium and, unfortunately, the person in front of you is very large and is wearing a big hat as well. You cannot even see the batter at the plate! You watch the pitcher throw the ball and hear a loud crack but you never see the batter actually hit the ball. The ball goes high over the center field fence and out of the ballpark for a home run.

Although you did not see the batter hit the ball, there are two things of which you can be quite certain: The batter hit the ball pretty much "squarely," and he hit very hard! What we have done by observing the direction and distance the ball was hit was to make an assumption about what direction and with how much force the bat was swung—without ever seeing the bat.

You may be wondering what this has to do with the Doppler. Believe it or not, Doppler principles can be understood with this analogy. We essentially send an ultrasound wave into the blood vessel (the pitched ball), observe the signal returning (the hit ball), and make an assumption about the force and direction.

Doppler Shift

The *Doppler shift* provides the vascular specialist with information about blood flow. The shift is dependent on how the received signal is different from the signal that was sent into the blood stream. In essence, the piezoelectric crystal sends an ultrasound signal into the blood stream and then listens for the returning echo. The system then displays the difference between what was sent and what was received; that is, the frequency of what goes in minus what comes out equals the Doppler shift. If the signal was sent into the blood stream at 5 MHz (5 million hertz) and was received back at 5.002 (5 million and 2 thousand Hertz), the Doppler shift would equal 2 kHz.

Doppler at 0 Degrees Versus 90 Degrees

If you could take your Doppler transducer, miniaturize it, and place it directly inside the blood vessel, you could then aim the ultrasound beam directly at the oncoming red blood cells. The results would be the ideal angle (0 degrees) to obtain the best Doppler shift; it is like a direct pitch to a solid swing of the bat. The farther this angle is moved away from 0 degrees, however, the less directly the ultrasound strikes the moving cells and the lower the Doppler shift. At the extreme, if one aims the Doppler beam directly at the blood stream at 90 degrees to the horizontal, there will be no Doppler shift at all (Fig. 5-11).

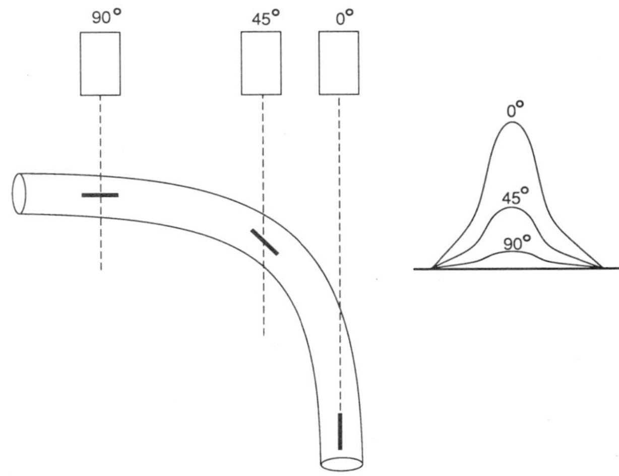

Fig. 5-11. At 90 degrees to the vessel the Doppler shift is virtually nonexistent. At 45 degrees, the shift is improved. At 0 degrees the Doppler shift is maximum.

If the blood cells are not moving fast, you won't get much of a Doppler shift (a bunt). If the blood flow were moving in a different direction, the Doppler shift would be in the opposite, or negative, direction (the batter fouls the ball back toward the catcher). If the Doppler hits the blood cells on an angle and not directly, the shift will be smaller (foul ball).

In sum, the Doppler shift is increased by two factors, assuming the fundamental frequency of the Doppler is the same:

1. Increasing the speed at which the red cells strike the incoming ultrasound beam
2. Decreasing the angle between the direction of flow of the red cells and the direction of the ultrasound beam

Frequency Versus Velocity

If we use a continuous-wave Doppler (discussed later) to obtain a signal from an artery, we do so knowing the constant of velocity through tissue (1,540 m/sec) and the fundamental frequency of the Doppler transducer (4 MHz, 8 MHz, etc.), but how do we know the angle of the ultrasound beam to the flowing blood cells? For the most part we assume the vessel is running parallel to the skin and attempt to keep an angle of 45 to 60 degrees. This is only an assumption, however, and in fact, many times the vessel is nowhere near to being parallel. In this case (blind continuous-wave examination), we cannot utilize the Doppler formula for velocity but are often forced to look at frequency shifts alone.

With duplex ultrasound, on the other hand, the vascular specialist is able to see the vessel he or she is evaluating and assume that blood flow is indeed parallel to the vessel walls (Fig. 5-12). Therefore, by steering the "flow cursor," one tells the system what the angle theta is for the Doppler equation, and the system can subsequently convert frequency to velocity.

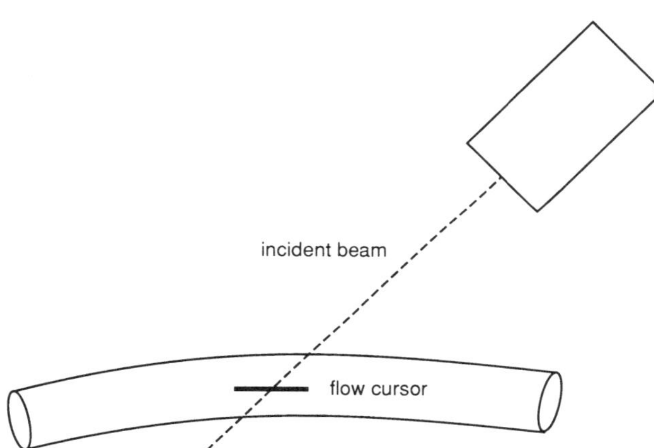

Fig. 5-12. The flow cursor in relation to the incident beam.

Whether frequency or velocity is the more accurate parameter to use when categorizing vascular disease is still being debated. There are two points of controversy. First, because one truly does not know the angle of blood flow to the vessel wall, the assumptions of flow are subject to error. Second, add to this the increased error associated with angles greater than 60 degrees, and the prospect for inaccurate figures increases. Both of these sources of error can have an effect on frequency measurements as well as calculated blood velocities. Before angle-corrected velocities were routinely available, early diagnostic criteria were developed based on frequency shifts. Subsequently, equivalent velocity criteria have been determined. At this point in the debate, the conventional standards for categorizing disease include both velocity and frequency parameters.

Doppler Instruments

There are two main types of Doppler used in vascular technology:

1. The continuous-wave Doppler
2. The pulsed-wave Doppler

Continuous-Wave Doppler

The *continuous-wave Doppler* (CW Doppler) has two piezoelectric crystals, one to send and another to receive. Because there are two crystals, each sending crystal can emit or receive ultrasound continuously (Fig. 5-13).

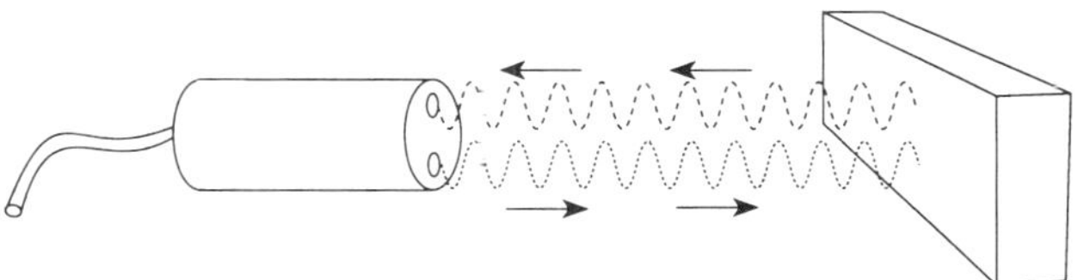

Fig. 5-13. The continuous wave Doppler contains two crystals: one to (continually) send and one to (continually) receive ultrasound signals.

The sending and listening crystals are usually aimed at a fixed depth; otherwise, the listening crystal beam would never intersect with the sending crystal beam and, therefore, would not be able to "hear" the returning signal. The region where the beams overlap is called the *zone of sensitivity*. It is important to know the sensitivity zones of various CW Dopplers in order to determine whether a blood vessel will be in the appropriate range for the Doppler. For example, a 5-MHz Doppler is likely to have a deeper zone than a 10-MHz Doppler. If you attempt to listen to a superficial vessel with a lower frequency Doppler probe, you may miss the vessel.

A primary concern with CW Doppler is the lack of ability to listen to a specific anatomic area, such as one single vessel. In other words, the zone of sensitivity for the CW Doppler defines a fairly large area, which may include more than one artery or vein. The results are sometimes confusing because you will hear both arterial and venous flows within the same signal. And if you think your ears are confused, the spectrum analyzer is equally baffled. The term used to define the inability to listen to just one location is referred to as *range ambiguity*.

On the positive side, CW Dopplers are ultrasensitive to frequency shifts because they send and listen *continuously*. Because they are constantly on, they won't miss very high frequency signals or alias as pulsed Dopplers do on occasion (more on *aliasing* later).

Pulsed-Wave Doppler

The *pulsed-wave Doppler* (PW Doppler) is somewhat more complicated than the CW Doppler. As mentioned earlier, the CW Doppler has difficulty determining the specific vessel location in terms of depth. If an artery lies next to a vein, and they normally do, you will have great difficulty in putting the CW Doppler into one vessel only. The results are a confusing signal from an undetermined depth (Fig. 5-14).

The pulsed wave Doppler differs from the CW Doppler in that it has only one crystal, which both sends and receives ultrasound signals (Fig. 5-15). To do so, it sends out a signal in a short burst, or pulse, and then listens for the signal to return. In a sense, the "mouth piece" becomes the "ear." Keep in mind that these are extremely short time intervals and the PW transducer is sending and listening thousands of times a second.

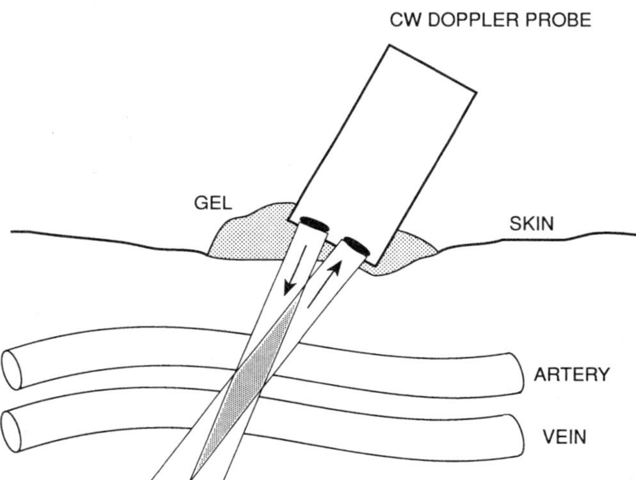

Fig. 5-14. Here the CW Doppler is picking up signals from both the artery and the vein. This can be confusing!

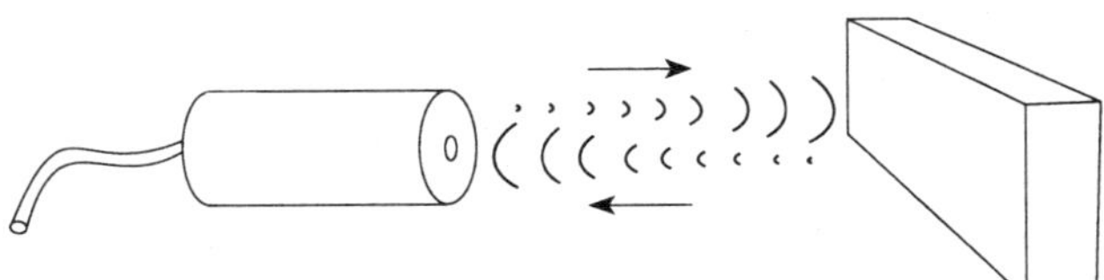

Fig. 5-15. The pulsed wave Doppler contains one crystal, which first sends a signal, then electronically switches to listen to the reflected signal.

The specific advantage of the PW transducer is that, unlike the CW transducer, you can listen to a specific anatomic location. Because you can see vessels with imaging ultrasound, you can decide not only which vessel you want to hear, but also *where* in that vessel you want to interrogate. To understand this, we need to review some previously covered physics.

You recall that ultrasound travels through tissue at a constant speed (1,540 m/sec). Because you can measure the precise location and depth of a vessel of interest, you can perform some calculations. These calculations utilize the single-gate pulsed Doppler system and are based on what you do know: *how deep* the vessel is and how fast ultrasound travels in tissue.

$$\text{Time} = \frac{\text{Distance}}{\text{Speed}}$$

Single-Gate Pulsed Doppler

Let's say you send a friend to the store, which is a mile away, to buy some much needed ultrasound gel. You are very busy and do not want to be disturbed before your friend gets back. You figure that your friend walks at a constant speed of 2 miles an hour, so the round trip should take just about an hour. After 15 minutes have elapsed, a salesman knocks on the door, but you don't answer it because you know it is not your friend; it's too early for her to have made the round-trip journey. Another 15 minutes pass, and you hear another knock—this time a different friend coming to pay a visit—but you don't answer it, knowing it still is too early for your friend to have made the round trip. After an hour, you get up from your desk and open the door just as your friend walks up the steps with the ultrasound gel. Your timing was perfect!

Pulsed Doppler works in somewhat the same way. The system knows how far the ultrasound wave has to travel because you have moved a cursor to a particular part of the artery and the system therefore automatically measures the distance. The system then takes into account that the ultrasound beam must make a round-trip journey from the transducer to the vessel and back again, so it doubles the distance. The system also knows how fast the ultrasound wave travels in tissue (1,540 m/sec) because that has been programmed into the system.

Subsequently, once the pulse of ultrasound is emitted, the transducer calculates how long it should take for the beam to make the round trip, then "opens the door" at just the right moment to let the desired "friend" in. The desired friend could be the Doppler information in the internal carotid artery and not the transverse facial vein, which is lying right next to it.

Sample Volume

When listening to a specific point in the vessel, how large or small is the area? There are a few factors that will determine this.

First of all, as mentioned, the pulsed Doppler system sends and then listens to a signal, but how long does it listen to that signal before it sends out another? If we listen to only the shortest time possible, we are listening to only a very small area in the vessel. This is due to listening to signals "timed" from that very small particular anatomic site. If we "open the door" and listen a little longer, we might get more information than we had intended to hear.

This area being listened to is the sample volume. The larger the size of the sample volume, the longer we are listening to that one specific area. There are two other factors, however, that influence the *sample volume size*.

1. The length of the pulse we are transmitting. A longer pulse length offers longer sampling times and increases the sample volume size.
2. The beam width affects the lateral sample volume size; the larger the beam width, the larger the lateral sample volume size (Fig. 5-16).

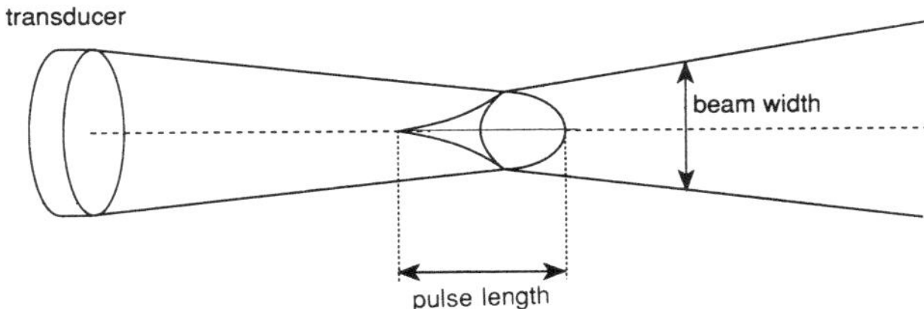

Fig. 5-16. Pulsed Doppler sample volume size is determined by the beam width and pulse length.

Pulse Repetition Frequency (PRF)

The pulsed Doppler system sends a pulse of ultrasound signal, then turns the probe into a listening crystal. As mentioned earlier, it does this very fast. In fact, the speed at which the PW Doppler turns on and off is measured in kilohertz, because it is often thousands of times per second. The number of times a pulsed Doppler repeats these pulses is called the *pulse repetition frequency* (PRF).

The faster the PRF in a system, the greater its ability to send and then listen to a wide range of Doppler frequencies returning from the vessel. Keep in mind that ultrasound must wait for the round-trip journey of the signal before it can send another signal. Subsequently, the farther the signal must travel, the longer the transducer must wait for the returning signal, and the lower the PRF (Fig. 5-17).

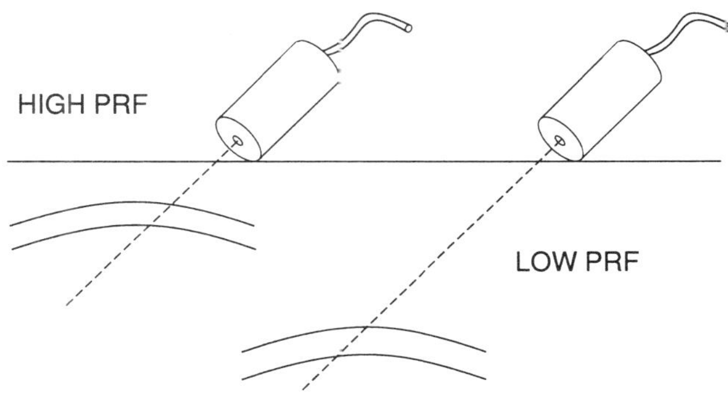

Fig. 5-17. The deeper the vessel, the longer the round trip of the ultrasound signal, and the lower the PRF.

To be as accurate as possible, vascular specialists should obtain as much information as possible as often as possible. If blood flow is moving very fast, we have to sample very quickly in order not to miss any information. Subsequently, we need to turn the Doppler on and off (increase the PRF) as quickly as possible to ensure sensitivity.

There are, of course, physical limitations regarding how quickly we can turn the Doppler on and off. First of all, ultrasound travels through tissue at a constant speed; we simply cannot make it go any faster. Second, we must wait for a signal to return before we can send out another burst of ultrasound. Otherwise, it would be like asking a question and not waiting for an answer before asking another question! In ultrasound, the farther the wave has to travel, the longer the PW has to wait for the signal to return, and the lower the PRF.

The Nyquist Limit (Aliasing)

How do we determine the physical limit (known as the *Nyquist limit*) of a pulsed Doppler system? In other words, at what point do we know when the pulsed Doppler is not going to be able to turn on and off fast enough to capture all the frequencies returning to the transducer?

Using our knowledge of the pulsed Doppler system, we can understand that in order for a transducer to detect a frequency, it must transmit at a PRF at least twice that of the frequency being assessed. Why twice? Because of another inescapable law of physics; that is, to accurately measure a frequency such as a Doppler signal, you must access the signal at least two times for each cycle.

If the PRF of your system is 10 kHz, you will be unable to reliably detect any Doppler frequencies over 5 kHz. While the pulsed Doppler is waiting for a signal to return, some very fast moving cells flow by undetected. Missing high-frequency information due to low Doppler PRF is referred to as aliasing (Fig. 5-18). The rule in pulsed Doppler sampling is that the highest Doppler frequency that can be sampled without aliasing is one half of the PRF. Expressed mathematically,

$$Fmax = PRF/2$$

where Fmax = maximum frequency that can be detected and PRF/2 = one half of the PRF.

Figure 5-18 demonstrates aliasing. Each dot represents a pulse from the PW transducer. The waves represent the frequency of the blood cells. When the frequencies from the blood cells are generally low, the pulses are able to detect the various points along the wave, as seen in the upper two tracings.

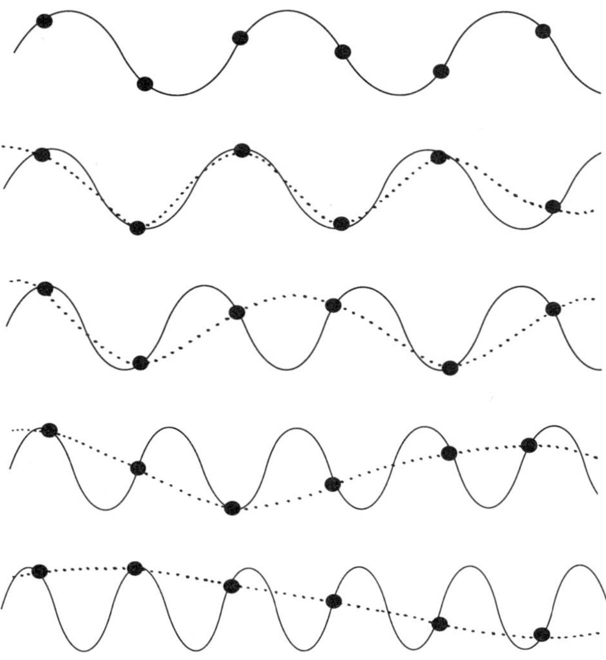

Fig. 5-18. If the reflected frequency (*solid line*) is greater than the PW Doppler's frequency (*dots*), the frequency will be interpreted as a low frequency (*dotted line*).

By connecting the dots, one is able to obtain a representation of the waveform. The more pulses (dots) the more accurate the waveform representation. All of the waveforms in Fig. 5-18 are sampled by seven pulses; notice, however, what happens when the frequency (number of waves over the same period of time) starts increasing. If you connect the dots on the third, fourth, and fifth tracing, you will get a waveform that is dramatically different from the frequency that actually exists. The blood cells are moving faster than the pulsed Doppler's ability to repeat the pulses. That is aliasing!

Effect of Transmitting Frequency on Doppler Frequency Shift

The Doppler shifted frequency is based on the difference of what was sent out compared with what was received back. Trying to make sense of received frequencies alone, without comparing them to what was sent out, simply does not mean much at all.

If you are comparing two different banks for investment, and a friend tells you, "I made $100 by putting my money in my bank," that may sound good, but the real question is how much money did your friend put in the bank initially? If your friend put $1,000 in, then the interest would be pretty fair. If your friend put $100,000 in the bank and only received $100 in interest, however, he'd better go back to Accounting 101! The importance here is not what he got back but the difference between what he put in and what he got back. The more you invest (given a stable rate of return), the more you should get back.

The amount of the Doppler frequency shift also is determined by what was put in. The higher the fundamental frequency of the Doppler transducer (the frequency of your Doppler probe), the higher the Doppler shift contained in the received signal. Given a constant incident Doppler angle, the frequency shifts shown in Table 5-2 are all equivalent and only vary due to the difference in the transmitted frequency used for the examination.

Table 5-2. Normal and Abnormal Doppler Frequency Shifts

Doppler Frequency (MHz)	*Normal (Hz)*	*Abnormal (Hz)*
3	2,000	4,500
5	3,300	7,500
8	5,300	12,000

Effect of Insonation Angle on Doppler Frequency Shift

Remember the baseball park when the batter hit a home run? Although we could not see the ball, we were quite certain the batter hit the ball "dead on" in order to force the ball out of the park. If we could construct the ideal Doppler, it would sit in the middle of a blood vessel and be able to hit the blood cells dead on. In that way, we could get the best frequency shift and therefore the most reliable information. Cardiac technologists are able to accomplish this in some views by being able to aim the Doppler beam at 0 degrees to the oncoming red cells. This dead-on approach sends the ultrasound waves right into the oncoming red cells in order to give a maximum Doppler shift.

Unfortunately, we cannot always aim the Doppler at 0 degrees and are therefore resolved to try for an angle usually between 45 and 60 degrees. Once we go beyond 60 degrees, the information becomes too unreliable to use. In fact, at 90 degrees, the ultrasound provides no Doppler shift because the blood cells are moving across the beam and not toward or away from the Doppler probe. Once the Doppler goes beyond 90 degrees, it again can see the cells moving either toward or away and therefore provides a Doppler shift (Fig. 5-19).

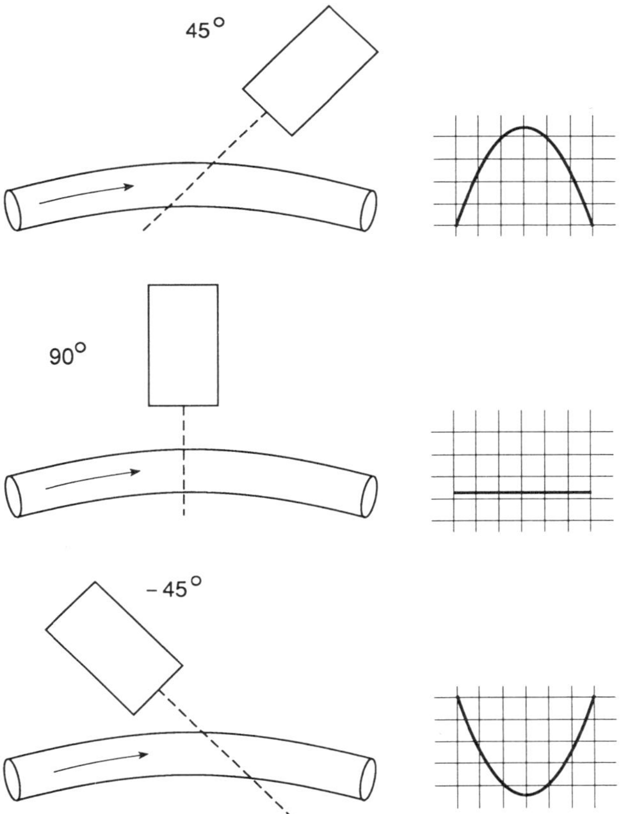

Fig. 5-19. At 45 degrees toward the oncoming blood cells, the Doppler shift is above the baseline. At 90 degrees, there is no Doppler shift. At 45 degrees away from the blood cells, the Doppler shift is negative.

Extracting the Doppler Signal

The block diagram of the Doppler instrument's organization (Fig. 5-20) can appear rather intimidating, but if we break down the components and look at their functions individually, using information we have already learned, the whole picture will start making a lot more sense. Let's start with the CW Doppler instrument.

Continuous Doppler System

As mentioned earlier, a CW transducer (TR) has two separate piezoelectric crystals: one to transmit and the other to receive. What the engineers usually do is take a single crystal and split it in half so that each has a separate function. In Fig. 5-20, T indicates the transmitter, which sends the ultrasound signal, and R refers to the receiver, which receives the reflected frequency. The signals coming back are first channeled to a receiver (R) and then to the comparator (C). The comparator essentially looks at the difference between what was put in and what was received back—the Doppler

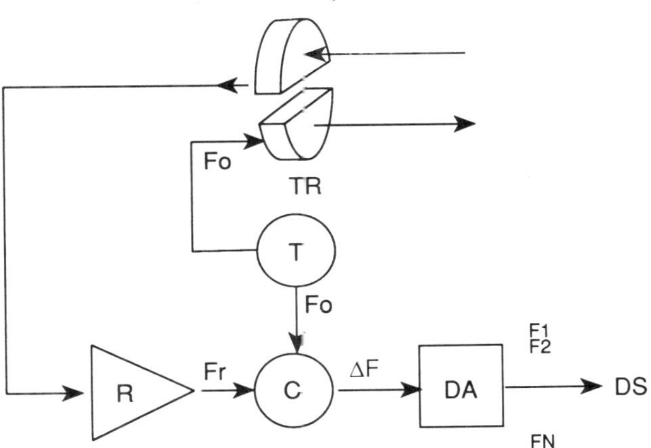

Fig. 5-20. The CW block diagram. R, receiver; T, transmitter; C, comparator; DA, analysis; DS, monitor; TR, transducer. Fo, transmitted frequency; FN, range of frequency components; Fr, received frequency; ΔF, the difference between the transmitted and the received frequency.

shift. These components are then analyzed (DA) as to *phase* (direction), *amplitude* (strength), and *frequency*, and then are displayed on a monitor (DS).

In a factory, you have a similar organization. There is a shipping department, which sends items out; a receiving department, which receives items in; and an accounting department, which compares how much came in with how much went out. The information is analyzed by the corporate heads, and the results are displayed on a chart.

Pulsed Doppler System

The pulsed Doppler system is, unfortunately, not so straightforward (Fig. 5-21). First of all, there is a *master oscillator* (MO), which feeds the ultrasound signal through the *gated transmitter* (GT). The GT is a "gatekeeper" that allows only a certain number of pulses to be emitted at one time. Otherwise, the ultrasound would be transmitted continually, in the same manner as that of a CW Doppler.

While the transmit gate is closed, a certain segment of the returning waves corresponding to the placement of the sample volume is allowed to return, and is then channeled into a receiver (R). From the receiver, the signal enters the quadrature phase detector (QD), which determines which direction the flow is going (forward or reverse). The forward and reverse components are then fed into the Doppler detector (DD). Here, the Doppler shift (ΔF) information is extracted (the difference between what went out and what came in), and that information is sent to the Doppler analyzer (DA), which either displays (M) the phase, amplitude, and frequency or provides the listener with an audible signal (A).

This instrumentation, although more complicated than the CW organization, would be more similar to a one-person business than to a factory. The factory (CW organization) sends and receives items constantly, but the one-person business can send items out only after it receives payment for what it has shipped. The MO watches what went out, then stops further shipments until they have been paid for!

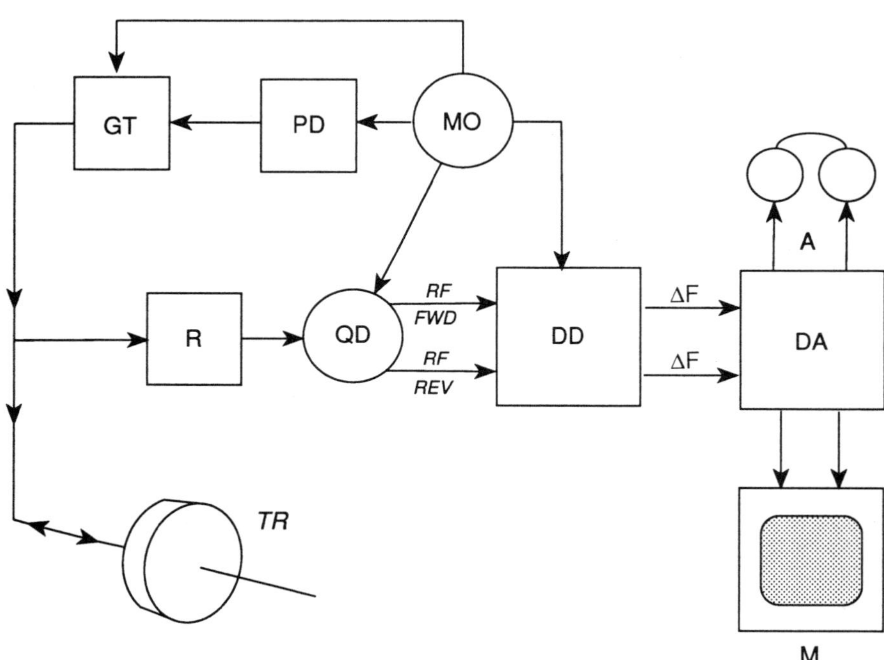

Fig. 5-21. The PW block diagram. MO, master oscillator; GT, gated transmitter; R, receiver; QD, quadrative phase detector; DD, Doppler detector; DA, Doppler analyzer; M, monitor; A, audible signal; PD, pulsed Doppler; TR, transducer; ΔF, the difference between the transmitted and received frequency.

Audible Doppler Signal Analysis

Audible Doppler signal analysis occurs at the end of the Doppler organization. Because the phase quadrature detection has separated the signal into forward and reverse components, this information can be channeled through amplified stereo speakers or headphones. Then the vascular specialist can determine the direction of flow, depending in which ear the signal is heard.

It can be said that the ear is a very good spectrum analyzer. In fact, many vascular specialists can determine adequately the approximate Doppler-shifted frequency values of blood flow simply by listening. Listening is subjective, however, and it is not always suitable for quantifying subjective information.

Analog Doppler Signal Analysis

Zero-crossing Detector

One of the most common early devices used for documentating Doppler signals was the zero-crossing detector. With this type of circuit, a trigger is set each time the input signal crosses through zero in a positive direction and is reset when the signal crosses zero in a negative direction. Counting the number of times the trigger is set for each second in time gives an estimate of the Doppler frequency, or cycles per second.

The zero-crossing detector does not extract the true mean (halfway between the highest and lowest frequency detected); instead, it detects a frequency somewhat higher than mean. These systems tend to cost less than spectrum analyzers but are subject to erroneous signals due to

1. poor probe-vessel angle
2. a broad spectrum of frequencies
3. vessel wall motion
4. a combination of arterial and venous signals
5. weak Doppler signal

In peripheral arterial Doppler testing, an analog signal from a zero-crossing detector will often suffice, providing an adequate representation of direction and amplitude of blood flow. For more accurate information, however, the Doppler spectrum analyzer provides far more specific and accurate data on the complete range of frequencies present.

Spectral Analysis

The term *spectrum* means the entire range or full extent of something. Spectrum analysis of blood flow indicates the ability to analyze how all the red blood cells are moving at a particular point in time.

Instead of having to describe a finding by saying, "Wow, this blood flow sounds weird," or "I think there is something wrong with this internal carotid artery," we are provided with an instrument that allows us to evaluate the blood cells' movement objectively and display that movement on a graph. The graph is essential for displaying information such as frequency, velocity, direction, and turbulence.

If you were in a traffic helicopter flying over a major road leading to a city, you could provide computers with information about the traffic conditions. First, you would report the direction and speed of the cars on the highway; second, the time of day the speed was recorded; and finally, the number of cars on the highway at the time of the report. As the speed of the cars and time of day is plotted on the graph, a pattern begins to appear (Fig. 5-22). We can see that at 8 A.M., there are a number of cars traveling on the road, but they are going quite slowly. By noon, there are many fewer cars on the road, but the speed of those cars has increased significantly. Finally, at 4 P.M., the traffic begins to build up again, and the speed begins to slow down. In addition, you note that a number of cars are going both fast and slow in the afternoon—typical rush hour traffic!

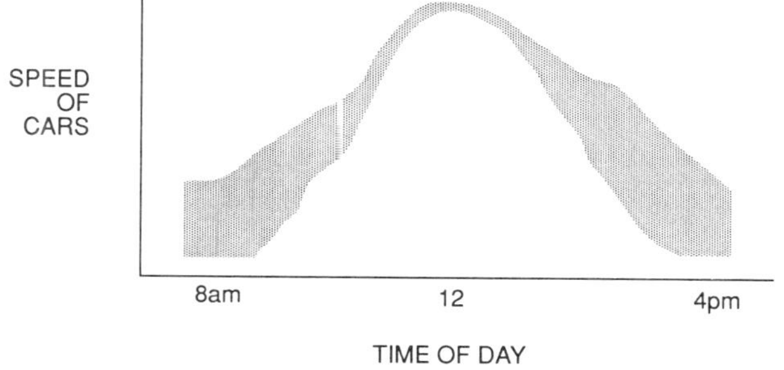

Fig. 5-22. The graphic traffic analyzer.

Spectral Trace

The spectrum analyzer uses the Doppler signal information to plot the frequency or velocity of blood cells in very much the same way the traffic helicopter provides detailed information about the cars on the highway. When a group of blood cells are detected, they are assigned their frequency at a point in time on the graph. As the dots begin to accumulate, a pattern is often recognized in the form of a waveform, indicating the systolic and diastolic portion of the cardiac cycle. Within that waveform, other information becomes available. At what time of the cardiac cycle are the blood cells moving the fastest? Are most of the blood cells moving pretty much at the same speed, or is there a wide range of frequencies? If there is a wide range of frequencies, where in the cardiac cycle does this occur?

If all the blood cells in a vessel always traveled at the same frequency or velocity, a spectrum analyzer would probably be less helpful. In fact, when the blood cells are first ejected out of the left ventricle, they do travel at a relatively uniform rate; the resistance of the vessel walls has not had a chance to slow down the red cells away from the center of the stream. In addition, if the heart were not a pump and all the blood flowed like water from a hose, there would be no systolic and diastolic component of the flow; it would just flow in a steady stream. If we were to have such a system where all the blood cells traveled at the same frequency, and the heart was not a pump but provided a steady flow of blood, an analysis of the flow would look something like Fig. 5-23. If we were to look at flow that is truly laminar, and the red cells near the vessel walls were moving slower than the red cells in the middle, the spectrum would look something like Fig. 5-24.

Because the heart is a pump, however, with a systolic and diastolic component, the spectrum looks more like Fig. 5-25.

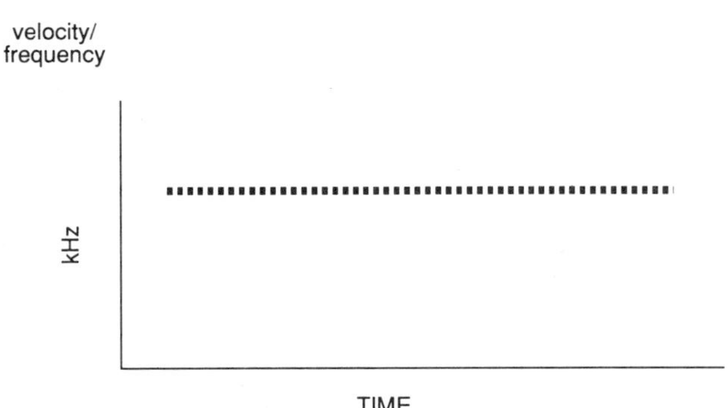

Fig. 5-23. Steady flow at all the same frequency.

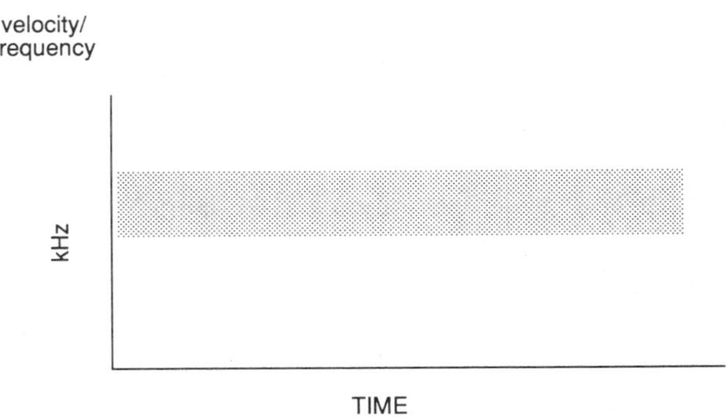

Fig. 5-24. Steady flow with different frequencies.

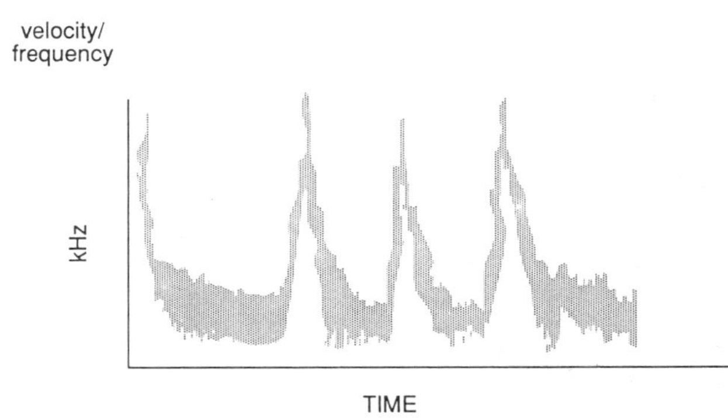

Fig. 5-25. Pulsatile flow with various frequencies in systole and diastole.

Fast Fourier Transform

The fast Fourier transform (FFT) is a mathematical, computerized technique used in real time that analyzes short segments of the Doppler signal into a series of spectra. In other words, FFT provides a lot of information in a very short period of time in the waveform.

The FFT is analogous to the photo finish of a horse race. You may have seen a spectacular horse race in which three or four of the horses seem to cross the finish at exactly the same time. It is difficult even for the observer at the finish line to truly tell who came in first and second. At the finish line, however, there is a camera that takes a photograph directly across the finish line at the exact moment a horse's nose reaches that point. Judges can look carefully at the picture and determine which of the horses was one or two inches over the finish line and subsequently the winner.

In a way, FFT takes hundreds of "photos" along the course of the spectral waveform during the cardiac cycle to provide the vascular specialist with a detailed snapshot of the spectrum at various points in time. This information includes the peak and the lowest frequency detected, the range between the highest and lowest frequency, where in the frequency profile the bulk of cells are traveling, and at which part of the cardiac cycle this "photo" occurred.

The abundance of research performed on spectral analysis provides ample information regarding the significance of these changes. Certain frequencies or velocities may fall into normal categories, and elevated frequencies or velocities will indicate certain levels of disease. The criteria for interpreting these data will be discussed in detail in chapter 6.

Duplex Ultrasound System

Duplex ultrasound implies two instruments within the ultrasound probe: one for imaging and the other for Doppler. The advantage of duplex is that imaging provides anatomic information and Doppler provides physiologic information. The simultaneous combination of this information is far more advantageous than using one instrument alone. Thus we are able to image the vessel we want and, for the most part, place the pulsed Doppler in an exact place to assess the blood flow.

One of the earliest duplex systems utilizes a rotating mechanical sector probe with three rotating transducers. These transducers are sequentially activated as they pass by the skin surface, generating real-time images at 30 frames per second. When an area of interest is imaged for physiologic Doppler information, the rotating scan is stopped and one of the transducers is "switched" to function as a pulsed Doppler.

Another type of duplex transducer uses an "outrigger" Doppler, which is attached to one end of the imaging probe. This Doppler is independent of the imaging transducer and can therefore be steered into the field of view without affecting the image. The advantage of this type of duplex instrument is that it allows the vascular specialist to obtain optimal angles (i.e., closer to 60 degrees or less).

With the advent of linear-array imaging transducers, acquisition of the Doppler mode became a little more complicated. The linear array transducer assigns a certain group of imaging elements to function as a pulsed Doppler in between imaging. The size of this group of elements is referred to as the *aperture*. Through a series of electronic delays and focusing, a pulsed Doppler beam is formed and directed by the operator into the blood vessel (Fig. 5-26). In this manner, real-time pulsed Doppler and imaging is obtained.

Several problems surface with this method of duplex, however. First, we know that imaging is best obtained at an angle 90 degrees to the reflector, and Doppler information is best obtained at 0 degrees to the reflector. The sensitivity of the Doppler is diminished due to the electronic steering necessary to obtain a Doppler angle. Second, the relatively wide aperture necessary to form the Doppler elements results in a multiple of angles intersecting the blood vessel, each of which displays a different Doppler shift. This results in spectral broadening not generally seen in a single-element transducer.

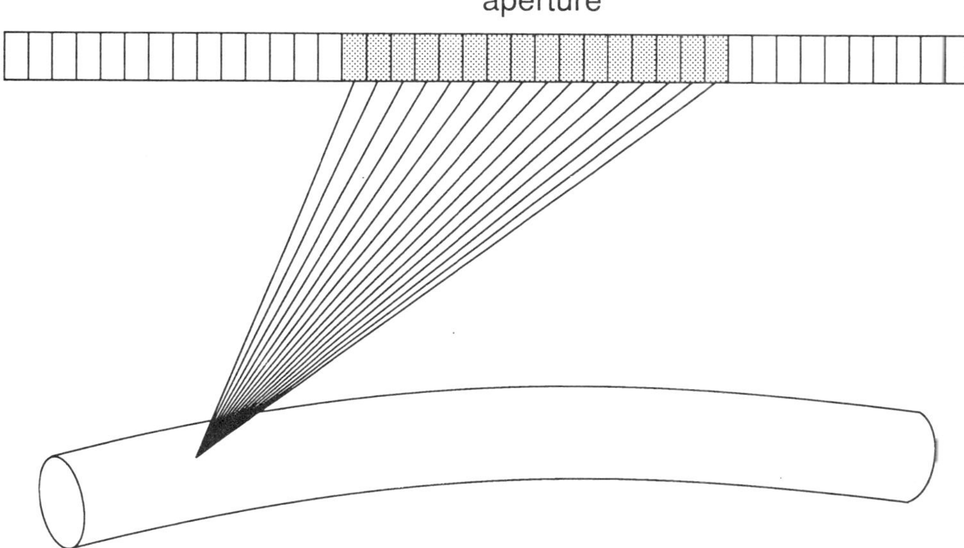

Fig. 5-26. Several elements are focused to form a Doppler beam.

Review Exercise

1. The Doppler formula states

$$Df = \frac{2FV(\text{Cos }\theta)}{C}$$

a. Df = ______________________________

b. 2FV = ______________________________

c. Cos θ = ______________________________

d. C = ______________________________

2. There are three pieces of information that you want from your Doppler instrument:

a. ______________________________

b. ______________________________

c. ______________________________

3. What questions reflect the information provided in Review Exercise 2?

a. ______________________________

b. ______________________________

c. ______________________________

4. The Doppler shift is dependent on how the ______________ ultrasound signal is different from the one that was ______________ into the blood stream.

5. The ______________________________ transmits an ultrasound signal into the blood stream and then listens for the returning echo.

6. If the emitted ultrasound signal is the same as the received signal, the Doppler shift will be

a. increased
b. decreased
c. zero
d. reversed

7. If the blood flow were moving in the opposite direction from the emitted ultrasound signal, the frequency of the received signal will be

a. increased
b. decreased
c. not changed
d. reversed

8. If the ultrasound beam is moved to hit the blood cells on an angle (45 degrees) instead of zero degrees, the Doppler shift will be

   a. increased
   b. decreased
   c. not changed
   d. reversed

9. The closer the Doppler angle is to ______________ degrees, the greater the Doppler shift.

10. The closer the Doppler angle is to ______________ degrees, the lower the Doppler shift.

11. Theoretically, there is no Doppler shift at

    a. 0 degrees
    b. 45 degrees
    c. 60 degrees
    d. 90 degrees

12. The Doppler shift is increased by two factors:

    a. ______________________________

    b. ______________________________

13. The Doppler-shifted frequency is based on the ______________________ of what was sent out, compared with what was received back.

14. The higher the fundamental frequency of the transducer, the

    a. more reliable the information
    b. better the sensitivity
    c. higher the Doppler shift
    d. lower the Doppler shift

15. By aiming the Doppler beam directly at the oncoming blood vessels (0 degrees), the vascular specialist obtains the ______________ Doppler shift.

16. Practical Doppler angles for vascular ultrasound are usually

    a. between 0 and 45 degrees
    b. between 45 and 60 degrees
    c. between 60 and 90 degrees
    d. more than 90 degrees

17. Once Doppler angles go beyond 60 degrees, the information becomes

    a. more reliable
    b. less reliable
    c. more sensitive
    d. less sensitive

18. At a Doppler beam angle of 90 degrees, the ultrasound shift is

    a. maximum
    b. moderate
    c. minimal
    d. zero

19. There are two basic types of Doppler used in the vascular lab:

    a. ______________________________

    b. ______________________________

20. CW Dopplers utilize _____________ crystals.

21. One crystal of the CW Doppler _____________ and the other crystal _____________.

22. The CW beams intersect at the

a. mid zone
b. end zone
c. ozone
d. zone of sensitivity

23. Lower frequency CW Doppler transducers have (closer/more distant) zones of sensitivity than do high-frequency Doppler transducers.

24. The advantage of CW Doppler over PW Doppler is that the CW signal won't _____________.

25. The disadvantage of CW Doppler is

a. aliasing
b. range ambiguity
c. lack of sensitivity
d. lack of penetration

26. The PW Doppler has _____________ crystal(s).

27. A PW Doppler sends a signal out in short

a. pulses
b. amplitudes
c. timing
d. all of the above

28. The specific advantage of the PW transducer is that

a. it won't alias
b. it is location-specific
c. it has two crystals
d. it has a better signal than CW Doppler

29. Because you can see vessels with imaging ultrasound, you can decide not only _____________ vessel you want to hear, but also _____________ in that vessel you want to interrogate with PW Doppler.

30. Pulsed Doppler knows how far the ultrasound wave has to travel, because of the position of the

a. crystals
b. a and c
c. transducer
d. range gate

31. The transducer takes into account the fact that the ultrasound beam must make a _________________________ journey from the transducer.

32. Once the pulse of ultrasound is emitted, the transducer calculates _________________________ is required for the beam to make the round trip.

33. The region a pulsed Doppler system listens to is called the

a. range gate
b. sample volume
c. field of view
d. all of the above

34. The larger the size of the sample volume, the

a. higher the frequency shift
b. lower the frequency shift
c. longer the listening time
d. shorter the listening time

35. There are two factors that influence the sample volume size:

a. ______________________________

b. ______________________________

36. The speed at which the PW turns on and off is measured in ______________________________.

37. This number of times a PW pulses in a second is called

a. Nyquist limit
b. aliasing
c. pulse repetition frequency
d. transducer frequency

38. The higher the PRF in an ultrasound system, the greater its ability to send and then listen to ______________________________ frequencies returning from the vessel.

39. The frequency at which the pulsed system cannot reliably detect any higher frequencies is referred to as the ______________ limit.

40. Aliasing occurs at a Doppler shift frequency

a. of twice the PRF
b. of one half the PRF
c. of the frequency of the Doppler
d. only with CW Doppler

41. At what frequency will the following transducers alias?

a. PRF = 10 kHz ______________________________

b. PRF = 5 kHz ______________________________

c. PRF = 8 kHz ______________________________

d. PRF = 3.8 kHz ______________________________

42. Define the components of the following formula:

Fmax = PRF/2

Fmax = ______________________________

PRF/2 = ______________________________

43. The quadrature phase detector (QD) determines ______________________ of the ultrasound signal.

44. Audible Doppler signal analysis occurs at the beginning of the Doppler instrumentation organization scheme. True or False?

45. The phase quadrature detection separates the signal into ____________ and ____________ components.

46. The "trained" ear is a reasonable good spectrum analyzer. True or False?

47. Fast Fourier transform (FFT) is a mathematical technique used in real time that analyzes short periods of Doppler signal into a ______________________________.

48. A zero-crossing detector is as good as spectral analysis, only less expensive. True or False?

49. Analog recorders take the ____________ frequency and display it on a strip-chart recorder.

50. FFT looks at large segments of a waveform to analyze the spectral data accurately. True or False?

DUPLEX AND COLOR DOPPLER IMAGING

In this section, we will review the fundamental principles of duplex and color Doppler imaging (CDI). Imaging and Doppler ultrasound are rapidly becoming the primary technologies in most vascular laboratories. In many cases, duplex and CDI have outdated much of the previous indirect methods of studying blood vessels.

Key Terms

Aliasing
Aperture
Average frequency
Axial resolution
Color Doppler imaging
Duplex imaging
Frame rate
Lateral resolution
Lines of site
Pulse repetition frequency
Sample volumes
Sensitivity
Steering

We have discussed the benefits of both imaging and Doppler ultrasound. We noted that imaging was beneficial for providing anatomic information and identifying vessels, disease, and plaque characteristics. Doppler, on the other hand, provides the critical physiologic information of blood flow. Now we get to combine imaging and Doppler technology into duplex ultrasound to enhance the advantages of combining anatomic and physiologic information.

Prior to the development of duplex technology, assessing arterial and venous structures was sometimes difficult and time consuming, even in the hands of the best technologists. Performing imaging alone, although beneficial for looking at vessels, failed to provide specific information about blood flow. In addition, the more severely the vessel was diseased, the more difficult was it to evaluate the vessel. Doppler, on the other hand, although helpful in providing physiologic information, was relatively insensitive to low or moderate disease conditions and provided no information about plaque morphology or surface characteristics. In addition, being unable to see the vessel position and direction of blood flow made accurate velocity calculations quite difficult. The marriage of the two technologies resolved many of the limitations encountered by the use of one instrument alone.

Mechanical Sector Duplex

The first type of duplex employed a separate Doppler transducer attached to the housing of the imaging probe. Some of these Dopplers were fixed, making them impossible to steer within the imaging field. Other "outrigger Dopplers" allowed movement by a small lever connected to the Doppler transducer, in order to place the sample volume in the vessel, and more important, at the required angle.

Linear Array Doppler

With the increasing popularity of linear arrays for vascular imaging in the mid 1980s, a new problem and opportunity developed for *duplex imaging*. Linear array crystals could be assigned different tasks in order to allow the transducer to function in various ways. By delaying a group of crystals, the beam could be *steered* in order to better view various tissue interfaces (Fig. 5-27). Another task that could be assigned to linear array crystals was that of making a certain group of elements temporarily stop functioning as imaging crystals and start functioning as a pulsed Doppler during the duplex mode.

This group of crystals could also be steered, although with some difficulty, to obtain reasonable angles for Doppler analysis. Keep in mind that by using elements that are, for the most part, aimed at 90 degrees to a vessel, we have to steer a great deal to obtain a 60-degree (or less) optimal angle. Increased steering by electronic means results in a greater loss of Doppler *sensitivity*, however, so when you are wondering why your linear array may not be getting as crisp a Doppler signal as your old mechanical sector, think about the electronic contortions the linear array is performing. It is the difference between looking at something directly in front of you and glancing at it from the corner of your eye.

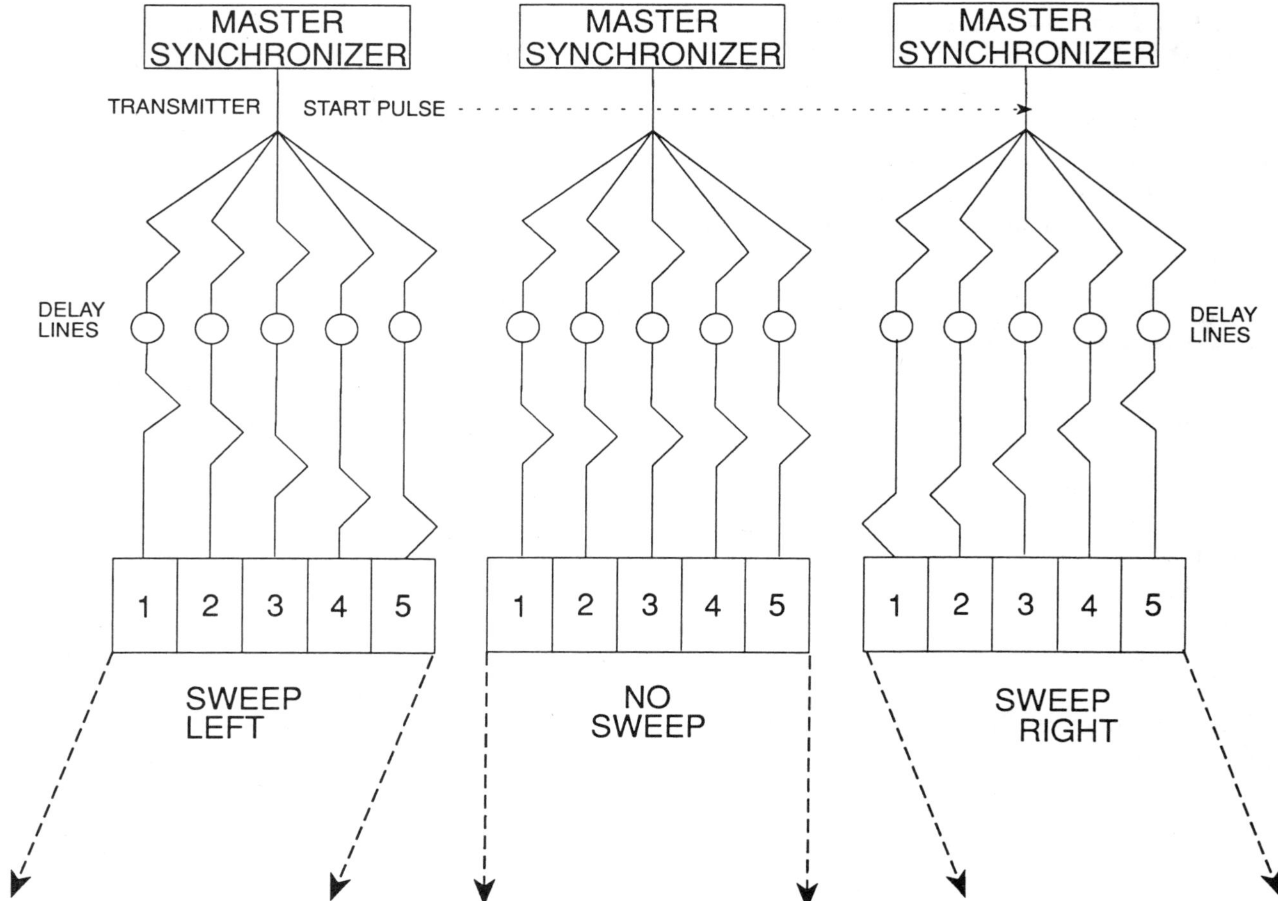

Fig. 5-27. Steering an ultrasound image to the left, center, or right using electronic delays. This enables the user to aim the imaging beam at 90 degrees to the interface.

Color Doppler Imaging

As duplex technology revolutionized vascular technology in the early 1980s, so did color technology a few years later. Although originally designed and manufactured for cardiac ultrasound, color rapidly became extremely popular for vascular applications. Today *color Doppler imaging* (CDI) systems are found in nearly all of the major vascular ultrasound labs.

An ultrasound system used for vascular applications has two primary functions: to detect whether disease is present and, if there is disease, to determine the extent of it. The detection of the presence or absence of disease often can be laborious and difficult. Even thin necks in young patients can prove to be difficult examinations, depending on vessel anatomy and location of the disease. Pulsed Doppler is helpful in finding potential trouble by acting like a spotlight to search the vessel segment from wall to wall and distally to proximally. Once a suspicious area is detected, an appropriate Doppler spectral display can analyze blood flow objectively and provide data to determine the extent of the disease.

Whereas pulsed Doppler acts like a spotlight, CDI functions like a floodlight on the vessel. In essence, color insonates the imaging field with several Dopplers at the same time, each of which looks for phase, amplitude, and frequency (or direction, strength, and speed, respectively) at different points in the vessel. CDI then interprets each of these parameters and assigns a color to each. CDI then overlays this information onto a grayscale image. Sound like a lot of work for an ultrasound system? You are absolutely right. Let's take a look at just how your system performs these many complicated tasks in such a short period of time.

Linear array remains the transducer of choice for CDI for two main reasons. First, linear technology provides large-*aperture* focusing techniques (activating a large number of crystals) in order to obtain varying depth within the imaging field. Mechanical fixed-focus transducers cannot meet these criteria. Second, because linear array allows many imaging *lines of sight* from its number of individual crystals, color Doppler imaging can more easily be applied to those crystals to provide several Doppler lines of listening.

In the previous section, we discussed how different crystals within the linear array transducer could be assigned different tasks. For example, by delaying some crystals at the end of the transducer and gradually lessening that delay down the series of crystals, images can be steered to obtain the optimum tissue interface. If a vessel does not lie perpendicular to the imaging probe, the beam can be steered to that vessel in order to intersect the vessel interface at 90 degrees. In another application, a linear array transducer assigns a few imaging crystals to function separately as a pulsed Doppler. Again, delays allow us to steer this Doppler at somewhat limited angles in order to obtain a suitable Doppler shift.

In the comprehensive vascular examination, a good part of our goal is to obtain an understanding of blood flow—not at one particular point in the vessel, but at the entire segment of the vessel. In the carotid bifurcation, for example, it often is necessary to move the Doppler sample volume through several areas of the vessel to get an understanding of the flow profile and to be certain that subtle abnormalities are not missed. Studying a patient with a large neck and diffuse disease can be difficult and time consuming. So let's construct a transducer that will assist in making this task easier.

First, let's add several additional *sample volumes* along the Doppler line of site (Fig. 5-28). In this case, we are receiving several pieces of information back from a single slice in the vessel. This incoming information from the several sample sites is causing a considerable burden on the system's computer; it is having difficulty performing a complete FFT on each one of the several sample volume sites. So you compromise Let's not do a complete FFT on all the sample volumes; let's just look at the average frequency detected by each one of the individual sample volumes. By doing so, you have relieved the microprocessor of a considerable workload. But there is another problem; it is difficult to look at the number of individual Doppler signals as they come and go with each cardiac cycle and movement of the Doppler. How can we make this a little easier to look at and evaluate?

Let's assign a color-coded pixel to each one of the individual Doppler sample volumes. If the signal is toward the transducer and therefore above the Y axis, we will assign that signal red, and if it is away from the transducer, we will assign it the color blue. In addition, the lower frequencies will be assigned a different hue, or shade, of color. The lower forward-flow frequencies will be assigned a darker hue, or deeper red, and the higher forward-flow frequencies will be assigned a lighter hue of red. Now that we have direction and average frequency, all we need is amplitude; that will be provided by the intensity of the color.

You are still not quite happy, however. Yes, you have a nice sampling site along the Doppler axis, but you want to get a better sense of what is going on around

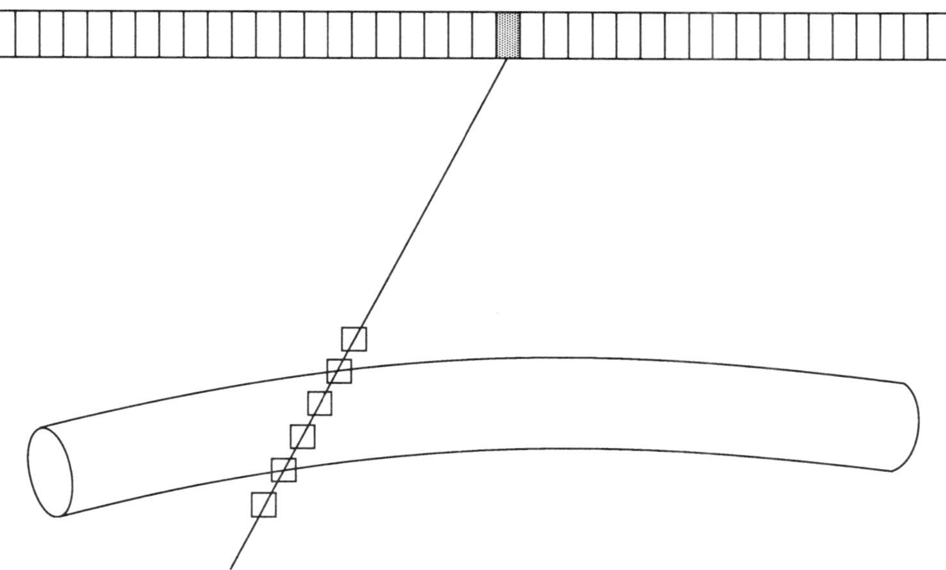

Fig. 5-28. Multiple sample volumes along a single line.

the whole area of the segment, not just a slice! To do so, you will have to ask your transducer to compromise again, and this time you are asking a lot. Perhaps we can shut down the imaging crystals for a frame and just do Doppler. Then we can put in a number of Doppler signals along the entire imaging area (Fig. 5-29). Sure, the image will suffer due to a lower frame rate, but you only want to look at Doppler here and you are willing to make the sacrifice.

Now, you have a number of crystals functioning as Doppler with not one, but several, sample volumes flood-lighting the entire segment of the vessel. After your sweep with Doppler, the crystals electronically switch back to their imaging mode and give you a frame of gray scale. Once that is completed and displayed, the crystals switch back to their Doppler mode and perform their multi-gated color Doppler imaging functions. Although your imaging frame rate has been reduced, all of this is happening so fast that the color Doppler imaging appears to be happening at exactly the same time as the gray-scale imaging.

At this point, there seems to be no end to what you can ask your color Doppler duplex ultrasound system to do, but there is! For one thing, you noticed that the frame rate of your color Doppler has begun to slow down when you add the multiple Doppler lines. The color image appears a little choppy and flow isn't going very smoothly. What can be done to improve the frame rate?

Imagine the ability to have a conversation with your ultrasound system and ask, "Just what's going on? Listen, I want you to perform real-time gray scale at 30 frames per second and in between the sweep of gray scale, I want you to perform one hundred lines of color Doppler, each with one hundred different sample volumes. Then, display amplitude, direction, and frequency as color in various intensities and shades of red and blue. Oh, one more thing. Do this all at about 20 frames per second, so I don't get that choppy look!"

Your system's response will not be what you hoped to hear: "You have got to be kidding! Do you have any idea how much work you're asking me to do in such a short period of time? Even if I had a separate computer to handle just the color alone, it would be difficult. Give me a break!"

You suggest, "O.K.! Let's try this. Because I only need to look at color in the vessel and not in the entire field of view, why don't we reduce the area in which you perform color to a smaller area and only perform the color Doppler imaging in a color box (Fig. 5-30)?"

The computer replies, "That will help, but if you want to keep the frame rate up, you'll have to sacrifice something more!" To which you reply, "Well, maybe I don't need to perform color on every line, perhaps only on every other line. But fewer lines means poorer *lateral resolution* (Fig. 5-31)!" Your system replies, "Too bad! That's your problem, not mine. Keep going."

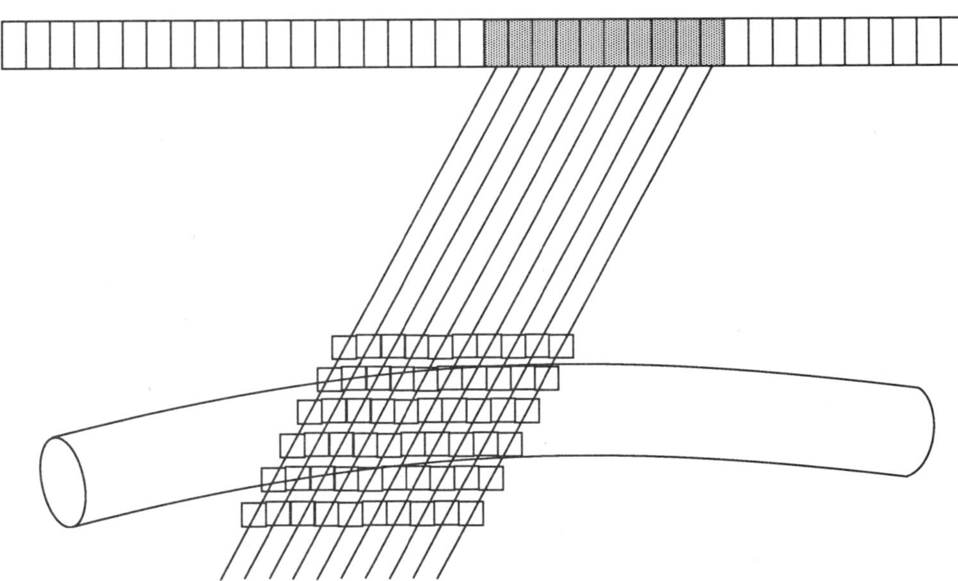

Fig. 5-29. Multiple sample volumes along multiple, different lines.

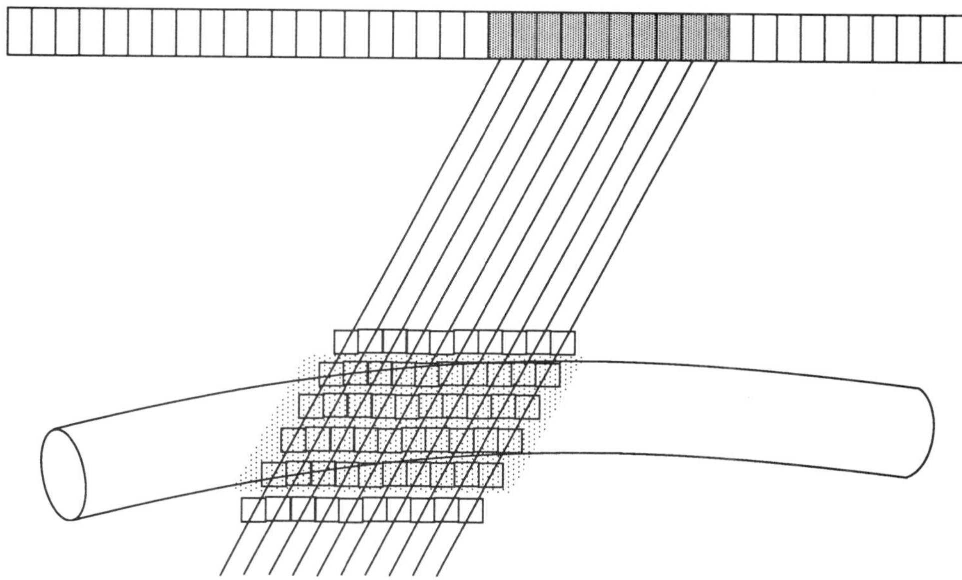

Fig. 5-30. The color Doppler imaging area of interest (*shaded area*).

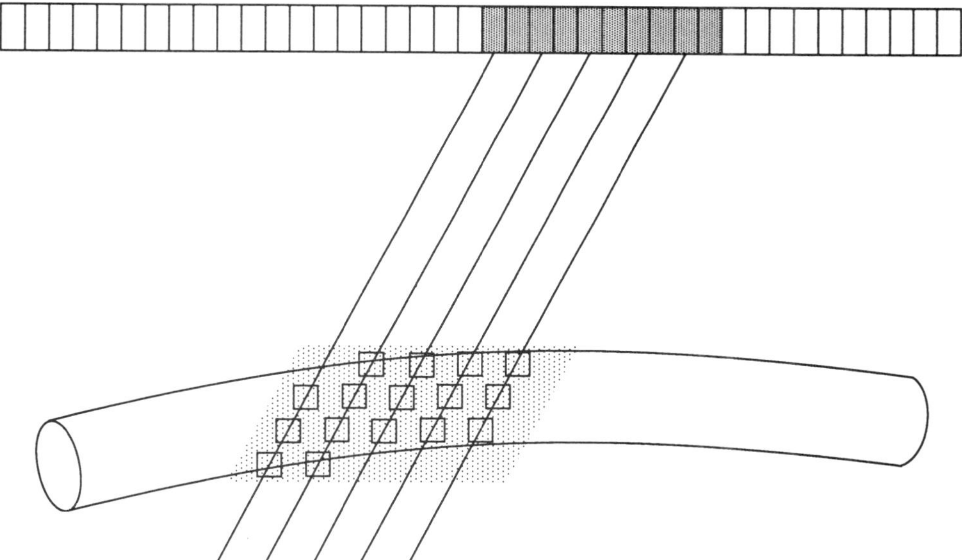

Fig. 5-31. Reduced color Doppler scan lines.

"All right," you bemoan, "I'll decrease the number and the size of the sample volumes, so there is less time listening there, but that will cut down on my axial resolution!" Your system replies, "Now you're talking! Now you can get the frame rate you wish!"

Just when you believe you have the situation under control, you are confronted with yet another problem. Your next patient is one with suspected venous disease and you know that you will need to use lower Doppler frequencies to detect the low-amplitude flow. Low flow, however, requires lower *PRF*. Lower PRF means a longer waiting time between firing, and longer waiting time means slower frame rate.

In summary, color flow requires—first and foremost—a basic understanding about how color is acquired. It is not necessary to go into great depth here about the technology and physics, but it is important to understand the principles and avoid common misunderstandings. Although there are various types of systems producing color flow, the most common method is the phase-shift color Doppler imaging. When using the phase-shift method, remember the following points.

1. Color information is an *average frequency* shift, not a velocity shift. There is no angle correction and subsequently no velocity-flow information.
2. Color changes can occur for several reasons:
   a. Change in direction of flow
   b. Change in vessel angle
   c. Increased frequencies secondary to a stenosis
   d. Aliasing
3. Increasing frame rate may require sacrifices:
   a. Reduced sensitivity (fewer pulses per line)
   b. Reduced lateral resolution (fewer color imaging lines)
   c. Reduced axial resolution (larger sample volume size)
   d. Reduced flow rate detection (increased PRF)
4. Reduced PRF for low-flow states requires more time for the round-trip pulse journey. Frame rates are subsequently lower.
5. Increase PRF for high-frequency flow states to avoid *aliasing*. Frame rates will be higher, but low velocities may not be detected.

Recording Devices

There are various recording techniques used by vascular ultrasound laboratories. What's best for one lab may not be good necessarily for another; it depends entirely on the individual needs and likes of any given department. What is certain is that clear and concise documentation of the examination is important. This is true for primary reasons: first, to ensure that the interpreting physician has ample data to make a confident interpretation, and second, to ensure that recorded data are sufficiently clear to share with other laboratories and departments, as the need arises.

Multiformat X-ray film is common among radiology departments because of the familiarity of the format and accessibility to film development. Black-and-white print paper, usually of a heat-sensitive type, is economical and provides high-quality reproductions. Video tapes are particularly beneficial in that they provide a real-time image as well as real-time pulsed Doppler and color flow Doppler information. In addition, the interpreting physician can listen to Doppler signals while viewing the tape and have the benefit of the vascular specialist's narration of the examination. Finally, color print paper is essential for color flow imaging where video is not available.

Review Exercise

1. Duplex refers to both ______________ and ______________.

2. Duplex allows the acquisition of both ______________________________ information from imaging and ______________________________ information from Doppler.

3. Performing imaging alone, in general, fails to provide specific information about

   a. increased velocities
   b. plaque morphology
   c. turbulent flow
   d. a and c

4. Performing Doppler alone, in general, fails to provide specific information about

   a. increased velocities
   b. plaque morphology
   c. turbulence
   d. disturbed flow

5. The marriage of the two technologies resolved many of the ______________________________ encountered by the use of one instrument alone.

6. Name the two types of transducers most commonly used by vascular specialistss.

   a. ____

   b. ____

7. By delaying a group of crystals, the beam of a linear array transducer can be ______________ in order to better view various tissue interfaces.

8. Imaging is best obtained at ______________ degrees.

9. Doppler is ideally assessed at 0 degrees but realistically between ______________ and ______________ degrees.

10. Although originally designed and manufactured for ______________ ultrasound, color Doppler rapidly became extremely popular for vascular applications.

11. Whereas pulsed Doppler acts like a spotlight, CDI functions like a ______________________________ on the vessel.

12. In essence, color Doppler imaging insonates the imaging field with ______________ Dopplers at the same time.

13. Color Doppler imaging primarily displays

    a. ______________________________, or the direction of a signal

    b. ______________________________, or the strength of a signal

    c. ______________________________, or relative speed of a signal

14. Traditional CDI overlays color information onto a gray-scale image. True or False?

15. Linear arrays remain the transducer of choice for CDI for two main reasons:

    a. ____

    b. ____

16. Color Doppler imaging looks at the ______________________________ shift detected by each of the individual sample volumes.

17. Phase-shift CDI is mean frequency because one cannot obtain the ______________ of blood flow.

18. Color changes can occur for several reasons:

    a. ____

    b. ____

    c. ____

    d. ____

19. List three sacrifices that may be necessary in CDI to increase frame rate.

    a. ____

    b. ____

    c. ____

20. Reduced PRF for low-flow states requires more time for the ______________________________ pulse journey.

21. Lower PRF usually results in lower ____ rates.

6
Vascular Testing

In this section, we will discuss the various noninvasive vascular tests available to vascular specialists. This is not intended to provide the in-depth instruction necessary to perform all aspects of a thorough study. This section is intended to serve as an overall review of the principles of a good history and physical examination combined with the fundamentals of a noninvasive cerebrovascular, peripheral arterial, or venous study.

TESTING FOR PERIPHERAL ARTERY DISEASE

Key Terms

Acute arterial ischemia
Allen test
Ankle brachial index
Arteriography
Biphasic waveform
Chronic arterial insufficiency
Claudication
Functional assessment
Ischemic rest pain
Penile brachial index
Peripheral arterial disease
Plethysmography
Segmental blood pressures
Stress testing
Triphasic waveform

History of Present Illness

Peripheral arterial disease (PAD) is far more common in the lower extremities than the upper. The expanding role of the vascular lab, however, has allowed for a variety of studies of the arms and digits as well. In general, PAD refers to disease of the arteries in either the arms or legs, but technically may include the carotid arteries and aorta because they both lie outside of (peripheral to) the heart. For the purposes of this section, however, we will focus on testing of the upper and lower extremities only.

Claudication

A common complaint from patients suffering from PAD is pain in either one or both of the lower extremities. Pain is subjective and patients will express their symptoms in many different ways—not always as the classic "pain" that you may often think. In fact, the origin of the term *claudication* comes from the Greek word meaning "to limp."

Many times, patients with arterial insufficiency of the lower extremities will describe their symptoms as a dull ache or cramping pain that is predictably brought on by exercise and relieved with rest. Claudication always occurs in the large bulky muscles of the buttocks, thighs, or calf, but never in the foot. The location of the pain helps to localize the disease. For example, pain in the buttocks or thighs usually indicates aortoiliac disease, whereas pain in the calf usually is due to occlusive stenosis of the superficial femoral artery.

The vascular specialist must learn to ask the right questions in order to determine important information about that pain. Understanding pathophysiology will help determine, first of all, whether the pain is vascular in nature or due to other problems that may mimic a vascular disorder, such as a herniated lumbar disc or arthritis of the hip. The pain from a herniated disc is often associated with back pain that "radiates" down the leg. Pain associated with arthritis of the hip or degenerative joint disease may start with walking but actually ease as the patient walks on. If the leg pain is secondary to vascular insufficiency, the patient often will be able to describe the discomfort in such detail as to suggest which artery or arteries may be involved. In fact, it has been said, "A good history is 90% of the diagnosis!"

Acute Arterial Ischemia

A less common presentation of vascular disease is *acute arterial ischemia*. This vascular disorder is a surgical emergency. Acute arterial ischemia most often develops from an embolus, usually from the heart (cardioembolus). Thrombosis is another, although less common, causative factor. Typically, thrombosis originates from an occluded graft, atherosclerotic plaque, or an aneurysm. Patients with acute arterial insufficiency most often will present with what is referred to as the "six P's":

1. Pain
2. Pallor
3. Pulselessness
4. Paresthesia
5. Paralysis
6. Poikilothermia (coolness of the extremity)

The pain of acute arterial ischemia is often sudden in onset and severe in nature. Patients may complain of paresthesia and/or paralysis. The foot often will be pulseless and cold (poikilothermic), especially when compared with the opposite foot. Finally, the leg often will be pale due to the lack of arterial blood flowing into it.

Chronic Arterial Insufficiency

Chronic arterial insufficiency is a far more common presentation of PAD. It stems from long-standing vascular disease that progresses over time. At first, patients will adjust to its limitations by being less aggressive in their physical activities. Perhaps they stop to rest more often or take time to look at shop windows while allowing their claudication pain to subside. In the more severe cases, the patients gradually and continually limit their activities until they perform only minimal walking activity. Once again, the location and extent of the disease often can be identified by a good history!

Where Does It Hurt?

It is important to ask patients where it hurts. Does the pain occur in one leg or both? If it is both, does one leg hurt more than the other? Where in the leg does it hurt: the calf, thigh, or buttocks? (You will find that patients will have little difficulty in either pointing to one area, such as in the calf or ankle, or rubbing the buttocks, demonstrating that the entire muscle hurts.)

How Long Have You Had These Symptoms?

In order to differentiate between chronic and acute vascular insufficiency, it is essential to find out how long the symptoms have occurred. It is not beneficial, however, to have patients tell the vascular specialist that they have had pain for a long time. To some, a long time can mean several days, while to others it can mean weeks, months, or years. Ask specific questions!

What Does the Pain Feel Like?

Is the pain sharp or dull? Does the limb feel heavy or tired? Pain can be throbbing, knife-like, or burning. Some patients with PAD will complain of vague weakness or fatigue in the affected limb. The nature of the pain can help the interpreting physician correlate the test results with those symptoms. For example, a patient complaining of knife-like pain radiating from the back, but having a normal vascular test, might lead the physician to consider a neurologic problem. On the other hand, a patient complaining of dull and aching calf pain in the presence of an abnormal vascular study might suggest a vasculogenic disorder.

What Makes the Pain Worse?

What makes the pain occur: sitting, standing, or bending? Usually, a patient with PAD will complain of pain when walking a certain reproducible distance. Ask how far: in a block, two blocks, or half a block? Does the pain come on gradually or slowly? Pain of PAD typically builds up gradually, especially when patients have to walk up a hill or stairs.

Has the Pain Gotten Better, Stayed the Same, or Gotten Worse?

Peripheral arterial disease is most often a progressive disorder that gradually gets worse over time. Patients will often alter their activities to compensate for the pain, however. Ask patients if their discomfort keeps them from playing nine holes of golf or walking to the mail box. The symptoms of peripheral vascular disease may stabilize or get worse. Most patients don't require surgery and may get better by quitting smoking, losing weight, and exercising. In fact, only about 10% of patients with claudication will progress to a limb-threatening situation.

Ischemic Rest Pain

We have learned in our early studies of pathophysiology that the symptoms of claudication occur when the exercising muscle's demand for oxygen exceeds the artery's ability to supply that muscle with blood. Ischemic pain, you will recall, occurs when the muscles' demand for oxygen exceeds the artery's ability to supply the affected muscle with blood, even at rest.

It is especially important, therefore, to ask if the pain occurs at night and, if so, what do patients do to relieve those symptoms? Most patients with PAD state they will hang the leg over the edge of the bed to get some relief from the pain. This is called *dependency*. In this position, gravity can help blood move to the affected limb. Some patients will say they need to get up and walk around a bit, which doesn't immediately make a lot of sense. When you think about what they are really doing, however, you realize they are increasing their cardiac output while keeping their leg dependent. In addition, walking vasodilates the vessels in the leg, allowing for some minimal increase in flow, at least enough to help relieve the pain. That does make sense!

What Makes the Pain Feel Better?

One of the most important questions you can ask patients, other than what makes the pain worse, is what makes it go away? If a patient tells you his leg pain goes away after taking a couple of aspirin, it is probably not PAD. If a patient tells you her leg feels better if she raises it up in the air, it is probably not arterial disease. Raising the leg in the air will further drain arterial blood from the limb and cause the opposite effect that dependency produces. If the symptoms are relieved with rest, you need to know the length of rest required. And, does the pain stop immediately or gradually after resting?

Functional Assessment

It is very helpful for the interpreting physician to know how much the symptoms interfere with patients' life style. Some people who complain of severe leg pain are still able to work at their jobs full time, but others may not be able to walk to their cars in the morning without having to stop three or four times!

Past Medical History

Related Illnesses

Vascular disease rarely affects only one part of the arterial system. It is not uncommon to see patients with a number of vascular problems, including coronary artery disease or cerebrovascular disease. Ask the patient about these conditions.

Risk Factors

Diabetes Mellitus

Diabetes mellitus (DM) affects 5% of the United States population. Many diabetics are able to control their conditions by watching their diets and keeping their weights under control. On the other hand, uncontrolled diabetes primarily affects the small arteries of the body and may result in blindness, kidney disease, and severe ischemic changes in the toes or fingers.

Cigarette Smoking

It is well known that people who smoke are prone to vascular disease. It is important to document not only whether the patient smoked but also for how long? The term for tobacco use is often called *pack years*. If a patient smokes one pack of cigarettes a day for 10 years, then it is referred to as 10 pack years. If a patient smokes two packs of cigarettes a day for 10 years, it is referred to as 20 pack years.

Hypertension

Because of the relationship between PAD and hypertension (HTN), it is important to document the presence or absence of that disorder. It is also helpful to note the medications a hypertensive patient is taking.

Hyperlipidemia

Most people are well aware of the relationship between elevated cholesterol and vascular disease. In fact, a cholesterol profile is usually included in a physical examination. Ask patients if they have ever had a problem with cholesterol and most likely they can tell you their numbers. Documenting a positive history is usually sufficient, however.

Family History

It is well established that patients with vascular disease often have parents or siblings with the same disorder. Peripheral vascular disease, coronary arterial disease, and diabetes are typical familial disorders that are passed on through generations. Ask whether parents have had any vascular surgery performed or whether members of their families had similar vascular disorders.

Past Surgical History

Prior vascular surgery is particular important in the history, but all major surgical procedures should be noted. Ask patients specific questions: "Have you ever had an operation on the blood vessels in your legs or heart?" Keep in mind that many patients with peripheral vascular disease may be older and a little confused. If some patients claim not to have had any vascular surgery, but you point out scars on their legs, then they might remember: "Oh yeah! I had my veins stripped 20 years ago!"

Physical Examination: Lower Extremities

Inspection

By taking a few brief minutes prior to the noninvasive examination, the vascular specialist will gain valuable information simply by looking at the patient. As mentioned, does the patient have any scars suggesting previous vascular surgery? If so, note them. Is there an absence of hair in the lower extremities? Patients with PAD often have a notable absence hair on the affected feet. What about the color of the feet? Are they deep red (rubor)? Are they particularly pale or demonstrate pallor? Are there any signs of infection? Are ulcers present? These are all signs of vascular disease that are important to note.

Tissue Loss

The progressive stages of PAD typically go from claudication to rest pain and finally to tissue loss. The most common sites for nonhealing arterial ulcers are the toes, the heel, or other pressure points of the foot. Ulcers on the gaiter area are most often associated with venous disease. The gaiter area, as you recall, is the medial aspect of the ankle just above the medial malleolus.

Palpation

While looking at the lower extremities, take a few moments to feel the legs and feet. You may find the back of your hand or fingers are more sensitive to temperature changes than is the palm of your hand. When feeling for pulses, use your fingers, not your thumb; it's too easy to pick up your own pulse in the fleshy pad of that first digit. Train your hands to feel for the location of pulses that will later help direct the positioning of your Doppler probe. Above all, if you don't feel pulses, don't think it's because you are not a good vascular specialist. Accurately palpating pulses is an art that many clinicians will admit is quite difficult to master!

Auscultation

The term *bruit* is a French word that means "noise." Bruits suggest turbulent blood flow in the blood vessel and are often discovered during the physical examination when the physician uses a stethoscope to listen over an artery. Many patients are sent to the vascular laboratory by the referring physician for evaluation of a bruit. If you are feeling pulses in the groin of a patient with suspected peripheral venous disease, take a quick listen in that area. It may be one more piece of information that will help to determine the nature of the patient's symptoms.

Doppler Examination of the Lower Extremities

Prior to beginning the examination, explain to the patient exactly what you are going to do. Many people are unaware of noninvasive testing and some may believe they are going have an invasive arteriogram! A few moments of simple explanation will put the patient at ease and help you obtain a more cooperative situation. In addition, it is a good idea to allow at least 15 minutes after the patient has done any walking or stair climbing.

Be sure the examination room is warm and comfortable. Keep in mind that just because you are warm from running around all morning doing studies, it doesn't mean your patients feel the same. Warm cotton blankets will be appreciated by your older patients and help keep their blood vessels from constricting.

Continuous-Wave Doppler

After palpating for pulses, place a small amount of acoustic gel over the maximum pulse sites, which are located at areas where the arteries are close to the skin. Very firm tissue or bone lies just beneath the artery, making it easier to feel. These areas include the groin, popliteal fossa, the area just behind the medial malleolus, and the dorsum of the foot (Fig. 6-1). Using a high-frequency continuous-wave (CW) Doppler (8 MHz), obtain wave-

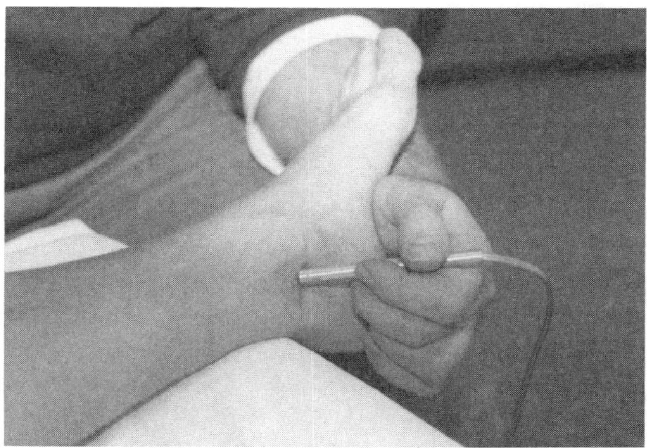

Fig. 6-1. Proper Doppler technique for the posterior tibial artery.

forms of the distal external iliac, common femoral, superficial femoral, popliteal, posterior tibial, and dorsalis pedis arteries. Attempt to maintain a 60-degree angle (or less) to the skin. You will find that slight movements in angle and position either increase or decrease the quality of your signal. Listen carefully while watching the Doppler waveform on your scope. Adjust the gain and speed appropriately.

Once you have obtained the best audible signal, start the strip-chart recorder or if you have an automated system, press "run" on the monitor. Record at least four good waveforms, making sure that you have not cut off either the top or the bottom of the signal. Once you have completed the Doppler analysis, label the waveform and continue to the next vessel.

Interpretation

Interpretation of Doppler waveforms on a zero-crossing detector is subjective. Keep in mind that the zero-crossing detector represents mean frequency and not peak frequency information. In addition, because the vessel angle is unknown, velocity information is unattainable. The patterns of the Doppler signal, however, will provide the vascular specialist with particular information that is extremely valuable in the early stage of the arterial examination.

PHASICITY

Doppler signals are described in phasic terms. Phasicity refers to the direction of blood flow. As you will recall from the section on physiology, peripheral blood vessels normally display a highly resistant flow pattern; blood flow "bumps into" the branches of the terminal arteries and actually "bounces back" a little. In addition, the healthy elastic blood vessel, now filled with arterial blood during systole, contracts again, propelling the blood forward once again. All of these phases are represented audibly and on the zero-crossing detector as direction of flow.

TRIPHASIC WAVEFORM

Subjective analysis is used widely in the evaluation of CW Doppler signals. The normal Doppler waveform is characterized as triphasic, which means consisting of three separate components (Fig. 6-2). An experienced vascular specialist will be able to hear the triphasic audible Doppler signal. A distinct and rapid "one-two-three" sound can be heard, and the recording of that signal reveals a forward, reverse, and another forward component to the signal.

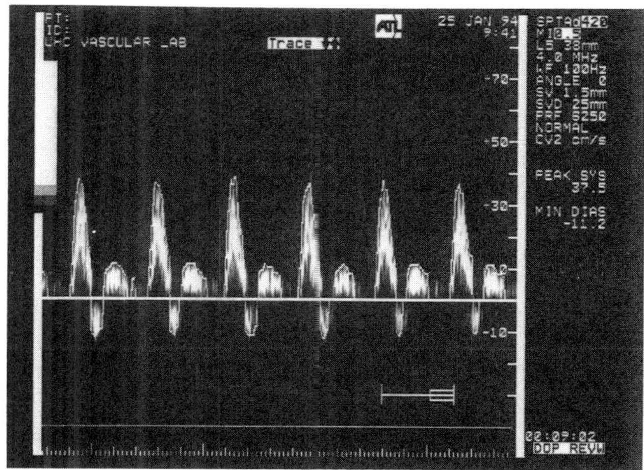

Fig. 6-2. Triphasic waveform.

BIPHASIC WAVEFORM

The initial effect on a waveform in the presence of an arterial obstruction is the change from triphasic to *biphasic*. The second component, representing flow reversal, is lost. The vessel audibly sounds more like a "one-two" instead of the classic "one-two-three" (Fig. 6-3).

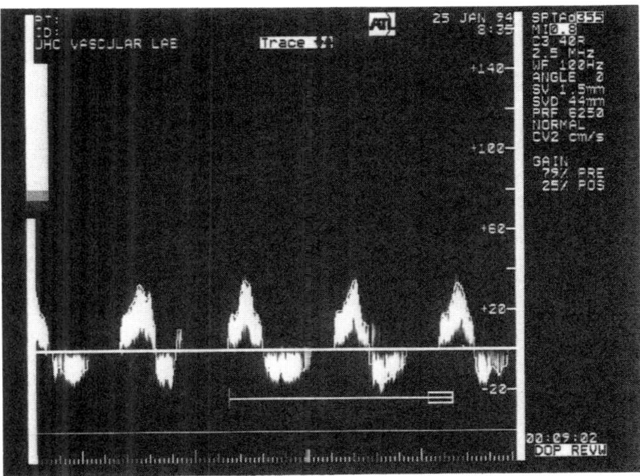

Fig. 6-3. Biphasic waveform.

MONOPHASIC

Next, as disease progresses, the Doppler waveform loses its second phase and becomes *monophasic*. Again, the experienced vascular specialist will hear that change and be able to analyze it before looking at the recorded signal. The monophasic signal simply has one component and sounds more like "one" instead of the biphasic "one-two" or triphasic "one-two-three" (Fig. 6-4).

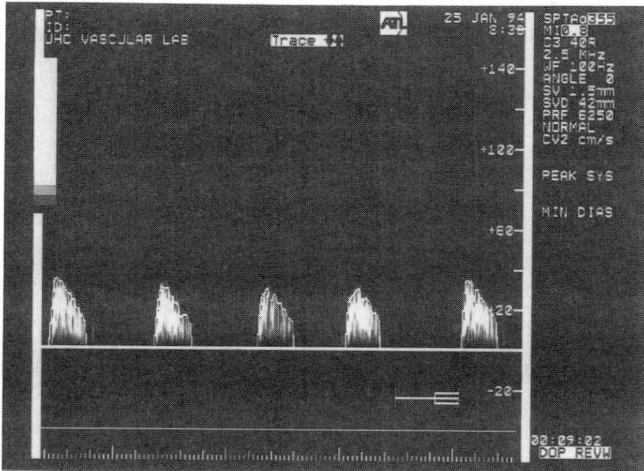

Fig. 6-4. Monophasic waveform.

Segmental Blood Pressures

With the patient on the bed or examining table, apply a brachial blood pressure cuff on each arm. The cuff bladder size for the arm should be 12 × 40 cm. It is recommended that the width of the cuff be at least 1.2 times larger than the diameter of the limb being measured. If your patient has a very large arm or leg, you will need to use a larger bladder. If, on the other hand, your patient has an exceptionally small arm or calf you may want to use a 10 × 40-cm cuff to compensate.

Apply the cuff to the upper arm, ensuring that the cuff bladder is situated against the artery. Palpate the brachial artery pulse in the antecubital fossa (the area where the front of the arm creases). Once you find that pulse, apply a small amount of gel in that area. Holding a high-frequency Doppler (i.e., 8 MHz) in your hand as you would a pencil, lightly place the probe over the brachial artery at approximately 60 degrees (or less) and obtain the best signal possible. Inflate the cuff to slightly beyond where the signal disappears (about 10 mmHg). At this point, slowly release the pressure in the cuff until the signal reappears and note the number on the sphygmomanometer. Record the findings and repeat this procedure for the other arm.

Next, apply the thigh, calf, and ankle cuffs. There are two methods of cuff placement for the lower limbs: either high and low-thigh method or a single larger thigh cuff. The single larger thigh cuff compensates for the larger muscle mass, but many labs prefer using the high/low-thigh method. For the purpose of this lesson, we will use the high/low-thigh method.

Place four cuffs around each limb: Keeping in mind that larger cuffs are necessary for the thighs, put a large 12-cm cuff at the levels of the high-thigh and low-thigh regions. Place a 12-cm cuff around each calf at the area of greatest muscle mass and a 10-cm cuff around each ankle.

Be certain that the cuffs are tight enough. A simple test for this: When two fingers are inserted between the cuff and the skin, they should fit snugly (Fig. 6-5). This may not be as important for taking blood pressure as it will be for the pulse volume recording, but because you will most likely use the same cuffs for the procedure, do it right the first time!

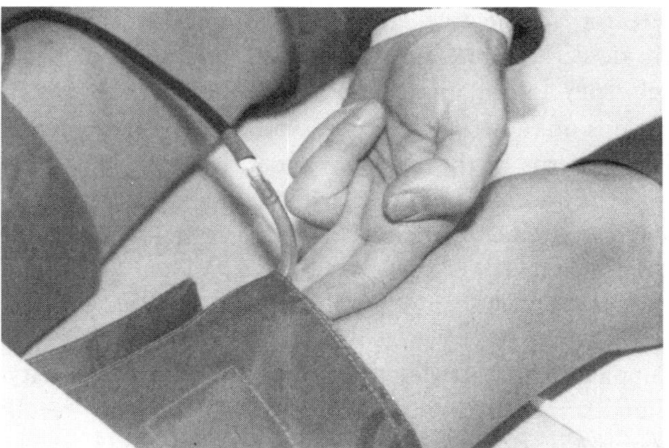

Fig. 6-5. Proper fitting of leg cuffs. Two fingers should fit snugly between the cuff and the thigh.

To find a Doppler signal at the dorsalis pedis artery, take a pressure measurement of the ankle in the same fashion as for the brachial pulse. Repeat the ankle pressure again, this time using the posterior tibial artery, which is found just posterior to the medial malleolus. You may also obtain a measurement from the peroneal artery, which is found just anterior to the lateral malleolus. This is not customary, however, and whether to perform this added procedure is up to the lab director. On the other hand, in an extremely ischemic limb, the peroneal artery may be the only site at which a Doppler signal may be found. Record your measurements from each artery on both ankles.

Foot and Digital Arterial Pressures

Foot pressures can be obtained by placing a small 7-cm cuff around the transmetatarsal region, or mid-foot, and obtaining an arterial signal by either Doppler or photoplethysmography (PPG) (Fig. 6-6). Obtain your Doppler signal at the deep plantar artery. This vessel is an extension of the dorsalis pedis artery, and it courses between the first and second digit. If a signal is not found here with a Doppler, use the PPG method that is described next.

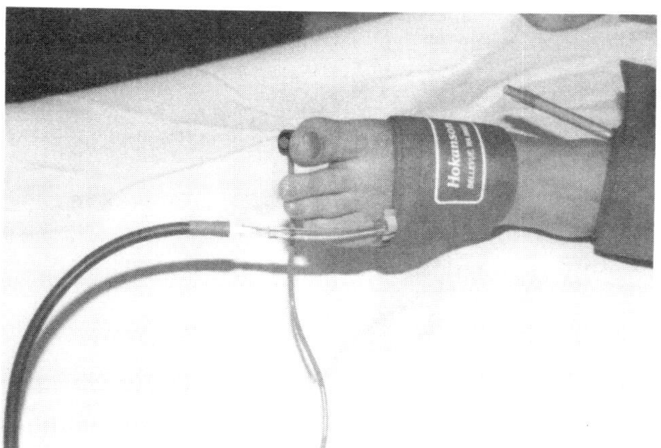

Fig. 6-6. Using PPG to assess foot pressures.

Arterial pressure with PPG is obtained by placing a small piece of double sticky tape on the fleshy pad of the distal phalanx (toe). First obtain a PPG signal, then inflate the transmetatarsal cuff in the usual fashion for obtaining a blood pressure until the PPG signal disappears. Gradually release the pressure and watch for the signal to reappear. Document the pressure at which your signal reappears.

Toe pressures are obtained by placing a 2.5-cm digital cuff around the base of the phalange. Place the PPG on the pad of the distal phalange using double sticky tape to secure it. Gently inflate the cuff, as it will not take too much air to fill it. Slowly release the pressure and document the pressure at which the PPG signal reappears.

Once the ankle pressures are obtained, you can proceed to the more proximal calf and thigh cuffs, repeating the same procedures that were done for the ankle pressure, with one exception. It is not necessary to take measurements of both the dorsalis pedis and posterior tibial at each level. Use only the vessel with the highest pressure in the foot.

You might be wondering why the vascular specialist wouldn't simply measure pressure from the brachial down to the thigh, calves and then the ankles. It would seem to be more orderly! If you find the pressures normal in the ankle, there is no need to continue measuring the other segments unless you think the vessel is noncompressible. (*Noncompressible* refers to the inability to compress the artery in a normotensive patient beyond 180 mmHg.) This condition is typical of diabetic vascular disease and is assumed to be secondary to calcinosis (heavy deposits of calcium) in the artery.

Interpretation

Normally, the thigh pressure is about 20 mmHg above the brachial pressure. This is due to the relatively larger muscle mass in the thigh when compared with the upper arm. In addition, most thigh cuffs, particularly when using the two-cuff method, are smaller than the recommended 1.2 times or 20% larger-than-limb diameter. If, however, one chooses the single larger thigh cuff, that pressure should be close to the brachial pressure.

The purpose of the two thigh cuffs is to attempt to differentiate between aortoiliac disease and superficial femoral artery disease. Because high- and low-thigh pressures are normally greater than brachial pressures, a finding of lower thigh to brachial pressures may indicate significant aortoiliac disease. Decreased thigh pressure, however, may also indicate proximal femoral artery disease when the profunda and superficial femoral arteries are affected. Finding a good Doppler signal at the distal iliac artery should further help to sort out this dilemma.

When the high-thigh cuff pressure is greater than the brachial pressure, but the more distal thigh cuff pressure is lower than the high-thigh cuff pressure, the superficial femoral artery may be diseased. If only the thigh cuff pressure of one limb is equal or lower than the brachial pressure, then the iliofemoral arterial system on that side should be suspected of having disease.

A 20-mmHg drop in pressure from the thigh to the calf suggests distal superficial femoral or popliteal artery disease. Finally, a 20-mmHg gradient between the calf and ankle suggests hemodynamically significant disease in the tibial and peroneal segments, which include the anterior and posterior tibial arteries and the peroneal artery.

Transmetatarsal cuffs can also give abnormally high pressures because the arteries in the foot are very close to the surface of the foot and are not necessarily easy to compress. In general, a pressure gradient from one cuff to another which is greater than 20 mmHg usually indicates significant disease in the intervening artery. When the pressure drops more than 40 mmHg, a total occlusion should be suspected.

Ankle Brachial Index

The *ankle brachial index* (ABI) is one of the most commonly used measurements for arterial sufficiency. It is simple to perform either in the office or on the ward. The ABI allows the vascular specialist to normalize the ankle pressure effectively, regardless of the brachial pressure. In other words, we use the brachial pressure as the norm and compare the ankle pressure to it. If both the ankle pressure and the brachial pressure are relatively the same, one can assume there is little or no peripheral vascular disease. An ankle brachial index is obtained by dividing the ankle pressure by the arm pressure.

$$\text{Ankle brachial index} = \frac{\text{ankle pressure}}{\text{brachial pressure}}$$

For example, if a patient had a brachial pressure of 150 mmHg and an ankle pressure of only 75 mmHg, the formula would read

$$\text{ABI} = \frac{75 \text{ mmHg}}{150 \text{ mmHG}}$$

$$\text{ABI} = 0.50$$

Calculate the following ABIs:

Brachial Pressure	Ankle Pressure	ABI
120 mmHg	100 mmHg	____
150 mmHg	150 mmHg	____
160 mmHg	20 mmHg	____

An interpretation of these figures is as follows:

≥ 9.0	Normal
0.75 to 0.9	Mild disease
0.5 to 0.75	Moderate disease
0.35 to 0.5	Severe disease
0.25 to 0.35	Consistent with rest pain/ischemia
< 0.25	Consistent with nonhealing

A somewhat simplified interpretation is as follows:

Ankle brachial index	≥ 9.0	Normal
Ankle brachial index	0.5 to 1.0	Suggestive of single-segment disease
Ankle brachial index	0 to 0.5	Suggestive of multilevel disease

Toe Brachial Index

Toe pressures normally are lower than ankle pressures. Subsequently, a toe brachial index is not considered abnormal unless it is below 0.64.

Limitations

Although segmental limb pressures and ABIs are two of the most common noninvasive studies performed in the vascular lab, they are not without limitations. One of the most typical pitfalls, previously mentioned, involves the noncompressible vessels found in the diabetic patient. The calcified vessels associated with diabetes prevent the blood pressure cuff from compressing the blood vessel. Subsequently, one can apply as much as 180 mmHg to a cuff without compressing the artery. Normally, if you reach a systolic pressure of 180 mmHg, you need not inflate the cuff any further. It won't compress.

If you have a patient with particularly large legs, and you use the standard 12-cuff size, blood pressures can be erroneously high. Always keep in mind the 1.2 times-greater-than-limb diameter rule.

Stress Testing

Claudication is one of the most common presenting symptoms in patients who have an evaluation of the lower extremities. The patient states, "When I walk a certain distance, my leg hurts." The cause of that pain, you recall from your studies of pathophysiology, results when the demand for blood to the muscle exceeds the artery's ability to deliver that blood to the legs during exercise. When the patient rests, the pain goes away, because the demand for oxygenated blood has lessened. To better understand this concept, let's review some fundamental physiology.

The blood vessels normally respond to a demand for greater blood supply during exercise by vasodilation. Vasodilation results in a decrease in peripheral resistance, thus allowing more blood to flow into the extremity. If a significant stenosis exists, however, the blood vessels will respond further by attempting to dilate the peripheral vessels even more in an effort to maintain a sufficient blood supply.

Most patients with significant vascular insufficiency will have abnormal findings of the segmental pressures and ankle brachial indices. A large number of patients, however, have borderline conditions in which the vascular disease is mild to moderate. Segmental blood pressures and ankle brachial indices performed on these patients may be normal. Does this mean that these patients do not have vascular disease or that they are faking? Neither!

Because these patients experience pain only during exercise, that is the time you need to evaluate their vascular status. If they do have vascular insufficiency, the ankle blood pressures will most likely drop during exercise. This is a type of stress testing performed on the muscles of the lower extremities. There are several methods used to stress muscles for testing:

1. Walking the patient
2. Toe ups
3. Treadmill testing
4. Reactive hyperemia

Walking the Patient

Perhaps the simplest stress test that can be performed is to walk patients until symptoms force them to stop. Patients who have pulses at rest may no longer have palpable pulses after exercise. This is referred to as the *disappearing pulse syndrome*. Blood previously flowing to the foot at rest is now being shunted to the muscles, and the foot pulses disappear! This technique also can be applied to noninvasive testing by obtaining a baseline study and then repeating that study after patients walk.

Toe Ups

One way to give your calf muscles a workout is simply to stand flat on your feet, rise up on your toes, and slowly drop back on to the flat of your feet (Fig. 6-7). Just try it! Vascular disease or not, you will find this quite stressful to your calf muscles. The same noninvasive technique described for walking may be applied here.

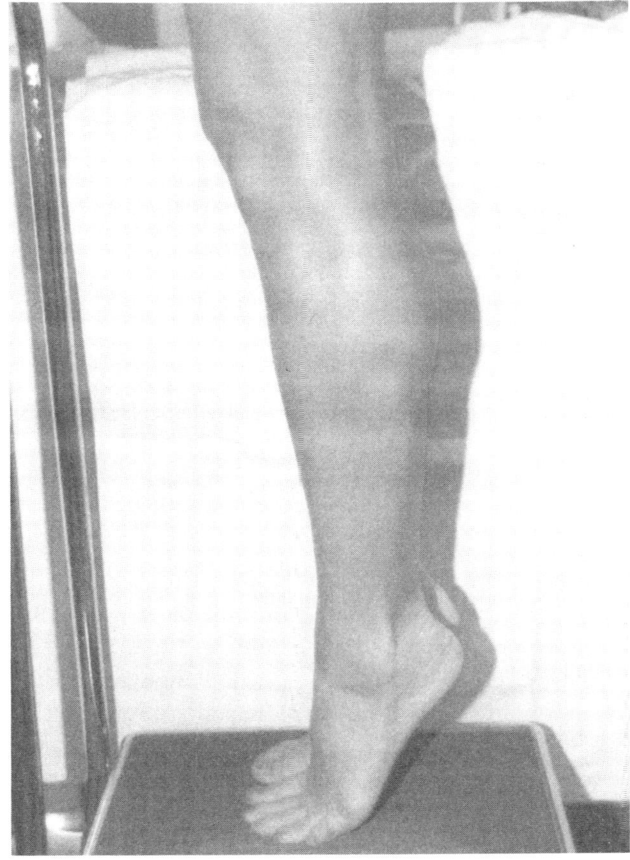

Fig. 6-7. Toe-up stress testing.

Treadmill Testing

One drawback of either walking the patient or performing the toe-up method is the lack of a standard with which to compare your results. Some patients clearly walk faster than others, and some patients may be less vigorous with toe-up exercise. The most controlled method for stressing muscles, therefore, is the use of a treadmill. This device allows the vascular specialist to measure time, distance, speed, and elevation (degree of difficulty). It also allows the patient to be in close proximity to the testing equipment.

An important consideration with treadmill testing is the physical layout of the laboratory. It would be ideal to measure the pressures continuously during treadmill exercise in order to time the immediate changes of pressures in the lower extremity. Because this is impossible with current systems, it is important to measure the findings as quickly after exercise stressing as is possible in order to document the physiologic changes that occur in relation to the patients' symptoms. Have Doppler, gel, and blood pressure cuffs neatly laid out in order to limit time between the end of the treadmill exercise and obtaining the results.

Another important consideration is EKG monitoring for patients over 50 years of age or for those with any symptoms of heart disease. Because arterial disease rarely is limited to only one arterial segment, the vascular specialist must be aware of cardiac conditions. If the vascular specialist is not trained in recognizing an abnormal EKG, however, monitoring may provide little benefit. In addition, if personnel are not trained in cardiopulmonary resuscitation, it may be wise to avoid stress testing altogether. It is best to consult with the medical director regarding your policy and procedures in this matter.

The standard set-up for treadmill testing is usually 2 miles per hour at a 12% grade. For some elderly patients the speed may be reduced to 1 mile per hour, if necessary, but be certain to note the speed change in reports. After obtaining a baseline study, explain the treadmill procedure to the patient. In some cases, it may help to demonstrate, because the abrupt whirring of the electric motor may be a little startling to some patients.

The stress test begins by having the patient step onto the moving treadmill while holding onto the support bar. There will be a tendency by some patients to lean on the bar; be certain to discourage this as it will adversely affect the test. The patient will be urged to walk up to 5 minutes, if possible. If, at any point, the patient expresses any chest pain or significant shortness of breath, do not hesitate to abort the test.

What we are looking for here is the pain that brought the patient to the vascular laboratory. Tell the patient to inform you of any symptoms he or she may be feeling during the test. If and when the symptom of claudication does occur, encourage the patient to walk a little bit further to ensure good test results. Then, stop the treadmill and quickly assist the patient over to the examining table.

As quickly as possible, apply the blood pressure cuffs to the ankles and take a blood pressure of the leg with the greatest symptoms first. Repeat this procedure every 30 seconds for the first 4 minutes and then every minute up to 10 minutes. If the values return back to the baseline at any time before the 10 minutes are up, it is unnecessary to continue this process.

Interpretation

There are three important findings that are essential for documenting the results of the stress test:

1. The length of time the patient was able to walk
2. The maximum drop in the ankle brachial index
3. The time required for the values to return to the baseline

Reactive Hyperemia

Some patients studied in the vascular lab, for one reason or another, find treadmill exercise impossible, or you may have decided that your department lacks the equipment and/or training to provide adequate EKG monitoring during exercise. Reactive hyperemia testing provides you with the ability to stress the lower extremities without having the patient perform physical exercise. Reactive hyperemia is a method that simulates the distal artery's response to exercise by temporarily decreasing blood supply to the lower extremities, thereby simulating vasodilation.

After taking a baseline ankle brachial index, two large thigh cuffs (19-cm wide) are placed around the thighs. The legs are then elevated to 45 degrees to drain them of venous blood, and at the same time, the thigh cuffs are inflated above brachial systolic pressure. The legs are then returned flat on the examination table and the pressure is maintained in the cuffs for a period of between 2 to 5 minutes, or as long as the patient can tolerate the procedure. At the end of that period, the cuffs are deflated rapidly and ankle brachial pressures are obtained every 30 seconds for up to 4 minutes, or until the pressures return to baseline. The normal response to stress testing would be an increase in pressures and waveforms. An abnormal test occurs when there is any pressure drop below the baseline study. As with treadmill testing, duration, pressure drops, and time to baseline must be recorded.

Plethysmography

Pulse Volume Recording

Segmental limb pressures provide relatively specific information about the major arterial branches of the lower extremity. By placing a Doppler over an artery and compressing it proximately with a cuff, one can assess the patency of the particular artery or arterial segment being examined. From those studies we assume blood flow for the entire limb segment.

As we have learned, however, pathological conditions such as arterial stenosis or occlusion alter normal arterial anatomy significantly. We know that an occlusion of a single artery does not necessarily mean a patient requires immediate surgery or is threatened with limb loss. Collateral vessels often adequately provide the necessary diversion for blood flow to the tissue of the affected limb. In addition, calcified vessels, common in patients with peripheral vascular disease, prohibit an accurate assessment of blood flow in the affected limb. So, how do we measure the blood flow in a limb? In these cases, *plethysmography* may offer important information about total blood supply in a given limb segment.

When you place your fingers on an artery to feel for a pulse, you make an assessment of not only whether the pulse is present or absent, but also the quality of the pulse. It may be strong or weak. You may classify it as 1+ or 4+. If you could place your hands around an entire limb and sense the subtle changes through your fingers of all the blood passing through the limb at each pulse and record those exact changes, you would be performing a form of plethysmography. Plethysmography refers to the blood volume change in a limb segment.

Technique

By using the same blood pressure cuffs for the segmental blood pressures, the vascular specialist can, with the proper equipment, perform pulse volume recordings (PVRs). The snugly fitting cuffs are left in place and the noninvasive equipment is changed to the PVR or volume pulse recording (VPR) mode. Air is injected into the cuff until a preset pressure of 65 mmHg is obtained. Be sure the patient is warm and comfortable and does not move during the test.

Transducers in the PVR system record the pulsatile volume changes at each cuff segment. Normally, blood flow rapidly fills a limb segment during systole. The limb segment filled with increased blood supply actually increases in diameter in order to accommodate the increased volume of blood. During diastole, the blood rapidly exits that limb segment and the limb size decreases. Those volume changes are recorded on either a strip chart recorder or an oscilloscope. The rapid filling of a limb segment is represented by a sharp rise in the waveform during systole and a rapid drop during diastole. In addition, the healthy elastic recoil of a normal artery reveals an extra blip on the diastolic downslope of the waveform. This is referred to as the *reflected dicrotic notch.* Recently developed systems store the waveforms and print them out on the final report: no cutting and pasting!

Interpretation

Amplitude

Most PVRs are interpreted qualitatively by evaluating the amplitude and morphology of the waveform. A good volume of blood in the limb will produce a good-sized waveform that is relatively consistent with the amplitude of the other waveforms. If there is a significant stenosis or occlusion of a major artery, the amplitude of that waveform will be diminished. Several other factors can affect PVR amplitude:

1. Ventricular stroke volume
2. Blood pressure
3. Vasomotor tone
4. Blood volume

PVRs are universally affected by exercise. As you will recall, the increased demands of muscles during exercise require an increase in blood volume. This occurs due to a decrease in peripheral resistance. Subsequently, the waveform produced after exercising will normally have a larger amplitude. Conversely, a significant arterial obstruction that impedes blood flow to the muscle will reflect a decreased PVR amplitude. Walking time, level of decrease, and recovery time are important to document.

The amplitude may be interpreted as

1. normal
2. diminished
3. blunted
4. flat

Morphology

The PVR contour also provides important information about the quality of blood flow in the limb. As described earlier, the waveform typically shows a rapid rise in the systolic upstroke followed by a somewhat slower fall in diastolic downstroke. In addition, the downstroke is briefly interrupted by a blip referred to as the reflected dicrotic notch (Fig. 6-8).

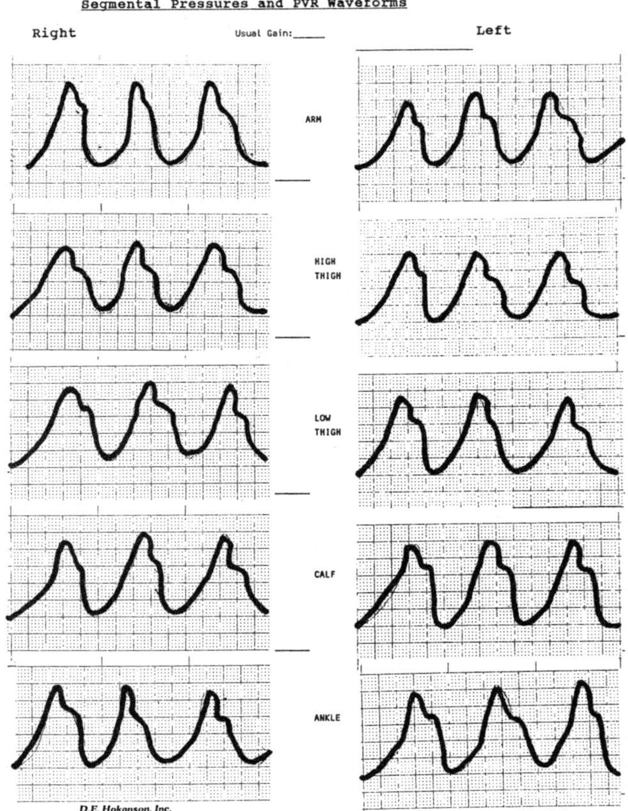

Fig. 6-8. Normal pulse volume recording waveforms.

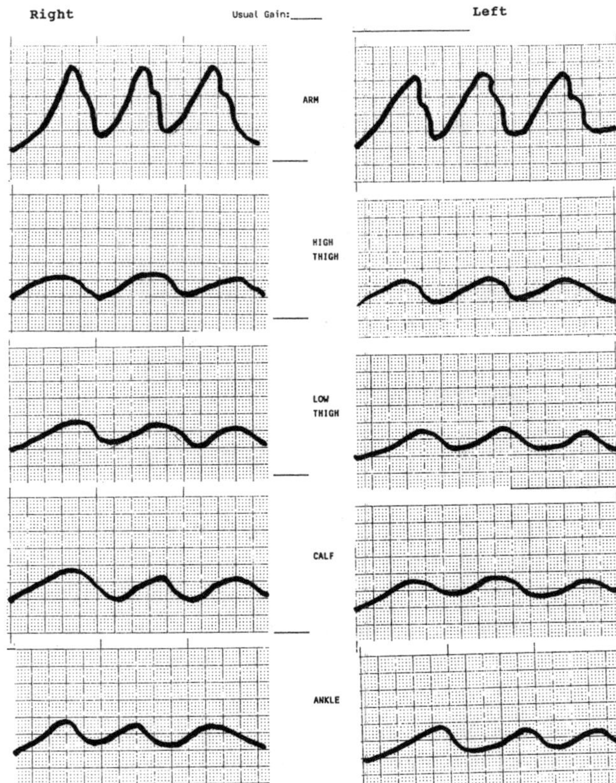

Fig. 6-9. Aortoiliac artery disease. All waveforms from the thigh down are markedly reduced bilaterally.

Abnormal PVRs

Arterial disease is reflected in the PVR when there is a deviation from the normal contour of the wave. The deviations are demonstrated by

1. absence of the reflected diastolic wave
2. slower rise of the systolic upstroke
3. rounding of the waveform crest
4. decrease in the fall of the diastolic downstroke

Tables 6-1 to 6-5 describe the PVRs for different sites of arterial disease. Figures 6-9 to 6-13, which correspond to the tables, show the associated waveforms.

Table 6-1. Aortoiliac Disease

	PVRs	
Arterial Segment Involved	*Right*	*Left*
Brachial	Normal	Normal
High thigh	Reduced	Reduced
Low thigh	Reduced	Reduced
Calf	Reduced	Reduced
Ankle	Reduced	Reduced

PVR = pulse volume recording.

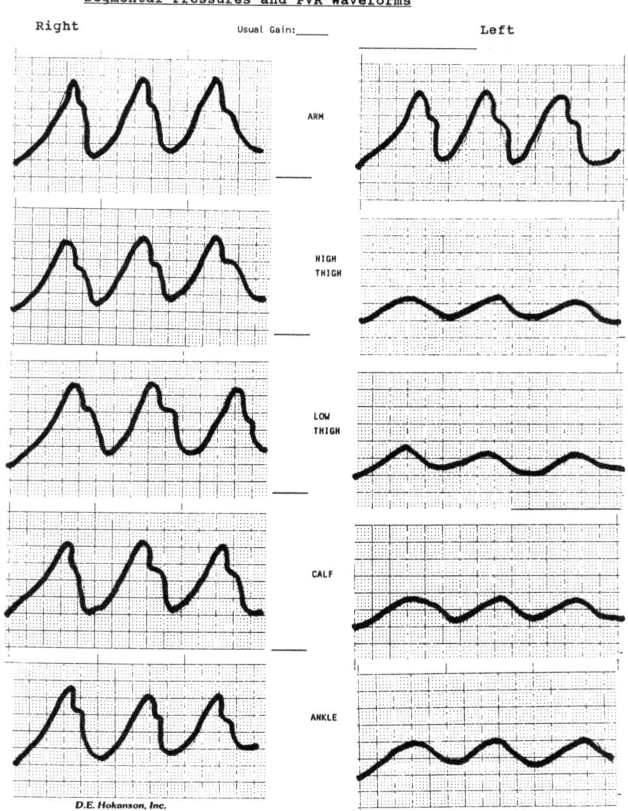

Fig. 6-10. Left iliac artery disease. All PVRs from the left thigh only are reduced.

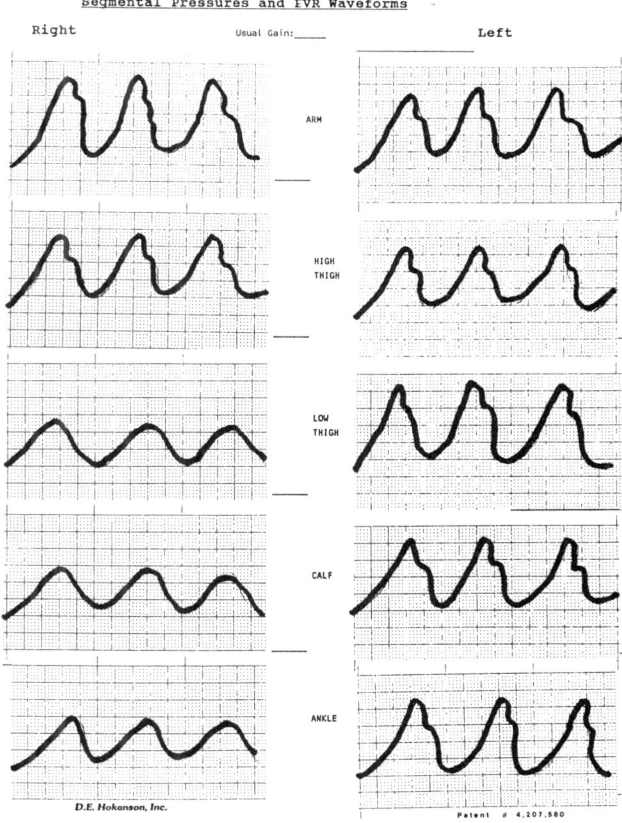

Fig. 6-11. Right distal superficial femoral artery disease. While the proximal right thigh PVR is normal, all waveforms distal to that are markedly reduced.

Table 6-2. Left Iliac Artery Disease

	PVRs	
Arterial Segment Involved	*Right*	*Left*
Brachial	Normal	Normal
High thigh	Normal	Reduced
Low thigh	Normal	Reduced
Calf	Normal	Reduced
Ankle	Normal	Reduced

PVR = pulse volume recording.

Table 6-3. Right Distal Superficial Femoral Artery

	PVRs	
Arterial Segment Involved	*Right*	*Left*
Brachial	Normal	Normal
High thigh	Normal	Normal
Low thigh	Reduced	Normal
Calf	Reduced	Normal
Ankle	Reduced	Normal

PVR = pulse volume recording.

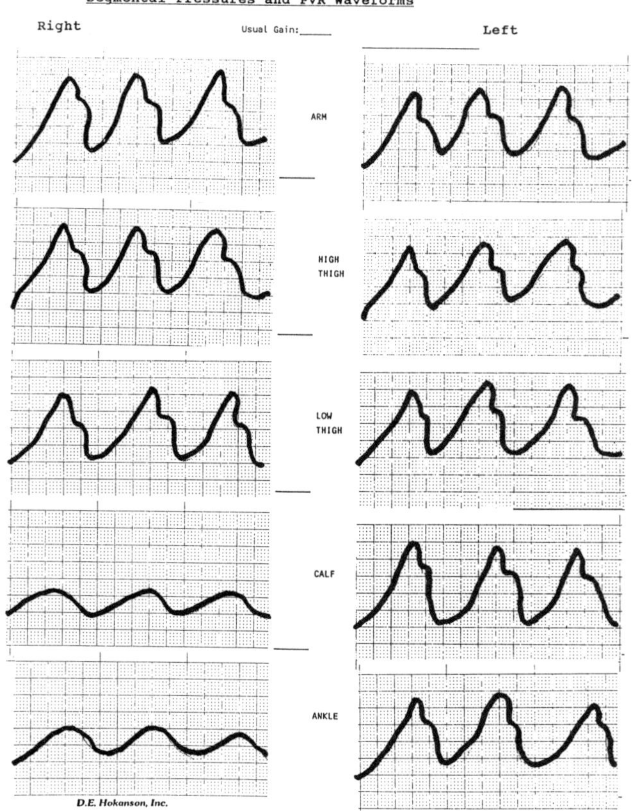

Fig. 6-12. Right popliteal artery disease. Markedly reduced waveforms from the calf to the ankle on the right.

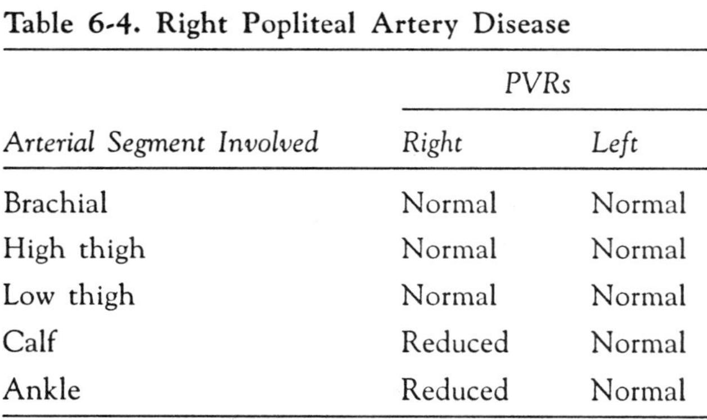

Table 6-4. Right Popliteal Artery Disease

	PVRs	
Arterial Segment Involved	*Right*	*Left*
Brachial	Normal	Normal
High thigh	Normal	Normal
Low thigh	Normal	Normal
Calf	Reduced	Normal
Ankle	Reduced	Normal

PVR = pulse volume recording.

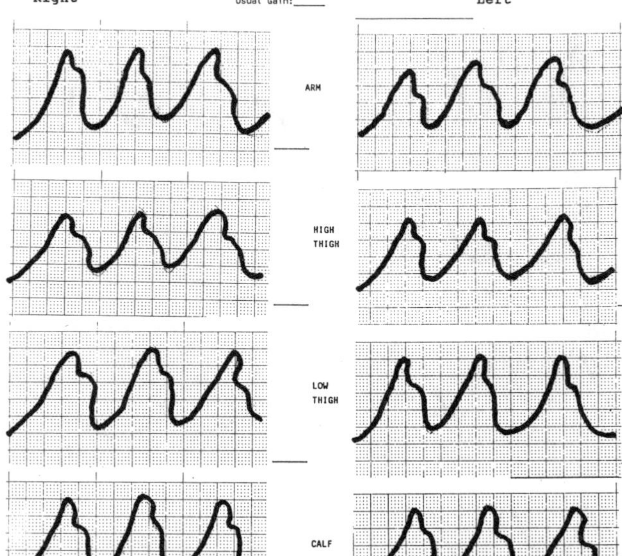

Fig. 6-13. Bilateral distal tibial artery disease. Ankle pressures are reduced bilaterally.

Table 6-5. Distal Tibial Artery Disease

	PVRs	
Arterial Segment Involved	*Right*	*Left*
Brachial	Normal	Normal
High thigh	Normal	Normal
Low thigh	Normal	Normal
Calf	Normal	Normal
Ankle	Reduced	Reduced

PVR = pulse volume recording.

Duplex of the Lower Extremity Arteries

Duplex ultrasound of the lower extremities is valuable in helping to localize and grade the severity of the disease. It is not considered beneficial as a screening device due to the time necessary to survey all of the peripheral arterial tree (1 to 2 hours). Used in conjunction with the traditional PVR and segmental limb pressures, however, duplex many times will offer more specific information for the interpreting physician. Duplex, in the hands of an experienced sonographer or vascular technologist, can be used to determine the appropriate interventional procedure.

Scan Protocol

1. Have the patient remove all clothing below the waist and cover the pubic area appropriately. Slightly flex the knee and externally rotate the leg so the medial aspect of the thigh is accessible. A pillow under the knee will help support the extremity. Apply gel along the course of the external iliac artery (EIA), common femoral artery (CFA), and superficial femoral artery (SPA).
2. Beginning high above the inguinal crease, identify the EIA by duplex while in the sagittal plane. The EIA rises anteriorly from the pelvis toward the probe. Obtain a Doppler sample of the vessel ensuring that you
   a. maintain a 60-degree angle, or less, to the vessel walls
   b. maintain the smallest sample volume possible
   c. survey as much of the vessel as possible
3. In real-time gray-scale or color Doppler imaging, proceed distally down the vessel taking velocity samples at the
   a. EIA
   b. CFA
   c. origin of the profunda
   d. SFA
   e. popliteal artery

Interpretation

The peak systolic velocity determined by Doppler ultrasound is an index of the percent diameter reduction in the artery tested. Table 6-6 describes typical Doppler findings for three progressively severe levels of reduction.

Table 6-6. Relationship of Peak Systolic Velocity Findings and Percent Reduction in Arterial Diameter

Diameter Reduction	*Peak Systolic Velocity*
0%–49%	> than two times that of the closest proximal normal segment
50%–99%	Two times the proximal adjacent segment, or > 200 cm/sec
Total occlusion	No flow in imaged artery

Waveform Criteria

The type of waveform observed depends on the severity of arterial diameter reduction. With a 0% to 19% reduction, a triphasic waveform is typically observed, with no appreciable spectral broadening. With a 20% to 49% reduction, a biphasic waveform appears, with mild spectral broadening. With a 50% to 99% reduction, a monophasic waveform is obtained, and there is significant spectral broadening. When there is total occlusion, no waveform is, of course, obtained, because there is no flow. A preocclusive thump may be heard proximal to the occlusion.

Color Doppler of the Lower Extremities

In general, color Doppler imaging (CDI) of the lower extremities provides only qualitative information about arterial flow. Pulsed Doppler should be performed during any arterial examination where quantitative information is required. It is well accepted that, with experience, your examination can be performed much faster and easier with CDI. Color Doppler imaging is valuable in "lighting up" potential trouble spots. When these areas are identified, pulsed Doppler spectral analysis can be performed to obtain velocity profiles.

General Considerations for Using CDI in the Lower Extremities

1. Use high frame rates and low velocity ranges to obtain the best visualization of triphasic color flow.
2. Use low wall filters
3. Maintain good beam-to-vessel angle.
4. Use color aliasing to identify flow acceleration.

Physical Examination: Upper Extremities

Arterial disease is less common in the upper extremities than in the lower extremities, but there are several vascular disorders other than atherosclerosis of which the vascular specialist must be aware. (These disorders are explained in depth in chapter 3.) The most common vascular disorders of the upper extremities are

1. thoracic outlet syndrome (TOS)
2. Raynaud's syndrome
3. trauma
4. complications from diagnostic arterial catheterization
5. cold sensitivity

The principle methods for upper arterial testing are similar to those for the lower extremities: pulses, Doppler, segmental pressures, PVRs, PPG, and digital arterial pressures using either PPG or strain-gauge plethysmography.

Pulses

Palpate the axillary, brachial, radial, and ulnar arteries. The axillary artery may be best felt by holding the patient's wrist and reaching high into the axilla region with the opposite hand. Keeping the patient's upper arm close to the body also may help.

Doppler

Obtain Doppler signals of the subclavian, axillary, brachial, radial, ulnar, and if appropriate, the digital arteries. The digital arteries are lateral to the phalanges and signals may be difficult to obtain. It is important to know that the arteries in the upper extremities may not display the triphasic-phasic flow typical of the lower extremities and flow varies between patients.

Upper Extremity Pulse Volume Recordings

Place a 10-cm cuff on each upper arm, forearm, and wrist and, again, make sure that the cuffs are fitting snugly. Inject enough air to maintain a *65-mmHg pressure* and obtain pulse volume recordings from upper to lower cuffs. Waveforms are interpreted in the same manner as is done for the lower extremities.

Upper Extremity Blood Pressures

Obtain a brachial artery signal and inflate the brachial cuff 20 mmHg higher than the point where the signal disappears. Slowly, release the pressure and mark when the signal reappears. Next, obtain a forearm pressure using both the radial and ulnar pulses. Record those pressures and repeat this process for the wrist cuff.

The digital arterial pressures can also be obtained by either Doppler, strain gauge, or PPG. Place a small 2.5-cm cuff around the base of the third digit, and if not using a Doppler, place a PPG or strain gauge on the fleshy pad at the distal end of the digit (Fig. 6-14). Slowly inflate the cuff until the signal disappears. Now slowly release the pressure and record the results. If individual digital arteries of the hand need to be evaluated, repeat this process for each digit.

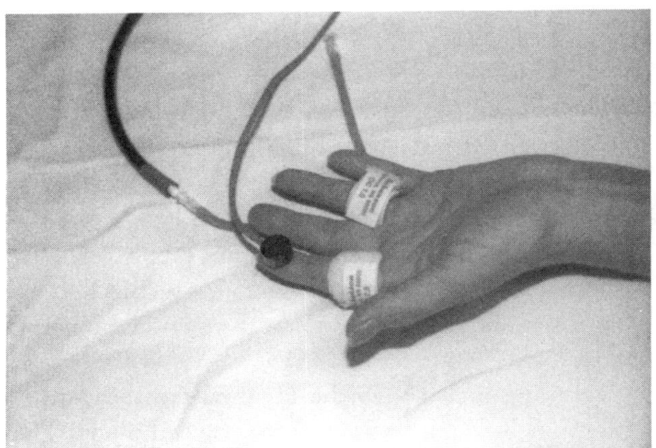

Fig. 6-14. Digital arterial pressures.

Cold Stress Test

Prepare the patient in the normal fashion by explaining the procedure, paying special attention to ensure that the room is warm and the patient is relaxed. Apply a PPG lens to the distal phalange and take a recording. Repeat this for each digit of the affected hand(s). Next, apply the 2.5-cm cuff around the base of each phalange. Using a PPG lens, take digital pressures of each hand. Pressures actually may be taken at the same time the PPG recording is made.

Remove the PPG and digital cuffs and submerge the patient's hands in ice cold water. The patient must keep her hands submerged in the ice water for a minimum of 5 minutes or until the patient can no longer tolerate the procedure. On termination of the cold immersion, note the length of time the patient was able to keep the hands submerged and the color of the digits once the hands were removed from the water. Blot-dry the hands in order to avoid any warming of the digits.

Quickly repeat the PPG recording on all the digits and obtain digital pressures on the second and third digits or the first and third digits. Record your findings.

Interpretation

Normally, digital pressures will drop 10 mmHg; a drop of more than 20% from the brachial arterial pressure, however, is consistent with Raynaud's disease. Cold stress testing has a 90% sensitivity and specificity.

Thoracic Outlet Syndrome Test

Explain to the patient the procedure you will perform and let the patient practice the maneuver before you actually perform the test.

1. Place a 10-cm cuff (12 cm for larger arms) just above the right elbow.
2. Obtain a resting PVR in this position.
3. Have the patient raise the arms to 45 degrees, abduct the shoulders, and internally rotate the arms. Take a PVR tracing for a minimum of five tracings.
4. Have the patient turn his head to the right, and obtain five waveforms.
5. Have the patient turn his head to the left, and obtain five waveforms.
6. Repeat this procedure on the left arm.
7. Obtain a bilateral blood pressure.

Interpretation

Arterial compression is present if any of the PVR waveforms go flat in any of the standard positions. As many as 25% of individuals compress arteries in at least some of the positions just outlined. It is therefore important to base therapy on the patient's symptoms, history, and other physical findings.

Allen Test

1. Have the patient sit with the arm to be examined in a relaxed position. The hand may be resting on a table or pillow at a comfortable height.
2. Take a systolic and radial blood pressure with a cuff on the lower arm.
3. With the patient's hand in a relaxed position with fingers upward, establish a baseline and perform PPG tracings on all digits. Adjust the waveforms and set.
4. Take a pressure of the thumb and little finger, representing the radial and ulnar artery, respectively.
5. With the 2.5-cm cuff on the patient's thumb, obtain a PPG recording. Next, occlude the radial artery with your fingers while the PPG is still recording.
6. With the radial artery still occluded, obtain a pressure of the thumb.
7. Release the pressure on the patient's radial artery and allow her to relax for 20 to 30 seconds.
8. Now, occlude the ulnar artery and repeat the PPG tracing and pressure on the little finger. Record the results.

Interpretation

Any diminution or loss of a pulse must be considered an abnormal test result. As with the thoracic outlet syndrome, however, the patient's symptoms, history, and physical findings must be correlated with the test findings.

Penile Vasculogenic Test

The arterial supply to the penis begins at the internal iliac artery, which branches to the internal pudendal and penile artery. The penile artery is a short vessel that divides into four different arteries. They are the

1. dorsal artery (feeding the skin and the glands)
2. urethral artery (supplying the corpus spongiosum and urethral tissue)
3. bulbar artery (feeding the urethral bulb and the bulbourethral gland)
4. cavernosa artery (supplying the erectile tissue of the corpus cavernosum)

Technique

The technique for performing penile impotence studies is basically the same as for the lower extremities. In fact, because one is essentially evaluating flow to the lower part of the body, a complete lower arterial study should be performed, with the exception of stress testing. CW Doppler signal analysis alone does not constitute a thorough study. By adding PVRs and a penile brachial index using the penile and the brachial artery, a more comprehensive study is performed. Some vascular laboratories are using duplex ultrasound with pre- and postpapaverine injections.

Penile Brachial Index

After first explaining the procedure to the patient, place the 2.5-cm digital cuff around the base of the penis. Locate the deep penile artery by using a high-frequency CW Doppler (8 MHz). Obtain a signal and slowly increase the pressure in the cuff to 20 mmHg above the point at which the signal disappears. Slowly deflate the cuff and record the pressure at which the signal returns. Obtain an index by dividing the penile pressure by the brachial pressure.

Penile Pulse Volume Recording

With the system switched to plethysmography, inflate the penile cuff to 65 mmHg of pressure. Record and document the PVR waveform.

Interpretation

Penile Brachial Index

The following is a list of diagnostic values for the penile brachial index.

Normal:	0.75 to 1.0
Compatible with vasculogenic impotence:	0.6 to 0.7
Abnormal:	<0.6

Arteriography and Interventional Radiology

Angiography is a technique by which radiopaque dye is injected into the blood, permitting visualization of the vascular system. The three primary objectives of arteriography are

1. to make a clinical diagnosis
2. to formulate a preoperative therapeutic plan
3. to provide anatomic information to reduce operative time.

Currently, the arteriogram is used primarily to aid in the formulation of an operative plan. Clinical diagnosis is made by the history and physical examination, and diagnosis may be confirmed by an arteriogram.

Technique

Angiography may be performed by several routes. The most common route is the femoral artery, which is located just above the inguinal ligament. If the femoral artery is stenosed, however, the axillary artery may be used. The axillary artery route is a little more difficult to access and may have greater risks in that the small size of the axillary artery may make catheter insertion troublesome. The approximation of the brachial plexus (a collection of nerves) also can increase the risk of this procedure. If neither the femoral nor brachial artery is available, a direct puncture into the abdominal aorta may be used through a translumbar approach. The major problem with this approach is that if there is any bleeding in the aorta, it is difficult to control because it cannot be compressed as the femoral and brachial arteries can.

Complications

Arteriography generally is a safe procedure with minimal complications. Those complications include

1. allergic reaction to contrast media, varying from rash to angiographic shock
2. AV fistula
3. formation of a pseudoaneurysm
4. distal embolization from dislodged plaque or clot
5. hematoma at the catheter insertion site

Angiography of the Lower Extremities

When visualization of the lower extremities is desired, an abdominal aortogram with visualization of the aortic bifurcation and iliac arteries is performed. When visualization of only one leg is needed, but disease of the femoral artery prohibits a puncture, the opposite femoral artery may be catheterized and fed around the aortic bifurcation.

Interpretation

Interpretation of arteriograms is made by measuring the lumen diameter where the contrast media shows a narrowing of the vessel. That measurement is then compared with a normal section of vessel. The narrowed lumen diameter is then divided by the normal lumen diameter to obtain percent stenosis (Fig. 6-15).

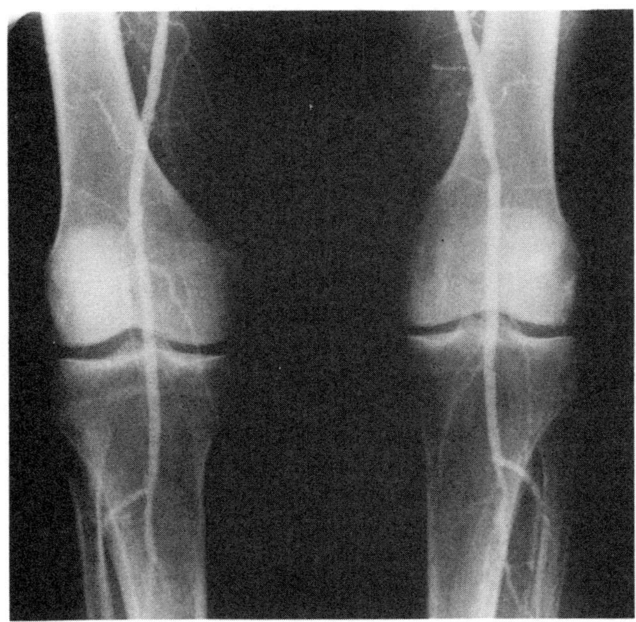

Fig. 6-15. Arteriogram of the distal femoral and popliteal arteries. Can you see the narrowing of the distal superficial femoral artery on the left leg?

Review Exercise

1. Peripheral arterial disease (PAD) refers to disease of the arteries in either the _____________ or _____________.

2. PAD is far (more/less) common in the lower extremities than the upper.

3. The most common complaint from patients suffering from peripheral arterial disease is

   a. pain
   b. numbness
   c. weakness
   d. nonhealing ulcers

4. Most often patients with arterial insufficiency of the lower extremities will describe their symptoms as a cramping pain that is associated with _____________ and relieved with _____________.

5. Acute arterial ischemia is very common. True or False?

6. Patients with acute arterial insufficiency will most often present with

   a. ____
   b. ____
   c. ____
   d. ____
   e. ____
   f. ____

7. The pain of acute arterial ischemia is often _____________ in onset and _____________ in nature.

8. Chronic arterial insufficiency is a far more common presentation than acute arterial ischemia. True or False?

9. Patients with chronic arterial insufficiency usually complain of

   a. unilateral calf pain
   b. bilateral calf pain
   c. buttocks pain
   d. either a, b, or c

10. Patients complaining of rest pain usually get their symptoms

   a. when resting after walking
   b. after standing too long
   c. at night
   d. none of the above

11. Patients with ischemic rest pain will typically do what to relieve their symptoms?

   a. Take aspirin
   b. Elevate the affected leg
   c. Apply heat
   d. Hang the leg over the bedside

12. List four risk factors associated with peripheral vascular disease.

   a. ______________________________

   b. ______________________________

   c. ______________________________

   d. ______________________________

13. The term *bruit* is a French word that means ____________.

14. An optimal CW Doppler for evaluating arteries in the lower extremities is

   a. 2 MHz
   b. 4 MHz
   c. 6 KHz
   d. 8 MHz

15. The best practical Doppler angle for assessing peripheral arteries is generally

   a. 90 degrees
   b. 180 degrees
   c. 0 degrees
   d. 60 degrees

16. A zero-crossing detector provides a ____________ frequency measurement.

17. Label the following waveforms and evaluate them from normal to most diseased.

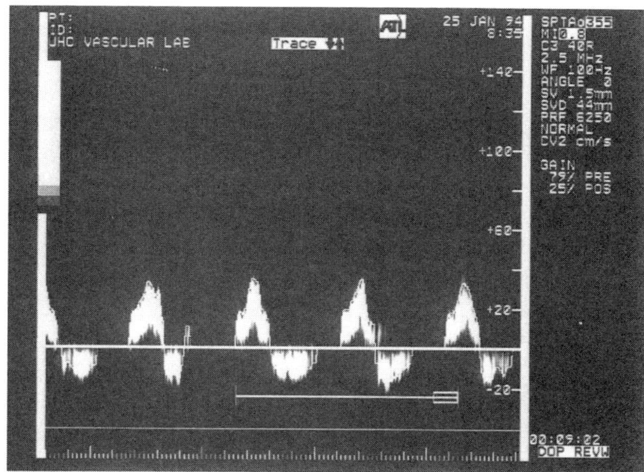

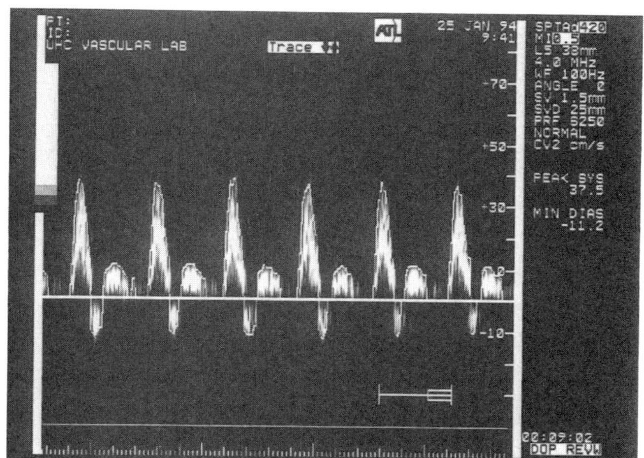

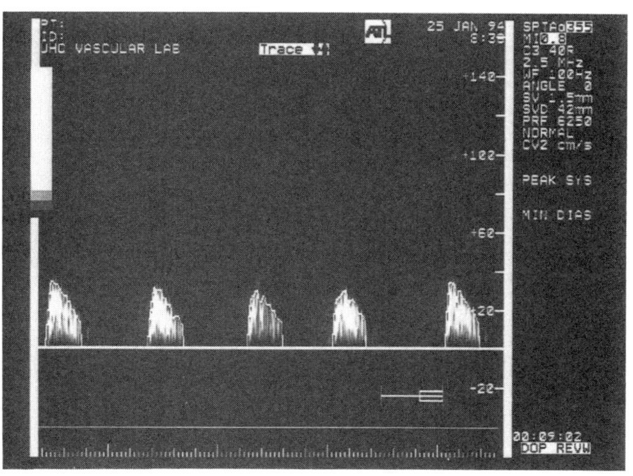

---

18. It is recommended that the width of the blood pressure cuff be at least ______________ times larger than the diameter of the limb being measured.

19. List the appropriate size of cuffs for the various limbs.

    a. Brachial ______________

    b. High thigh ______________

    c. Low thigh ______________

    d. Calf ______________

    e. Ankle ______________

20. Arterial pressure with PPG is obtained by placing a small piece of double sticky tape on the ______________ of the distal phalanx (toe).

21. Regardless of whether the ankle pressures are normal, it is necessary to measure both the calf and thigh pressures as well. True or False?

22. A significant pressure drop between a high-thigh and low-thigh cuff is

    a. 20 mmHg
    b. 10 mmHg
    c. 5 mmHg
    d. any drop at all

23. Write the formula for ankle brachial index.

24. List the values for the following ABIs.

    Normal ______________

    Mild disease ______________

    Moderate disease ______________

    Severe disease ______________

    Consistent with rest pain/ischemia ______________

    Consistent with nonhealing ______________

25. A toe brachial index is not considered abnormal unless it is below

    a. 1.0
    b. 0.9
    c. 0.6
    d. 0.3

26. It is common for a patient with diabetes mellitus to have

   a. disappearing pulse syndrome
   b. large vessel disease
   c. noncompressible vessels
   d. venous ulcers

27. If a patient has any peripheral vascular disease, the peripheral arterial examination at rest will always be abnormal. True or False?

28. List four methods of stress testing.

   a. ______________________________

   b. ______________________________

   c. ______________________________

   d. ______________________________

29. The standard set-up for treadmill testing is usually ____________ miles per hour at a ____________ grade.

30. There are three important findings that are essential for documenting the results of the stress test:

   a. ______________________________

   b. ______________________________

   c. ______________________________

31. Reactive hyperemia is a method that simulates the distal artery's response to exercise by temporarily decreasing blood supply to the lower extremities, thereby simulating

   a. vasodilation
   b. ischemia
   c. claudication
   d. rest pain

32. Plethysmography measures

   a. blood flow
   b. blood volume change
   c. blood pressure
   d. all of the above

33. Most PVRs are interpreted qualitatively by evaluating the ____________________ and ____________________ of the waveform.

34. List the other factors that can affect PVR amplitude.

a. ______________________________

b. ______________________________

c. ______________________________

d. ______________________________

35. The amplitude may be interpreted as

a. ______________________________

b. ______________________________

c. ______________________________

d. ______________________________

36. List four characteristics of an abnormal PVR waveform.

a. ______________________________

b. ______________________________

c. ______________________________

d. ______________________________

37. Various peripheral arterial disease states are listed below. Enter whether you would expect the waveforms to be normal or abnormal.

	Thigh	Calf	Ankle
Tibial vessel disease	______	______	______
No aortoiliac disease High SFA Disease	______	______	______
Small vessel disease	______	______	______
Aortoiliac disease	______	______	______
No aortoiliac diseasease Low SFA/popliteal disease	______	______	______

38. A Doppler signal at the CFA will help distinguish presence or absence of aortoiliac disease when thigh, calf, and ankle waveforms are abnormal.

39. List four conditions for which upper arterial testing may be required.

a. ______________________________

b. ______________________________

c. ______________________________

d. ______________________________

40. Testing digits in the upper extremities before and after cold water immersion is an examination for

a. Thoracic outlet syndrome
b. Raynaud's phenomena
c. Takayasu's disease
d. Allen's disease

41. A drop in ______________________________ after cold immersion is considered abnormal.

42. List the four positions necessary to perform a test for Thoracic outlet syndrome.

a. ______________________________

b. ______________________________

c. ______________________________

d. ______________________________

43. When performing the Allen test, it is necessary to compress which two arteries while performing a PPG?

a. ______________________________

b. ______________________________

44. The arterial supply to the penis begins at the ____________________ artery, which branches to the ______________________________ and ____________ artery. The penile artery is a short vessel that divides into four different arteries:

a. ______________________________

b. ______________________________

c. ______________________________

d. ______________________________

45. The diagnostic values for penile brachial index are

Normal	________
Compatible with vasculogenic impotence	________
Abnormal	________

46. Identify the following PAD velocity criteria for diameter reduction by duplex scan.

Diameter Reduction	**Peak Systolic Velocity**
0%—49%	________
50%—99%	________
	or
	________
Occlusion	________

47. Identify the following PAD waveform criteria for diameter reduction by duplex scan. (Provide both type of phasic waveform and degree of spectral broadening.)

Diameter Reduction	**Waveform Criteria**
0%—19%	________
20%—49%	________
50%—99%	________
Occlusion	________

TESTING FOR VENOUS DISEASE

Deep venous thrombosis (DVT) is one of the most common and most life threatening conditions seen by the medical and surgical practioner. There are an estimated 2,500,000 cases of DVT each year, resulting in more than 600,000 cases of pulmonary emboli and 200,000 deaths. Despite these staggering figures, DVT remains a difficult clinical diagnosis to make without the assistance of supportive tests.

Noninvasive vascular testing plays a critical role because DVT is such a difficult clinical diagnosis. Several direct and indirect methods of deep and superficial venous testing will be discussed in this section.

Key Terms

- Air plethysmography
- Augmented venous blood flow
- Coapt
- Compression
- Deep venous thrombosis
- Distal compression
- Echogenic
- Homan's sign
- Impedance plethysmography
- Induration
- Outflow plethysmography
- Phasic flow
- Postphletic stasis syndrome
- Proximal compression
- Stasis dermatitis
- Valsalva
- Valsalva maneuver
- Varicose veins
- Venous volume

Acute Deep Venous Thrombosis

Patient History

Deep venous thrombosis was discussed previously in chapter 3, but in essence, the patient most suspected of DVT is the patient at risk: the pregnant woman, the patient with major trauma or surgery to the lower extremity, patients with a previous history of DVT, cancer, and obesity, and patients who are on prolonged bed rest or who are immobile due to head trauma or stroke.

Patients who have symptoms generally complain of pain, swelling, and warmth of the calf. It is important to ask about trauma or previous history, even though patients may not offer that information initially. Ask patients to describe the pain, how long they have had it, and what aggravates or alleviates the symptoms.

Physical Examination

Look at the affected limb. Does it appear swollen or red? Do you notice any ulcers or bruises? Feel the affected area. Does it feel warm, and is it tender? Is it larger than the opposite limb? Many clinicians suggest measuring the calves for comparison. Ask patients to hyperextend (point the toes up) the foot or you may pull up on the toes to stretch the gastrocnemius (calf) muscles. Does that elicit pain? Pain upon dorsiflexion is called a positive *Homan's sign*. It is generally felt, however, that this is nonspecific for DVT because any inflammation of the calf muscles can cause pain. In general, the best clinical diagnosis is only 50% accurate.

Doppler Examination

Positioning

Proper positioning for the venous examination is extremely important. Because venous return is less dynamic than arteries, detecting flow may be significantly more challenging. Improperly positioned legs may easily impede venous return, giving you a false-positive test.

Phasic Flow

Make sure the patient is warm and comfortable. Have the patient remove any constricting underclothing as this may affect the accuracy of the test by artificially impeding flow in the groin. With the patient lying prone on the bed or examining table, bend the knee slightly and gently externally rotate the hip.

Using a low-frequency (4 MHz) Doppler, identify the femoral artery high in the inguinal region. Move the probe slightly medial to pick up the common femoral vein. Stop and listen carefully for the phasic "whoosh" of the femoral vein. The phasic quality of the femoral vein is characterized by the rhythmic changes as the patient breathes in and out. If you do not initially hear those phasic changes, you may want to ask the patient to take a big breath in and then let it out in order to accentuate the phasic changes associated with breathing. The absence of phasicity is one of the criteria suggesting the presence of a deep venous obstruction.

Valsalva Maneuver

Once you have identified the phasic flow of the femoral vein, ask the patient to hold his breath and bear down as if he is trying to blow up a balloon that won't inflate. This will temporarily impede the venous return to the right side of the heart. You should not hear any backflow during this bearing down because the healthy venous valves should prevent flow from moving backward. Next, ask the patient to exhale and breath normally. The subsequent release of pressure in the abdomen should normally cause a rush of venous return that sounds like a large "whoooooooosh." Place the Doppler on the opposite leg at the same level and listen. Are the qualities the same?

Distal Compression

Next, while listening to the phasic venous flow, reach distal to your Doppler probe and squeeze a large mass of muscle. This maneuver should essentially force the venous blood up the veins, causing an accentuated "WOOSSSHHH" as the venous blood rushes by your Doppler. Switch the probe to the opposite leg and repeat the maneuver. Is the quality of "whoosh" the same from one side to the other?

Proximal Compression

Now, slowly move the probe down the leg listening for the phasic changes in the superficial femoral vein and switching to the opposite leg periodically for comparison if necessary. As you move away from the groin, you may compress the muscle proximal to the Doppler probe and listen for backflow. Then reach across, distal to the Doppler, and squeeze the calf for the augmented "whoosh." Check the opposite side for comparison. Continue this procedure down the leg until you reach the distal superficial femoral vein. Release of proximal compression or having the patient *valsalva* normally results in an exaggerated "whooosh" similar to a distal compression.

Now, place the probe behind the knee and listen for the popliteal artery in the popliteal fossa. Move the probe slightly to pick up the popliteal vein. Perform a proximal and distal *compression*. Next, move the probe to the medial side of the calf to identify the posterior tibial artery. The vein may be so close to the artery you may have to listen to them simultaneously. Listen for the phasic flow and perform proximal and distal compressions, continuing this procedure as far distal as possible.

Interpretation

Doppler assessment of the deep venous system is a subjective procedure that is very technologist-dependent. The accuracy of this study by an experienced vascular specialist is quite good in the popliteal and femoral veins. The skills and experience of the vascular specialist will determine the accuracy of the study. Nevertheless, there are certain criteria that the examiner will find most beneficial in determining whether a deep vein thrombosis or external compression is present.

The first of these criteria is the loss of phasic venous blood flow. The signal may become monophasic and low frequency. You may hear a low rumbling sound or the signal may be absent altogether. This becomes especially apparent when you compare signals to that of the opposite side. Second, there is a kind of sluggishness in the augmented signal. As you perform the distal compression, the expected "WWHHOOSSHH" of the augmented venous blood flow is diminished to a dull and sluggish "chsch." Again, compare with the other side and be sure the patient's position is sufficient. The diminished or absent spontaneous signal combined with the diminished or absent augmented deep venous blood flow is a sensitive indicator of deep venous obstruction of external compression of the deep veins.

The purpose of performing a *proximal compression* is to assess venous valve competency. When squeezing the large muscle masses just proximal to the site you are listening to with the Doppler, blood is actually forced in both directions. Competent venous valves normally close during this maneuver, however, and blood is prevented from moving in a reverse direction. So, if you do hear blood flow with proximal compression, valvular incompetency should be suspected.

It should be noted that congestive heart failure can sometimes produce a continuous venous signal and phasicity therefore is lost. Also, mitral valve insufficiency can produce a pulsatile quality to a venous signal.

Venous Volume and Outflow Plethysmography

The use of plethysmography in assessing the deep venous system utilizes volume change to determine deep venous capacity and outflow. Venous capacity measures the amount of blood that fills an "empty" venous system. An empty venous system without blood or clot in it can be filled with a relatively large volume of venous blood. On the other hand, a deep venous system that is already filled with stagnant blood, particularly in the form of clot, will not be able to hold much more.

Venous capacity is measured by draining the deep venous system of blood and obstructing the venous return with a large blood pressure cuff, which is inflated between systolic and diastolic pressure, placed at the thigh. One can measure the volume increase of the venous blood as it "fills" the previously "empty" deep venous systems. This assumes that a deep venous system that is clear of major thrombus will show a marked increase in *venous volume* increase. A deep venous system that is filled with thrombus will not drain and therefore not show a volume increase when the venous return is occluded.

Outflow measures the volume change of venous blood passing through the deep veins. Outflow is the opposite of venous capacitance. By allowing arterial blood to flow into the limb, but preventing it from flowing out, the vascular specialist essentially builds a dam of venous blood in the leg. If one were to suddenly open all the large gates of that dam, the blood would normally rush out in a great torrent: a large "WHOOOOOOSSSHHH!" If the deep veins in the leg are filled with clot, however, there will be no rush of blood because clot won't flow. The flow will slow down as the venous blood behind the clot attempts to find its way around the obstruction through collateral pathways, as the outflow will be significantly slowed.

There are three principal plethysmographic methods of measuring venous capacitance and outflow. Each of these methods is based on the same principle: to apply an obstructing cuff around the thigh and a sensing cuff around the calf. The obstructing cuff functions as the dam and the sensing cuff measures the venous capacitance and outflow. The three *primary* methods for testing venous capacitance and outflow are

1. air plethysmography
2. strain-gauge plethysmography
3. electrical impedance plethysmography

Air Plethysmography

Air plethysmography utilizes a large cuff placed around the upper thigh. This cuff has a large, quick release valve that allows the cuff to deflate rapidly. A smaller sensing cuff is placed around the medial or posterior section of the calf and inflated with 20 mmHg of pressure. This is just enough pressure to sense the subtle changes that occur with venous capacity and outflow.

Technique

Proper positioning of the examined leg is extremely important for obtaining accurate results. To achieve the best position, place the limb on a pillow so that it remains above the level of the right atrium. This allows the venous blood to drain from the leg. Next, gently flex the knee and externally rotate (knee out, heel in) the leg. It may be quite helpful to ask the patient to roll slightly toward the leg being examined in order to ensure that the limb is not under any undue stress

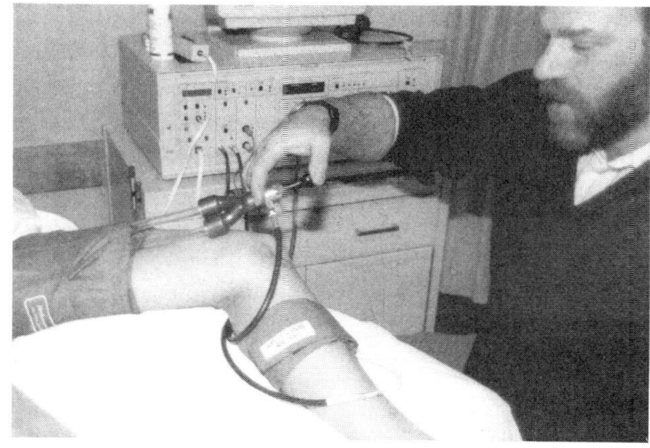

Fig. 6-16. Proper positioning and technique for air impedence plethysmography.

(Fig. 6-16). Taking time to position the leg properly cannot be stressed enough. Doing it right the first time will save you from doing the test over again.

With either the strip-chart recorder or scope on, obtain a tracing from the calf sensing cuff. Although it may be difficult to see the phasic changes of venous flow, you may be able to see small arterial oscillations of the tibial arteries. This indicates that your cuff is placed properly and functioning.

Next, inflate the thigh cuff to approximately 50 mmHg of pressure. This will effectively allow arterial blood to flow in but prevent venous blood from flowing out — in essence, the dam. Now the arterial blood is flowing into the leg but is unable to get out. So, what happens to the blood?

Remember from the anatomy and physiology section of this book that veins have much thinner walls and are able to change their shape and size much easier than are arteries. Subsequently, the veins start filling up like water in a balloon. Meanwhile, the sensing cuff on the calf is recording these changes. As the pressure in the veins starts increasing, the baseline from your tracing begins to rise. The more blood that fills the veins, the higher this line will rise.

As some point, the veins will reach their maximum capacity and stop stretching; the baseline will begin to level off. At this point, you know that all the venous blood that was able to fill the veins has done so. Now it's time to "bust open the dam," and this is done by rapidly deflating the thigh cuff.

With the sudden release of the thigh cuff pressure, the venous blood will, under normal conditions, rush out quickly. If you were listening over the vein with your Doppler, you would hear a loud

"WHHHOOOSSSHHH" as the blood returns up the deep venous system to the vena cava on its way to the right side of the heart. This sudden drop in pressure is sensed by the calf sensing cuff and it is reflected as a sudden drop in the tracing back to the baseline.

The amount of time it takes for the tracing to drop is crucial to interpreting the test. The less obstruction the venous blood meets after the thigh cuff is released, the faster venous blood will evacuate the deep venous system and the more rapidly the tracing will drop from its maximum height. If the venous outflow takes more than 2 seconds to bring the tracing back to baseline, a deep venous obstruction should be suspected. Keep in mind, however, that there are many "obstructions" that may cause a delay in the outflow, such as poorly positioned limbs, tight clothing, or pregnancy.

Mercury Strain-Gauge Plethysmography

Mercury *strain-gauge plethysmography* utilizes the same principles as air plethysmography, except that the sensing cuff is different. Instead of using a cuff filled with air, a mercury-filled silastic tube (refer back to your physics if this is not clear) is used to record the volume changes in the calf. The mercury-in-silastic is placed around the widest portion of the calf, and the length of the tube should reach 90% of the limb. As with the air plethysmograph, be certain not to place the strain gauge too tightly around the calf.

The interpretation of mercury strain gauge is based on the same principle as air plethysmography. After preventing venous return with the thigh cuff inflated to 50 mmHg, the mercury-in-silastic tube senses and records the increase in calf volume. Once the capacitance levels off, the thigh cuff is rapidly deflated and the outflow is recorded. The less-than-2-second rule also applies here. A decline in the outflow tracing that takes more than 2 seconds suggests an obstruction of the deep venous system.

Mercury strain gauge is extremely sensitive, which makes it responsive to the slightest movement. This may seem advantageous, but unless the patient is very still and cooperative, the tracings may be difficult to interpret. In addition, the shelf life for strain gauge is relatively short and it needs to be replaced on a regular basis.

Impedance Plethysmography

The principle behind *impedance plethysmography* (IPG) is based on Ohm's law (voltage = current × resistance). As you recall from the physics section, blood is a good conductor of electricity; the more blood in a vessel, the lower the resistance. Therefore, by measuring the electrical impedance of a limb, one can make an assumption about how much blood is in the limb. If the limb is elevated and venous blood is presumed "emptied out," one should expect to see high resistance in the limb. If, however, the leg is elevated and the IPG shows low resistance in the limb, the vascular specialist can assume that blood is retained within the deep venous system in the form of clot.

Technique

As with air impedance and strain-gauge plethysmography, positioning of the limb is very important. The knee should be slightly flexed, the limb should be externally rotated, and the calf should be elevated above the right atrium. An occlusion cuff is placed around the thigh, and the plastic band containing electrodes is placed around the largest portion of the thigh (Fig. 6-17). The thigh

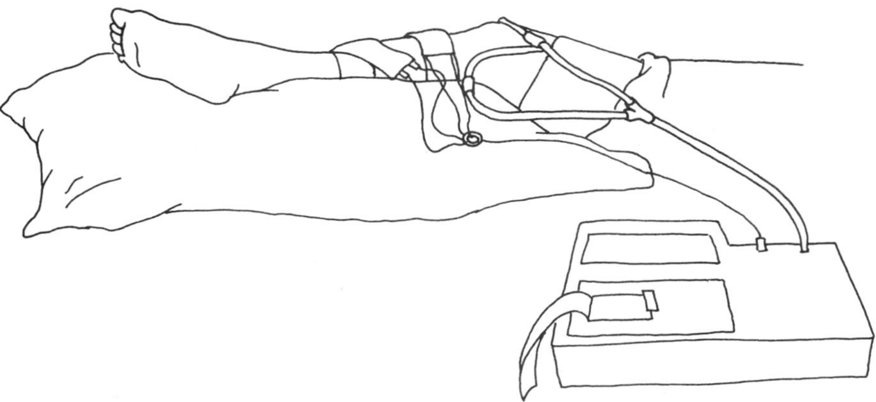

Fig. 6-17. Electric impedance plethysmography.

cuff is inflated and the venous capacitance is recorded. Once the capacitance levels off, the "plug is pulled" on the occluding cuff and the outflow time is measured. With the IPG method, any outflow greater than 3 seconds is considered abnormal.

Once an obviously normal study is obtained, the study may be terminated. Any equivocal or abnormal studies, however, must be repeated in order to ensure that there is no other outside factor influencing the results. These outside factors may include

1. calf muscle tension
2. tourniquet effect from tight clothing
3. bandages, casts, or traction devices
4. insufficient thigh-cuff release

Interpretation

The diagnostic criteria for impedance plethysmography involve plotting the venous capacitance (amount of venous blood that fills the deep venous system) versus the venous outflow (amount of venous blood that exits the deep venous system) over a period of time (usually 3 seconds). The principles of this interpretation are based on the assumption that

1. nonobstructed deep venous system will be capable of filling with an equal amount of blood when compared with the opposite limb
2. nonobstructed deep venous system will allow venous blood to rapidly exit the limb (<3 seconds) when the large thigh cuff is rapidly deflated

Figure 6-18 illustrates the principles of interpretation.

The accuracy of a properly performed IPG is approximately 90% for thrombi above the knee, but IPG is not sensitive for nonobstructive thrombi or calf clots.

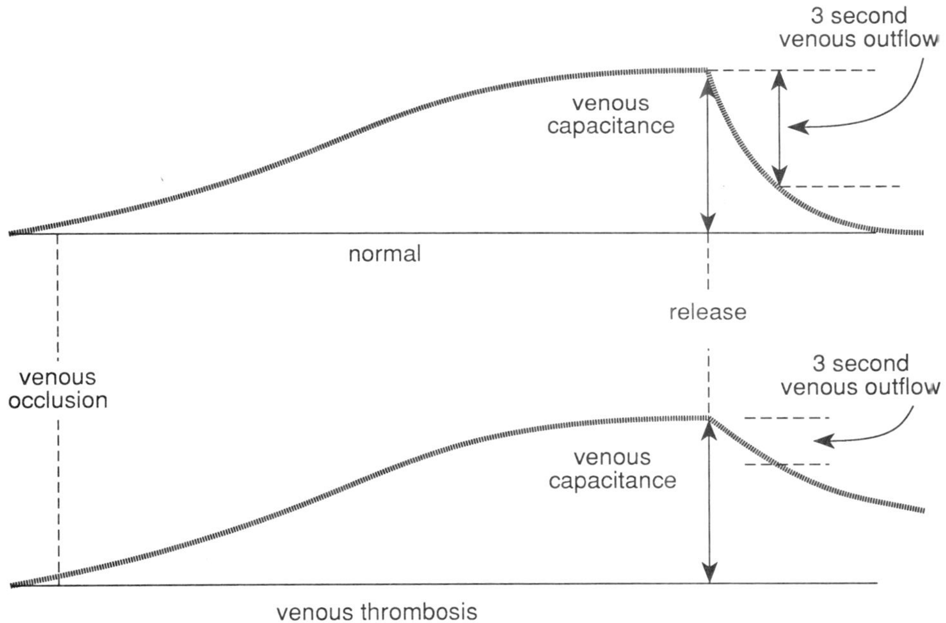

Fig. 6-18. Venous capacitance rises as the thigh cuff prevents venous return. Normally, when the cuff is released, the outflow tracing drops rapidly. With an occlusion, however, the outflow tracing decreases more gradually.

Venous Duplex Imaging

The advent of duplex ultrasound revolutionized deep venous testing in the vascular laboratory. Because direct assessment of the deep veins is possible by imaging and Doppler ultrasound, duplex generally has become preferred over other noninvasive studies. In fact, in many institutions, duplex has become the diagnostic study of choice over venography. It must be stressed, however, that duplex, like so many other noninvasive studies, is very technologist- or sonographer-dependent and accuracy is directly reflective of the skill and experience of the person performing the study.

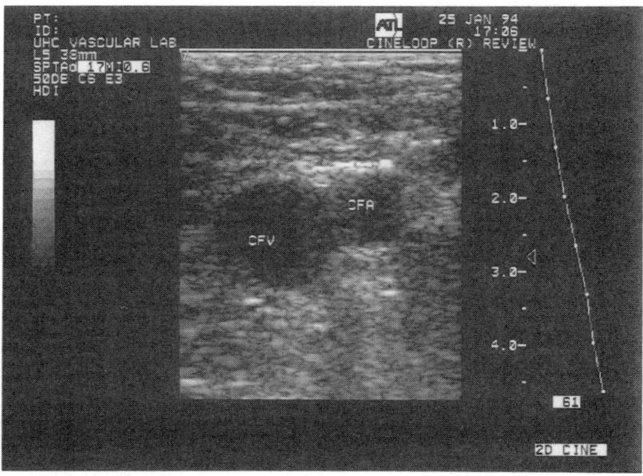

Fig. 6-20. The common femoral artery is on the right of the common femoral vein in this image. Note that the vein is larger than the artery and free of echogenic material.

Imaging Technique

Positioning, as with all venous studies, remains a very important factor for obtaining accurate results. After explaining the procedure, position the patient in the customary fashion of the previously mentioned impedance studies, with one exception. Instead of raising the calf above the heart, be sure the patient's heart is higher than the leg. This can be obtained by putting the examination table in reverse Trendelenburg (head up, feet down) and using hydrostatic pressure to fill the deep venous system. The reason for this switch in technique is that veins may be more difficult to image than arteries if drained of blood and collapsed.

Beginning with the transverse scan (Fig. 6-19), identify the distal external iliac vein if possible, or the common femoral vein high above the inguinal crease (Fig. 6-20), that fold in the skin when the thigh is flexed. The vein is usually medial to the artery. Firmly press the probe down until the vein fully compresses or *coapts*. Normally, a vein will fully compress with only a moderate amount of pressure (Fig. 6-21). If you find, however, that you need to apply so much pressure that the artery is beginning to compress, stop pushing! The vein is probably filled with clot.

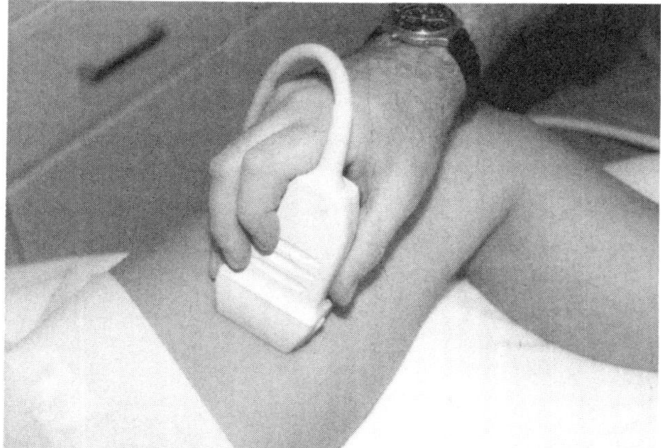

Fig. 6-19. Transverse scan of the superficial femoral vein.

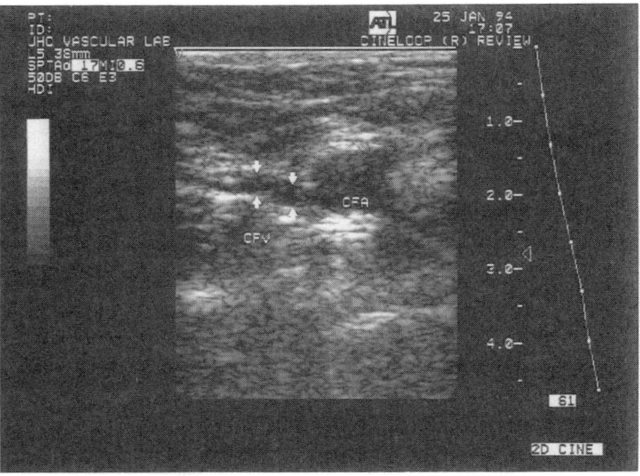

Fig. 6-21. This is the same examination as in Fig. 6-20, but this time with probe compression. Note that the vein is completely compressed between the arrows.

Continue scanning in transverse down the common femoral artery, compressing every centimeter or so. Be sure that the entire vein compresses before moving on to the next segment. Identify the saphenofemoral junction. Be sure that the first centimeters of the saphenous vein compress as well as the proximal superficial femoral vein (SFV). Continue down the SFV, using your other hand to support the thigh in order to get a good compression.

As you approach Hunter's canal, you will be faced with a dilemma. This is a common site for deep vein thrombus to form, and it is a difficult area to both see and compress. By adjusting your gain and depth setting, however, you should be able to get sufficiently distal down the SFV to both image and compress. In addition, by placing the ultrasound probe behind and high in the popliteal fossa, an adequate image of the distal superficial femoral artery can be obtained. Continue compressing every centimeter or so in the transverse scan plane to the distal popliteal.

Once you have completed the transverse compression scan of the deep veins above the knee, have the patient sit up on the examination table, if at all possible. This will provide additional hydrostatic pressure to the veins below the knee (tibial veins) and cause them to dilate just a little more. With the probe posterior to the medial malleolus, identify the posterior tibial veins. If you can't see anything, start compressing anyway. If you look into the tissue, you will see the vein "wink" with compression. Do your best to view the pair of posterior tibial veins (PTVs), and begin compressing proximally and medially up the leg every few centimeters or so. Remember to compress the veins completely to ensure that no isolated or nonocclusive thrombi are missed.

Once you begin to reach the gastrocnemius, you may begin to see the peroneal veins. Continue to compress the PTVs until you reach the popliteal vein. Once in the popliteal fossa, attempt to identify the peroneal veins and scan as far distally as possible, compressing every centimeter or so. The anterior tibial veins usually are not scanned because they do not drain venous blood from the venous sinuses and are therefore generally less susceptible to deep vein thrombus. Scanning protocol is determined by the medical director of your laboratory, however, not the author of this book.

Duplex Doppler Technique

Next, have the patient lie back on the table and position the extremity in the customary fashion, ensuring that the leg is lower than the heart. In the sagittal scan plane, identify the distal external iliac vein, if possible, or the proximal common femoral vein if not. With the proper Doppler settings (low wall filters and PRF), place the sample volume in the vein and listen. As with the Doppler venous exam mentioned earlier, you need to listen for the low phasic signal of the deep veins: "whhoooooooo" followed by a pause (patient breathes in and exhales; then you should hear another "whhoooooo" as venous blood moves through the patient's venous system (Fig. 6-22).

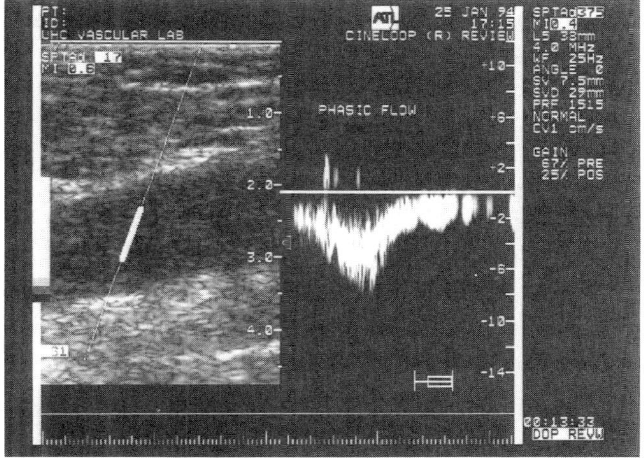

Fig. 6-22. This phasic venous flow increases as the patient exhales. This is the normal respiratory variation of venous flow.

The remainder of the Doppler aspect of the duplex examination is exactly the same as the regular Doppler examination. Have the patient take a deep breath and bear down to test valve competence. Next, perform distal compression to augment venous flow (Fig. 6-23). Moving down the deep venous system, continue the proximal and distal venous compression maneuvers to the popliteal vein. The assessment of the deep veins below the knee, once again, is up to the medical director's discretion.

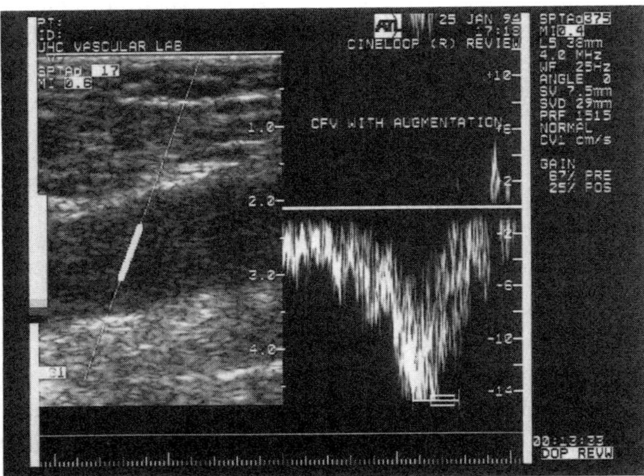

Fig. 6-23. By squeezing the limb distal to the Doppler, venous flow will normally augment, or increase, in the patent deep venous system.

Color Doppler Imaging of the Deep Venous System

Color Doppler imaging, as with all other aspects of noninvasive vascular testing, makes the examination easier and faster to perform. But easier and faster only comes after achieving the skills and comprehension of using color Doppler. At first, you may find yourself struggling and wondering if color is really an improvement at all, but stick with it. You'll find that color will help "light up" arteries, making it easier to find nearby veins that may be difficult to find in gray-scale alone. By imaging veins in color, phasic flow can be documented, making a real-time assessment possible.

INTERPRETATION

There are three major categories of identification and characterization of deep venous disease:

1. Thrombus-free
2. Nonocclusive thrombus
3. Obstructive thrombus

Thrombus-free

In the thrombus-free vein, no *echogenic* material is detected within the vessel lumen, nor is the lumen dilated. The vein is generally larger than the corresponding artery. The vein collapses completely in response to probe pressure, and the Doppler signal is phasic and augmentable. Color will fill the vein in response to distal compression.

Nonocclusive Thrombus

Echogenic material will be seen filling part of the lumen, and compression will be limited by the contained thrombus. The Doppler signal may be completely normal because the partially obstructing thrombus may not interfere with normal phasic flow or proximal and distal compressions. With a nonocclusive thrombus, color Doppler imaging will often demonstrate flow around the thrombus.

Obstructive Thrombus

With an obstructive thrombus, the vein is dilated and filled with echogenic material. The vein does not compress, and both audible Doppler and color Doppler signals are totally absent.

Observable Thrombus

Acute and chronic thrombus can be distinguished by certain observable characteristics of the imaged vein. Acute thrombus tends to be lightly echogenic and may even be indistinguishable from moving blood by image alone. The texture of the thrombus is spongy and the material is poorly attached. If the thrombus is totally obstructing the vein, the lumen will be dilated. Chronic thrombus, on the other hand, will appear brightly echogenic. The texture will be rigid and the thrombus well attached to the vein wall. The vein will be contracted, unlike that which is found with a fresh thrombus.

Note: Although deep venous disease of the upper extremity is relatively less frequent, when compared with the lower extremity, it is worth mentioning briefly. Swelling is the most common manifestation of venous thrombosis, and the patient may have a history of strenuous activity. This condition is referred to as *effort thrombosis*, which is due to compression of the subclavian vein. In addition, inpatients may have subclavian vein thrombosis due to catheterization lines. Although certain modifications must be made to adapt to the smaller circumferences of the arms, the principal Doppler and impedance techniques are essentially the same as for lower extremities.

Valvular Incompetence

Venous reflux refers to the retrograde flow of blood due to incompetent valves and is one of the major causes of chronic venous disease of the lower limb. Other diseases of valvular incompetence include

1. primary varicose veins
2. secondary varicose veins
3. postphlebitic stasis syndrome

The term *primary varicose veins* refers to a venous disease state in which the disorder is limited to the superficial venous system. The term *secondary varicose veins* refers to the venous disorder in which there is underlying deep venous incompetence and/or obstruction. Lastly, *postphlebitic stasis syndrome* with dermatitis and or ulceration is due to deep and perforating venous incompetence.

History and Physical Examination

The mechanism of venous incompetency is most often a result of deep vein thrombosis. Therefore, a history of that disease is common, although not always present. The typical physical picture of venous incompetence includes

1. ankle edema (swelling)
2. induration (hardening of the skin)
3. stasis dermatitis (dry, hyperpigmented or brown scaling skin with woody edema)
4. ulceration (a superficial shallow hole in the skin)

The importance of the history and physical examination and the noninvasive test is to determine whether the patient's symptoms are from chronic venous insufficiency or lymphedema, a swelling due to an obstruction of the lymphatic system.

Noninvasive Testing

There are several different tests available for evaluating venous insufficiency. The types that are discussed in this section include

1. photoplethysmography
2. Doppler
3. air plethysmography
4. duplex

Photoplethysmography

Photoplethysmography (PPG) uses infrared light to measure the changes in cutaneous (skin) circulation. In the AC mode, PPG is capable of sensing rapid arterial changes in the microcirculation. By employing DC coupling, the PPG transducer voltage output is filtered to provide a longer time constant so that the relative changes in the skin over time can be recorded. It is somewhat like a low PRF that allows essentially the slower and longer look that is necessary to monitor venous blood flow. The PPG transducer is connected to a strip-chart recorder.

Technique

Clean the pertinent area of the patient's skin with alcohol in order to remove any surface lotion, oil, or sweat. If the skin is particularly dry and scaly (eczematous), which is common with *stasis dermatitis*, you may need to use some tape to dab over the area on which you wish to place the PPG. The point being made here is that the PPG requires good solid contact with the skin. A poorly attached PPG will give erroneous results.

Have the patient remove her stockings and sit in a chair. Both feet should rest comfortably on the floor, evenly spaced apart. The PPG transducer is placed on the medial aspect of the calf about two thirds of the way down the leg (Fig. 6-24).

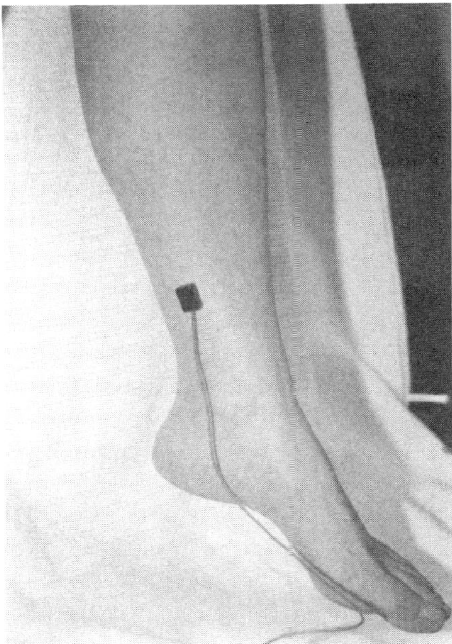

Fig. 6-24. Proper placement of photoplethysmography transducer.

There are several methods for attaching the PPG transducers, but double sticky tape seems to be the most preferred. A velcro strap, which is often provided with a PPG system, is also acceptable as long as too much pressure is not applied to the PPG. If the transducer is pushed into the skin, it will compress the microcirculation and prohibit accurate recording.

Try a practice run first, and then begin the test. The recording is started at 5 mm/sec. Once a baseline is obtained, instruct the patient to raise both heels off the floor and then relax, in order to actively contract the muscles in the calf. Ask the patient to repeat this maneuver five times. This will effectively squeeze blood out of the venous sinuses and propel it up the deep and superficial venous systems.

To assess the deep venous system and perforator veins alone, apply tourniquets either immediately above or below the knee. This will have the same effect as achieved with the Doppler examination. It will prevent any flow of blood through the superficial system, therefore assuring the examiner that the results obtained are from the deep system only.

Interpretation

Normally, the blood flow in the skin decreases significantly in response to the active calf-muscle contraction. Venous blood is propelled out of the area and normally will return only when the arterial inflow perfuses the capillaries to the venules and into the deep and superficial venous system. This assumes that the one-way valves are intact and that no reflux is present. The strip chart will reveal the five blips as the patient contracts the calf muscle, and the baseline will drop down as the venous blood is emptied. Then, very slowly, the line will begin to rise once again as the veins are filled from the arteries, until the tracing reaches the baseline once again.

In the incompetent venous system, however, blood will be propelled out of the veins, but as soon as the muscle relaxes, the venous blood falls back, unopposed by valves, into the venous system. The strip chart will reveal this rapid filling as a rapid return to the baseline.

In the more severe cases of valvular incompetence, the calf muscles won't be able to eject the venous blood out, and the baseline will reflect that disorder by not dropping the baseline at all (Fig. 6-25). Venous filling time of less than 18 seconds is considered abnormal and consistent with reflux.

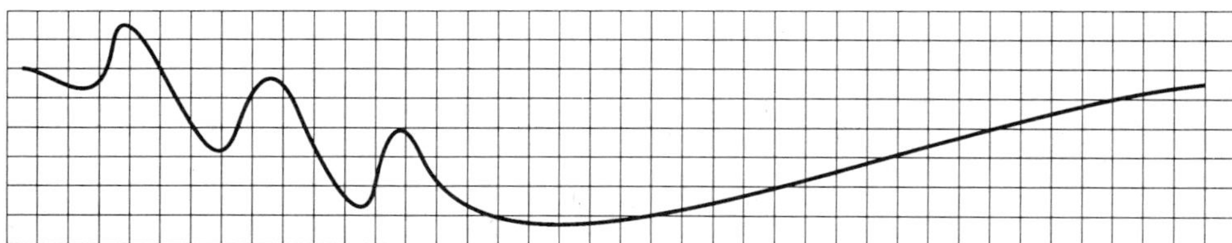

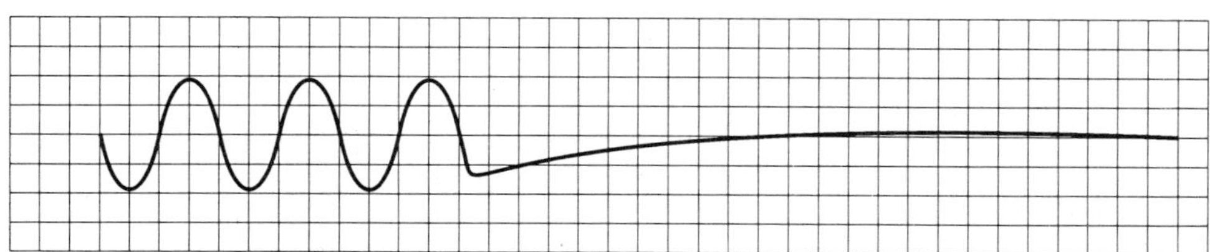

Fig. 6-25. The top recording is a graphic illustration of a normal PPG. Note that with each dorsiflexion of the foot, the baseline drops. The lower PPG shows that despite dorsiflexion, the calf is incapable of emptying out venous blood.

Doppler

In the previous section on DVT we have discussed that the proximal and distal compression maneuvers provide two pieces of information. (1) By compressing the limb distal to the Doppler probe, the vascular specialist augments the flow up the deep venous system, thereby determining patency. (2) By compressing the limb proximal to the Doppler probe, the specialist forces the venous blood flow in the opposite direction. This is referred to as *retrograde flow*. Competent venous valves will not allow blood to flow through, and you will hear no Doppler signal in the normal situation.

Saphenofemoral Junction

Have the patient stand facing away from you on a small stool, ensuring there is adequate means of support. Proper support will prevent movement or contraction of the calf muscle during the examination. Ask the patient to shift the weight to the leg opposite of the one being examined.

With either CW Doppler or duplex, insonate the femoral vein and obtain a signal, which may be somewhat difficult to hear while the patient is standing. To confirm that you are in the vein, squeeze the thigh just distal to the probe and listen for the "whhoosshh." Repeat this maneuver to assure proper Doppler placement, pausing between the distal compressions to allow for venous refill. As with the DVT examination, listen for the backflow. A brief split-second signal may indicate normal reversal as the vein fills and expands with blood. Any signal lasting longer than 1 second, usually 1 to 4 seconds, is indicative of reflux.

Differentiating Deep from Superficial Plethysmography

Because of your proximity to the saphenous vein, a reversal in flow longer than 1 second could be from the femoral vein or the saphenous vein. How can you be sure which vein has the incompetent valves? This dilemma can be resolved by using a tourniquet to occlude the greater saphenous vein about 5 to 10 cm below the inguinal crease. Be careful not to tie the tourniquet too tightly—just enough to prevent flow in the saphenous vein. Repeat the Doppler study, squeezing the thigh muscle just distal to the probe. Do you still hear reflux? If so, you know that, because you have occluded the saphenous vein, the reflux is originating from the common femoral vein.

Saphenopopliteal Incompetence

With the patient remaining in the standing position, place the Doppler probe over the popliteal vein. Briskly and firmly squeeze the calf muscle and listen for reflux of more than 1 second's duration. Now place the tourniquet about 5 cm below the knee to occlude the lesser saphenous vein. This will prevent any flow heard from the saphenous vein and ensure that any signal heard will be from the popliteal vein. Squeeze the calf while listening to the popliteal vein. Any reverse signal longer than 1 second in duration is consistent with reflux.

Air Plethysmography

Air plethysmography consists of a long tubular plastic air chamber that holds 5 liters of air. This plastic tube fits around the lower leg, extending from below the patient's knee to the ankle. With the patient lying in the supine position, the plastic tube is inflated with 6 mmHg of pressure to ensure proper contact without causing the patient discomfort. The cuff is then inflated with a specific amount of air and calibrated.

Next, the leg being tested is elevated at 45 degrees for approximately 20 seconds. This allows the venous blood to be drained. The patient is then guided to a sitting and then standing position with weight on the leg not being tested. The blood then fills the venous system, and the change is recorded by the change in volume of the attached air-filled tube. This is referred to as *venous volume*.

The patient is then instructed to shift the weight to the affected leg, raise up on the toes, and then return to the resting position. This maneuver causes the calf muscle to contract and eject the venous blood up the venous system. The toeups are repeated two or three times until similar ejections volumes are obtained.

Lastly, the patient is instructed to repeat the toe-up maneuver ten times and then return to the resting position. A diminished calf volume during exercise and the volume increase after the end of exercise are measured. This allows a determination of how well the calf muscle is able to pump out venous blood (calf-muscle pump function) and how quickly blood flow returns to the lower leg. The patient then returns to the bedside, the leg is elevated, and a new zero volume is recorded. The difference between the zero baseline and the volume after ten toeups is called the *residual volume*.

Interpretation

The changes in calf volume during the testing maneuvers provide quantitative information about the deep venous system. Because the plastic leg tube is standardized with a specific volume of air, the changes in that volume as the patient raises the leg, stands, and performs the calf muscle contraction maneuvers can be recorded and measured.

Duplex

Duplex and color Doppler imaging provide an excellent method to directly visualize venous blood flow during compression maneuvers. With the sample volume of the pulsed Doppler placed directly in the vein, proximal and distal compressions are performed. As with Doppler, flow should be augmented cephalad (towards the head) with distal compression, but no reversal of flow should be detected with proximal compression. Color flow, once again, will facilitate this technique by lighting up flow in either direction. Abnormal reversal of flow should be either taped or photographed with an assessment of how long the reversal of flow occurred.

Invasive Tests

Venography is performed far less because of the accuracy, cost efficiency, and safety of the aforementioned venous studies. Regardless, venography remains the "gold standard" for the evaluation of deep venous disease.

Venography is performed by introducing a needle into the dorsal vein of the foot. The examining table is then tilted between 45 and 60 degrees in reverse Trendelenburg (head up, feet down). Dye is then injected into the deep venous system and spot films are taken as the contrast travels up the deep venous system. Tourniquets may be used to exclude the superficial system from the contrast study.

Contrast venography complications are generally low but do include thrombophlebitis due to dye irritation of the venous endothelium. This complication may be reduced by a heparinized saline flush at the end of the study. Allergic reaction to the dye is the most common complication.

Interpretation

Using venography, acute DVT appears radiographically as a filling defect outlined by a rim of contrast medium. As the thrombosis organizes, it attaches to the vein wall, and the rim is lost. Complete occlusion subsequently follows. Once the vein recanalizes, thin stringy appearance occurs. At this point, collateralization and superficial varices develop.

Review Exercise

1. There are an estimated ______________ cases of DVT each year.

2. The patient most suspected of DVT is the

   a. pregnant woman
   b. patient with major trauma
   c. patient with a previous history of DVT
   d. all of the above

3. List the three common symptoms of DVT.

   a. ____

   b. ____

   c. ____

4. DVT is easily made by physical examination. True or False?

5. A technique to determine valve competency in the femoral vein is referred to as the ____________________________ maneuver.

6. By compressing the muscles distal to the Doppler probe during the venous examination, the vascular specialist tests for ____________________________ of the deep vein being examined.

7. By compressing the muscles proximal to the Doppler probe during the venous examination, the vascular specialist tests for ______________ of the deep vein being examined.

8. Doppler assessment of the deep venous system is a quantitative procedure. True or False?

9. The use of plethysmography in assessing the deep venous system utilizes ________________ change to determine deep venous capacity and outflow.

10. Venous capacity measures the ________________ of blood that fills an "empty" venous system.

11. An empty venous system without blood or clot in it can be filled with a ________________ volume of venous blood. On the other hand, a deep venous system that is already filled with blood, particularly in the form of clot, will fill with a ________________ amount of blood.

12. A deep venous system that is filled with thrombus will not drain and therefore not show a volume ______________ when the venous return is occluded.

13. There are three principal plethysmographic methods for measuring venous capacitance and outflow:

    a. ______________________________

    b. ______________________________

    c. ______________________________

14. Air plethysmography utilizes a large cuff placed around the upper

    a. calf
    b. thigh
    c. ankle
    d. none of the above

15. The smaller sensing cuff used in venous plethysmography is placed around the medial or posterior section of the calf and inflated with ______________ of pressure.

16. Proper ______________ of the examined leg is extremely important for obtaining accurate results.

17. The examined leg for a venous outflow study should be

    a. internally rotated
    b. straight
    c. below the level of the heart
    d. slightly flexed

18. As the thigh cuff is released in a normal venous outflow plethysmography examination, one would expect to see a sudden ______________________ in the tracing.

19. The time it should take for the tracing to return to normal is less than ______________ seconds.

20. As with the air plethysmograph, be certain not to place the strain gauge too ______________ around the calf.

21. Mercury strain gauge is extremely ______________, which makes it responsive to the slightest movement.

22. The principle behind electrical impedance plethysmography is based on ______________________.

23. Outside factors that may interfere with an IPG study are

a. ______________________________

b. ______________________________

c. ______________________________

d. ______________________________

24. In many institutions, duplex has become the diagnostic study of choice over venography. True or False?

25. Duplex, like so many other noninvasive studies, is very technologist or sonographer-dependent and accuracy is directly reflective of the ______________ and ______________________________ of the person performing the study.

26. Positioning for duplex is the same as with IPG. True or False?

27. A vein that can be compressed easily by moderate probe pressure is presumed to be ______________.

28. There are three major categories of identification and characterization of deep venous disease:

a. ______________________________

b. ______________________________

c. ______________________________

29. Venous reflux refers to the ______________________________ flow of blood due to incompetent valves.

30. Other diseases of valvular incompetence include

a. ______________________________

b. ______________________________

c. ______________________________

31. *Primary varicose veins* refers to a venous disease state in which the disorder is limited to the

a. greater saphenous vein
b. lesser saphenous vein
c. veins below the knee
d. superficial venous system

32. *Secondary varicose veins* refers to the venous disorder in which there is underlying incompetence and/or obstruction of the ________________.

33. List four typical physical findings of venous incompetence.

    a. ________________

    b. ________________

    c. ________________

    d. ________________

34. Photoplethysmography uses ________________ light to measure the changes in cutaneous circulation.

35. PPG is capable of sensing rapid arterial changes in the microcirculation in the ________________ mode.

36. By employing ________________ coupling, the PPG transducer voltage output is filtered to provide a longer time constant so that the relative changes in the skin over time can be recorded.

37. The strip-chart recording of PPG is started at

    a. 5 mm/sec
    b. 5 cm/sec
    c. 7.5 mm/sec
    d. 10 mm/sec

38. Normally, the blood flow in the skin ________________ significantly in response to the active calf-muscle contraction.

39. The changes in calf volume during the air plethysmography testing maneuvers provide ________________ information about the deep venous system.

40. Venography is performed by introducing a needle into the ________________.

41. Acute DVT appears radiographically as a ________________ defect outlined by a rim of contrast medium.

TESTING FOR CEREBROVASCULAR DISEASE

Cerebrovascular disease is the third leading cause of death in the United States, resulting in more than 200,000 deaths each year. Those who survive are often left with significant physical deficits. Cerebrovascular testing is therefore one of the most common and important noninvasive vascular evaluations that the vascular specialist will be asked to perform.

Key Terms

Asymptomatic bruit
Auscultation
Cerebrovascular accident
Direct tests
Duplex imaging
End diastole
Hypercholesterolemia
Oculoplethysmography
Ophthalmic artery pressure
Peak systole
Periorbital Doppler
Spectral broadening
Transcranial Doppler
Transient ischemic attack
Transient monocular blindness
Vertigo

Patient History

The specific pathophysiology of cerebrovascular disease was discussed in detail in the section on pathophysiology, but the important signs and symptoms of the disease are reviewed here.

Bruit

During a routine physical examination, the clinician will often examine the neck with a stethoscope. The reason for this technique is to auscultate (listen) over the area of the carotid bifurcation. Often, although not always, plaque in the carotid artery will cause turbulence and result in a bruit. About 50% of people with a bruit will have a significant ICA stenosis.

Although not always easy to do, it is important to distinguish a bruit from a transmitted heart murmur. For example, a murmur of aortic stenosis typically transmits up into the neck. A murmur will be loudest lower in the neck and diminish high up the neck. A carotid bruit will be loudest high up the neck and diminish as one listens low in the neck. The clinician needs to sort out the source of the bruit that is cardiac murmur versus murmur of aortic stenosis. Noninvasive cerebrovascular testing provides a safe and accurate alternative.

Transient Ischemic Attack

Many people don't realize that the brain is insensitive to pain. Only the dura, the brain's lining, can sense pain. Therefore, when there is an ischemic injury to the brain, the patient will not necessarily feel pain. Rather, the patient will most likely experience the neurological symptoms associated with the particular functional area of the brain that is affected (i.e., motor, sensory, or speech areas). For example, an injury to the left hemisphere affects speech in about 90% of right-handed people. Other symptoms are typically loss of sensation or strength in an arm and/or a leg, vertigo, and difficulty expressing words. The key difference between a transient ischemic attack (TIA) and a more severe event is that symptoms of TIA usually last less than 24 hours.

When talking to patients about a possible TIA, it is important to ask how long the symptoms last. If patients tell you the symptoms are brought on by particular physical movements, they are unlikely to be TIAs. If patients state that both arms and both legs get numb or weak at the same time, these symptoms also are not likely related to classic TIAs. It must be emphasized, however, that these are questions the physician, not the vascular specialist, must sort out to determine whether or not they are neurological.

Amaurosis Fugax, or Transient Monocular Blindness

You will recall from the anatomy section that the ophthalmic artery is the first branch off the internal carotid artery. An embolus traveling up the internal carotid artery from the heart or carotid bifurcation may lodge in the ophthalmic artery and interrupt blood supply to the eye. If this occurs, the patient may complain of transient visual loss in one eye (know as *transient monocular blindness*). This transient visual loss also is referred to as *amaurosis fugax*, which means "fleeting darkness," and usually resolves after a few minutes. Often the symptoms are described as gradual loss of vision in one eye "like a shade being pulled down."

Be sure to ask the patient how long the symptoms last and whether they occur in only one or both eyes. Again, the vascular specialist is not making the clinical determination of the patient's condition. She is obtaining information that will facilitate understanding of the problem so that the most thorough noninvasive vascular examination possible is provided.

Cerebrovascular Accident

A patient with a cerebrovascular accident most often presents with hemiparesis (weakness on one side of the body only) and/or dysarthria (difficulty articulating speech). In severe cases, the patient may be unable to respond to questions. For inpatients, the medical records will provide the best source of information regarding onset and nature of the stroke.

Vertigo

Dizziness is a common complaint, but it is generally not an acceptable indication for noninvasive cerebrovascular testing. On the other hand, it is important to distinguish dizziness from *vertigo* because the nature of these two problems has significant clinical implications.

If a patient tells you that he experiences dizziness, ask this question: "Do you feel like you are spinning around the room or does the room seem to be spinning around you?"

In general, patients with dizziness will complain that they are spinning around the room, whereas patients with vertigo feel the room is spinning around them. Vertigo *may* suggest vascular insufficiency of the vertebral and basilar arteries. Therefore, obtaining an accurate history will help the vascular specialist focus on the anatomic area that is likely to be the source of the problem.

Risk Factors and Contributing Disease

There are several risk factors/contributing disease associated with cerebrovascular disease. They include

1. hypertension
2. coronary artery disease
3. hypercholesterolemia
4. cigarette smoking

Physical Examination

The physical examination for the patient undergoing a cerebrovascular examination is primarily limited to

1. bilateral blood pressures
2. carotid auscultation

Bilateral blood pressures provide information about the subclavian arteries. For example, a significant stenosis of a subclavian artery would produce unequal blood pressures. This information is valuable to the interpreting physician when determining the possible location of disease other than the carotid bifurcation.

By listening to the carotid arteries in the neck, the vascular specialist may hear the turbulence associated with a carotid stenosis. In the past, there was an attempt to grade the stenosis based on the quality and duration of the carotid bruit. It is generally sufficient, however, to describe a bruit as either soft or loud and note the location, either low, mid, or neck.

Indirect Tests

Periorbital Doppler

In the case of significant internal carotid artery disease, the branches of the external carotid artery play an important role in supplying arterial blood flow to the brain. As described earlier, the external carotid artery provides blood primarily to the face and the scalp. The facial artery, which courses across the angle of the jaw and superiorly to the ocular orbit, normally terminates just lateral to the nasal bridge. The superficial temporal artery courses along the surface of the forehead where it communicates with the frontal and supraorbital arteries.

The nasal, frontal, and supraorbital arteries are branches of the ophthalmic artery (the first branch of the internal carotid artery). When there is a significant flow-reducing lesion of the internal carotid artery, blood flow in the external carotid artery is often increased, whereas flow in the ophthalmic artery is decreased. This causes an imbalance of pressure in the two vessels, and because blood seeks the course of least resistance, flow is forced through the terminal branches of the superficial temporal and facial arteries to the ophthalmic artery in the reversed direction. In this manner, blood is allowed to enter the internal carotid artery and supply the brain with blood.

Technique

By placing a high-frequency CW Doppler on the periorbital vessels, the quality and direction of flow can be assessed (Fig. 6-26). Care must be taken not to obstruct these superficial arteries with the transducer. If the direction of flow of one of the periorbital arteries is reversed, a high-grade stenosis or total obstruction of

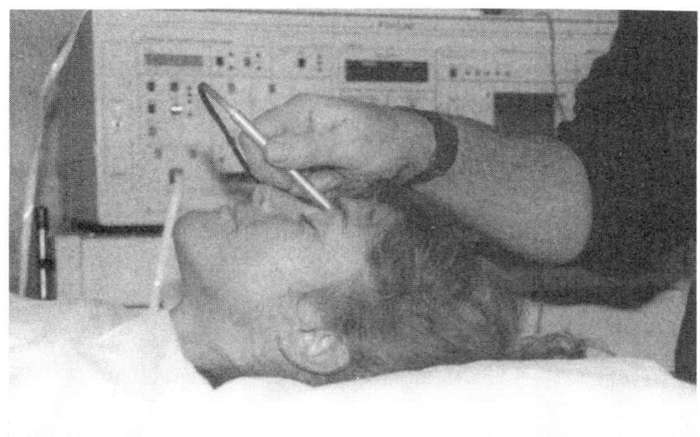

Fig. 6-26. The periorbital Doppler examination.

the internal carotid should be suspected. It is not possible, however, to distinguish between total and partial internal carotid artery occlusions. A more direct study, such as carotid artery duplex imaging, must be performed in an attempt to define the two conditions.

Pressure Oculoplethysmography

Prior to the advent of duplex imaging, *oculoplethysmography* (OPG) was considered the primary testing system for evaluation of the extracranial carotid artery disease in many of the vascular laboratories. Even today, many vascular laboratories still use this system. Historically, there have been two primary types of pneumoplethysmography: air (pneumoplethysmography) and water-filled OPG. Because the water-filled OPG currently is not considered an acceptable method of testing, only pneumoplethysmography will be discussed in this section.

Prior to the examination, a careful history should be taken, with particular attention to the eyes. Any patient with a history of retinal detachment, unstable glaucoma, recent eye surgery, lens implants, or conjunctivitis should be excluded from this examination.

Following a careful explanation of the procedure, the patient is placed in the supine position, and bilateral blood pressures obtained. The patient should be instructed to focus on a fixed point and avoid blinking. After placing a few drops of a topical anesthetic on the eyes, an eye cup is placed on the lateral sclera of each eye. The eye cups are held in place while a vacuum of either 300 or 500 mmHg is applied. The higher vacuum (500 mmHg) is reserved for hypertensive patients.

The vacuum essentially changes the shape of the eye globe, cutting off pressure to the ophthalmic artery. This results in a temporary loss of vision, which may sound brutal but is actually similar to the same effect of rubbing hard on your sleepy eyes in the morning. The patient may experience a temporary loss of vision, but it will return after a short time. By explaining this to the patient, one will avoid a sudden panic of this unexpected sensation.

After reaching the selected vacuum, the record switch is activated and the vacuum is automatically released in about 30 seconds. With the strip chart running at a relatively slow speed, the vascular specialist observes the return of the eye pulses, noting at what pressure they arrive. This, in a sense, is like taking a blood pressure of the ophthalmic artery. The vacuum in the eye cup cuts off flow to the ophthalmic artery, acting as a blood pressure cuff, and the return of the eye pulsations indicates the return of blood flow, just as your Doppler or stethoscope would.

Interpretation

Interpretation of this test is based on two primary criteria:

1. Pulse arrival time delay > 5 mmHg
2. Ophthalmic artery pressure below 0.66 mmHg

If the pulse arrival time of one eye, when compared with the other, is delayed by a gradient of more than 5 mmHg, that side is considered abnormal. Because the *ophthalmic artery pressure* is only 0.66 that of the brachial artery pressure, any drop below 0.66 suggests a hemodynamically significant stenosis of that ipsilateral (same side) internal carotid artery. As with the periorbital Doppler, however, differentiation between a hemodynamically significant lesion and a total occlusion is impossible (Fig. 6-27).

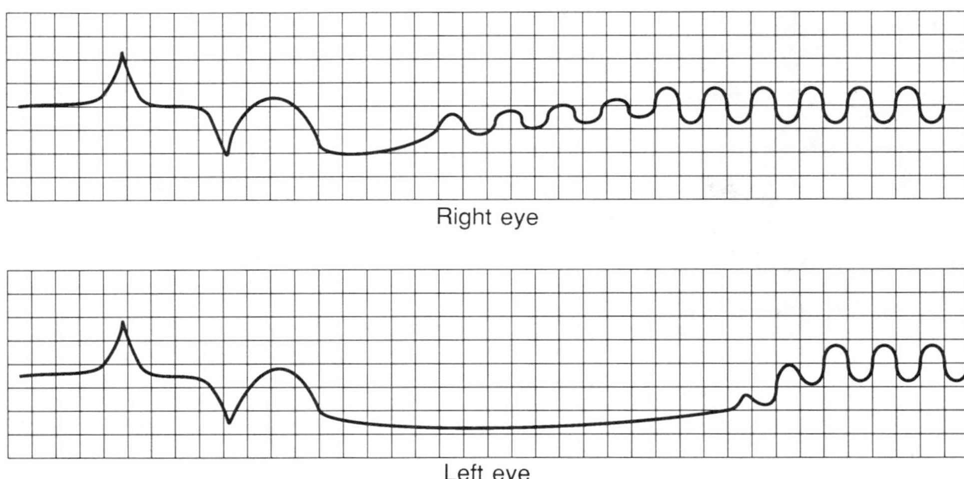

Fig. 6-27. These illustrations show delayed pulsations on the left eye when compared to the right side. This may indicate a hemodynamically significant lesion of the left internal carotid artery.

Direct Tests

Continuous Wave Doppler

Prior to the advent of OPGs and duplex imaging, continuous wave Doppler was one of the primary diagnostic tools available to the vascular specialist. The examiner's ear served as the primary spectral analyzer, and the identity of the vessel would be based on the audible signal received. In fact, many vascular specialists had developed such an astute ability to hear subtle changes in frequency shifts, their accuracy rivaled the results of the earlier duplex systems for hemodynamically significant disease.

An experienced vascular specialist using a CW Doppler alone could identify not only which vessel was being insonated but also the location and the level of disease in the carotid arteries. Their skill was based on knowledge of anatomy, flow physiology, and a keen auditory sense capable of detecting subtle frequency shifts.

You will recall from the section on physiology that the internal carotid artery primarily feeds the brain and the eyes. Because the brain, like the kidney, is so highly vascular, there is very little resistance to blood flow. That lack of resistance is reflected in a signal suggesting high diastolic flow. Therefore, the flow sounds like "whoooooooowhooooooowhoooo."

The external carotid artery primarily feeds the face and the scalp. This artery has several terminal branches, like the peripheral arteries in the legs, and flow is highly resistant. The blood flow runs into the terminal branches and bounces back a little, causing the blood to sound distinctly different from that of the external carotid artery. That signal sounds like "whitoooooowhitoooooooowhitoooooo."

When stenosis is present, the frequencies of the reflected signal are increased. The sound of that frequency shift is detected as a high pitched "SSSSSSSssssssSSSSSSSSssssssSSSSSSSSSs."

Obviously, despite the relative accuracy of the earlier Doppler pioneers of vascular technology, several drawbacks existed. Not being able to see the vessel being listened to made it too difficult to know where in the vessel you were evaluating. Angles and twists in the internal carotid artery caused increased frequency shifts that easily could be misinterpreted as stenosis. In addition, because CW Dopplers are not range-specific as are pulsed wave Dopplers, the zone one listened to often contained signals from the internal jugular or the transverse facial vein as well as the carotid artery. This mixture of signals made for some very frustrating examinations!

Waveforms

By adding spectral waveforms to the audible Doppler signal, the carotid artery examination is made more objective. The low-resistance signal of the internal carotid artery and the high-resistance signal of the external carotid artery can be identified and documented. Furthermore, the high-frequency shifts associated with hemodynamically significant disease can be evaluated by the interpreting physician.

By assuming a 60-degree angle, disease can be staged according to the maximum frequency shift and the presence of spectral broadening. The classification of ICA stenosis shown in Table 6-7 was made using a 5-MHz pulsed Doppler. As you will note, disease of less than 50% requires a subjective analysis of the amount of turbulence present. This may be difficult to discern because it requires exceptional skill on the part of the examiner to differentiate between minimal, moderate, and severe turbulence. It may be adequate to grade a disease without a peak systolic frequency shift of less than 4 kHz as less than 50% or nonhemodynamically significant.

Table 6-7. Classification of ICA Stenosis

Class	*Diameter Reduction (%)*	*Peak Systole (kHz)*	*End Diastole (kHz)*	*Spectral Broadening*
A	0	< 4	—	None
B	1–15	< 4	—	Minimal
C	16–49	< 4	—	Moderate
D	50–79	> 4	—	Severe
D+	80–99	> 4	> 4	Severe
E	100	NA	NA	No flow

NA = not applicable.

Cerebrovascular Duplex Imaging

The primary diagnostic equipment in most vascular laboratories is the duplex scanner. As mentioned earlier, *duplex* implies the combination of image for anatomic information and Doppler for physiologic information. The utilization of these two modalities, particularly in real time and with color Doppler imaging, makes the duplex system an extremely versatile and accurate noninvasive tool.

Duplex ultrasound has improved to such an extent in the past few years that it is often considered the *only* noninvasive study necessary for the screening of extracranial carotid artery disease. Although the technique for scanning the carotid vessels may vary from one vascular technology department to another, the fundamentals of the protocol remain the same. The following section describes a suggested scanning procedure.

Scan Protocol

After you explain the study, place the patient in the supine position in a warm quiet room. If necessary, provide the patient with a small pillow, although it is preferred that the patient's head not be elevated in order to avoid any bending of the neck. Sit at the head of the examining table, with the ultrasound system to one side or the other.

Gently lift the patient's chin up and turn his head away from the transducer. Using the appropriate amount of gel, begin the scan in the transverse plane, starting as low down in the neck as possible. Attempt, if possible, to identify the take-off of the common carotid artery from the right subclavian artery. On the left side, the common carotid artery originates from the arch, and it will be more difficult seeing the take-off. Document the presence or absence of disease, and then slowly begin scanning cephalad, or toward the head.

As you're scanning, identify your orientation and point out anatomic landmarks such as the thyroid (Fig. 6-28) and the jugular vein, as well as any disease that may be present in the common carotid artery. By videotaping the scan, you can provide the interpreting physician with an anatomical tour not only of what you are seeing but also by what you are hearing.

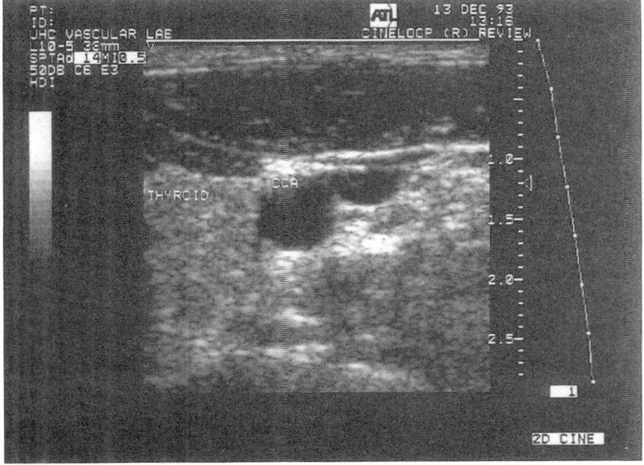

Fig. 6-28. Transverse scan showing thyroid to the left of the common carotid artery.

As you approach the carotid bifurcation (Fig. 6-29), pay particular attention to the vessel walls and the location of the internal and external carotid arteries. The internal carotid artery is usually larger, more lateral, and more posterior to the external carotid artery (Fig. 6-30). Repeat this imaging procedure in the sagittal view. If plaque is present, carefully document the location, surface characteristics, and plaque morphology. Surface characteristics of a plaque should be defined as either smooth or irregular, and plaque morphology as homogeneous or heterogeneous.

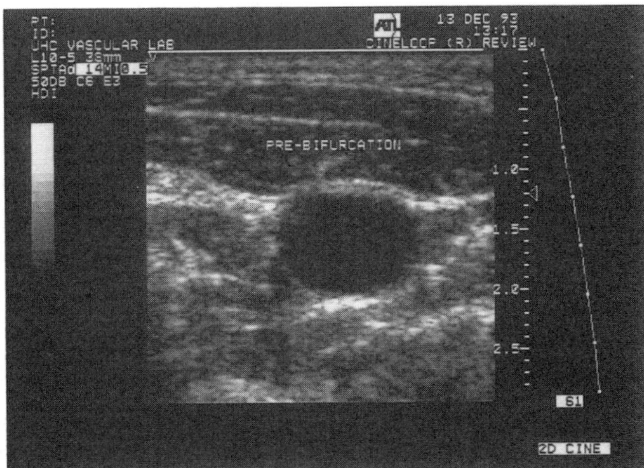

Fig. 6-29. The prebifurcation.

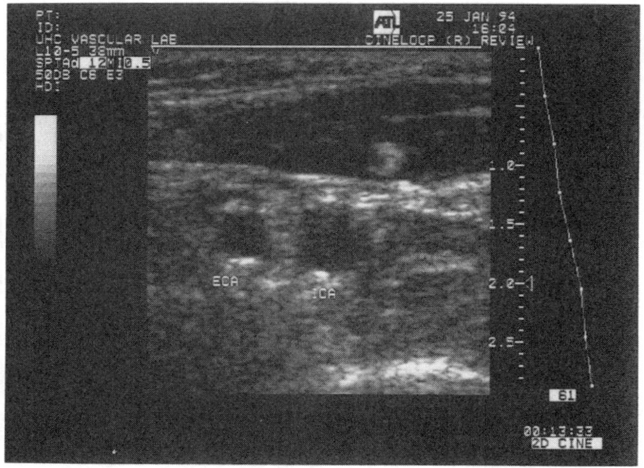

Fig. 6-30. The external carotid artery on the left (medial) and the internal carotid artery on the right (lateral).

Once you have completed the imaging in the transverse and sagittal planes, begin your Doppler evaluation in the sagittal plane low in the neck. Use color to highlight the vessel and identify any frequency shifts that may be a result of increased velocities. Ensure that the Doppler angle is 60 degrees or less and adjust your sample volume to about one third the vessel diameter. Listen and record on video the duplex examination from the proximal carotid to at least 3 cm beyond the origin of the internal carotid artery. Next, sample the external carotid artery and the vertebral artery and record on video.

Obtain all the necessary images and the *peak systolic* and *end diastolic* velocities of the

1. proximal common carotid arteries (Fig. 6-31)
2. distal common carotid arteries
3. proximal, mid, and distal internal carotid arteries (Fig. 6-32)
4. external carotid arteries (Fig. 6-33)
5. vertebral arteries

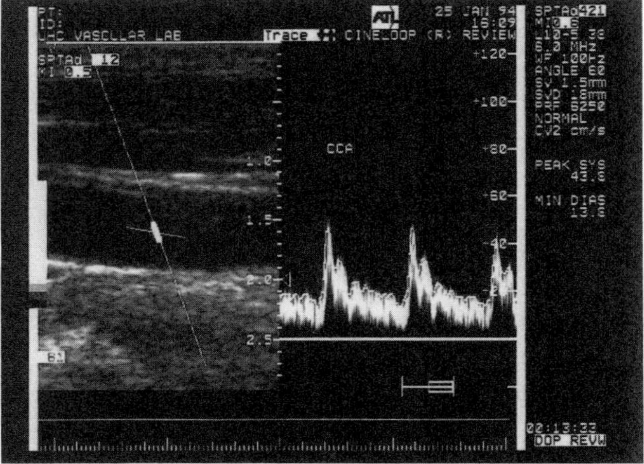

Fig. 6-31. Normal common carotid artery waveform.

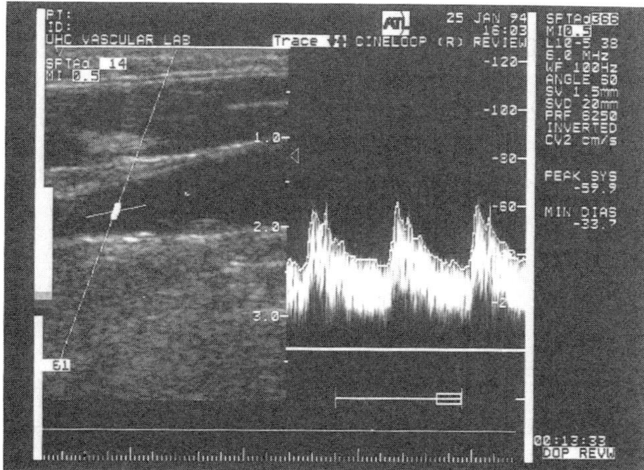

Fig. 6-32. Normal distal internal carotid artery waveform.

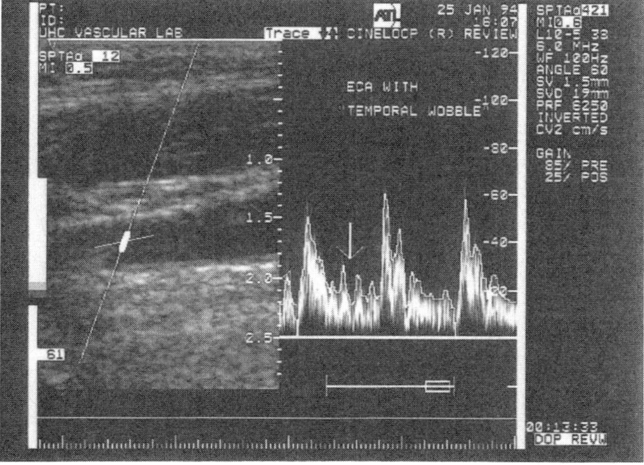

Fig. 6-33. Normal external carotid artery waveform. Note the temporal artery wobble obtained by gently tapping on the superficial temporal artery.

In addition, note any *spectral broadening*, particularly of the internal carotid artery. This will be graded as minimal, moderate, or severe.

Plaque Morphology and Surface Characteristics

The formulation of the data acquired by the vascular specialist is based on both imaging and Doppler information. First, in the presence of disease, the surface characteristics and plaque morphology must be defined:

Plaque Morphology	Surface Characteristics
Homogeneous	Smooth
Heterogeneous	Irregular

Don't be too rigid in the description, however. If you cannot adequately visualize the plaque due to calcific shadowing or other factors, say so. It is still considered professional to document the technical difficulty you may have encountered that might have resulted in a limited duplex examination.

Velocity Criteria

As carotid disease develops to a severe stage, the image becomes less reliable and the vascular specialist must rely almost totally on Doppler information. In addition, plaque isn't considered hemodynamically significant until it reaches a 50% diameter stenosis. At this point, velocities exceed the upper limits of normal in systole. Finally, it is important to understand how plaque in the internal carotid artery is affecting flow in relation to flow in the common carotid artery. In this way, we obtain a ratio that characterizes the differences of flow in these related vessels. Table 6-8 gives the diagnostic criteria for carotid artery disease.

Table 6-8. Evaluation of Internal Carotid Artery Disease

Class	*Diameter (%)*	*Peak*	*End*	*Flow Characteristics*
A	0	< 4 kHz < 125 cm/sec	—	No spectral broadening
B	1–15	< 4 kHz < 125 cm/sec	—	Minimal spectral broadening
C	16–49	< 4 kHz ≤ 125 cm/sec	—	Moderate spectral broadening
D	50–79	> 4 kHz > 125 cm/sec	—	Significant spectral broadening
D+	80–99	> 4 kHz > 125 cm/sec	> 4 kHz* > 140 cm/sec*	Severe spectral broadening
E	Total occlusion	NA	NA	No flow

Based on University of Washington, Seattle, WA, criteria.

*> 4 kHz, >140 cm end diastolic velocities are considered excessive by some laboratories. An end diastolic velocity of > 105 cm/sec may adequately meet the D+ (80–99%) stenosis criteria.

Velocity Ratios

Systolic Velocity		*Diastolic Velocity*	
(% Stenosis)	*(Ratio)*	*(% Stenosis)*	*(Ratio)*
Normal	< 2.0	Normal	< 2.0
50–79	2–4	50–79	2–4
> 80	> 4.0	> 80	> 5.6

NA = not applicable.

Transcranial Doppler

Transcranical Doppler is a noninvasive method to assess the intracranial vasculature introduced in 1982. The clinical indications for TCD are to

1. measure intracranial blood flow velocity
2. evaluate intracranial collateral blood flow
3. monitor hemodynamics during surgery
4. assess vasospasm in head trauma patients

Transcranial Doppler is performed by using either a 2-MHz pulsed Doppler stand-alone probe or a low-frequency (2 MHz) color duplex transducer. The intracranial vessels are insonated through "windows" via the temporal bone because of its relative thinness compared with the remainder of the skull. The major vessels of the circle of Willis that are accessible include the

1. middle cerebral artery
2. posterior cerebral artery
3. anterior cerebral artery
4. terminal internal carotid artery
5. Anterior and posterior communicating arteries (if they are functional)

Vertebral arteries and the basilar artery are insonated via the transforamenal approach at the base of the skull.

The limitations of transcranial Doppler vary by age, gender, and race. As many as 5%—10% of patients may have temporal bones too thick to allow adequate ultrasound penetration. Also, there are multiple anatomic variants that can make identifying "normal" anatomy difficult. In fact, only 50% of the normal (non-diseased) population has a complete circle of Willis.

Review Exercise

1. Stroke is the ______________ leading cause of death in the United States, resulting in more than 200,000 deaths a year.

2. The abnormal sound of blood flow heard in the carotid bifurcation with a stethoscope is called a

   a. bruit
   b. stenosis
   c. murmur
   d. hum

3. It is easy to distinguish a bruit from a transmitted heart murmur. True or False?

4. A transient ischemic attack is defined as a neurological symptom lasting

   a. less than 24 hours
   b. longer than 24 hours
   c. between 24 and 72 hours
   d. consistently

5. The ____________________________ artery is the first branch off the internal carotid artery.

6. An embolus traveling up the internal carotid artery may lodge in the ophthalmic artery, resulting in

   a. eye pain
   b. temporary blindness
   c. double vision
   d. total blindness of both eyes

7. Vertigo most likely suggests vascular insufficiency of the

   a. external carotid artery
   b. vertebral artery
   c. basilar artery
   d. both b and c

8. List four common risk factors of cerebrovascular disease.

   a. ____

   b. ____

   c. ____

   d. ____

9. The physical examination for the patient undergoing a cerebrovascular examination should include

   a. ____

   b. ____

10. In the case of significant internal carotid artery disease, the branches of the ______________________________ artery play an important role in supplying arterial blood flow to the brain.

11. The external carotid artery provides blood primarily to the __________ and the __________.

12. By placing a high-frequency CW Doppler on the periorbital vessels, the __________ and ____________________ of flow can be assessed.

13. List three contraindications to oculoplethysmography.

    a. ______________________________

    b. ______________________________

    c. ______________________________

14. OPG uses a vacuum of __________ mmHg in normotensive patients.

15. A patient having an oculoplethysmography may experience

    a. temporary loss of vision
    b. headache
    c. eye pain
    d. all of the above

16. Interpretation of OPG is based on two primary criteria:

    a. Pulse arrival time delay > __________ mmHg.
    b. Ophthalmic artery pressure below __________ mmHg.

17. The internal carotid artery primarily feeds the __________ and the __________.

18. The brain is so highly vascular, there is very little ____________________ to blood flow.

19. By adding spectral waveforms to the audible Doppler signal, the carotid artery examination is made more __________.

20. By assuming a __________-degree angle, disease can be staged according to the maximum frequency shift and the presence of spectral broadening.

21. Using a 5-MHz probe, a frequency shift over __________ is considered abnormal.

22. Surface characteristics of a plaque should be defined as either __________ or ____________________.

23. Plaque morphology of a plaque should be defined as ______________________________ or ______________________________.

24. Extracranial cerebrovascular peak systolic and end diastolic velocities should be obtained in

a. ______________________________

b. ______________________________

c. ______________________________

d. ______________________________

e. ______________________________

25. As carotid disease develops, the image becomes (less/more) reliable.

26. A plaque isn't considered hemodynamically significant until it reaches a ______________% diameter stenosis.

27. List the criteria for carotid artery disease.

Class	*Diameter*	*Peak*	*End*	*Flow Characteristics*
A	0%	< ___ kHz	—	______________________
		< ___ cm/sec		
B	1%–15%	< ___ kHz	—	______________________
		< ___ cm/sec		
C	16%–49%	< ___ kHz	—	______________________
		< ___ cm/sec		
D	50%–79%	> ___ kHz	—	______________________
		> ___ cm/sec		
D+	80%–99%	> ___ kHz	___ kHz	______________________
		> ___ cm/sec	___ cm/sec or ___ cm/sec	
E	Total occlusion	___	___	______________________

28. List the expected velocity ratios in the following disease categories.

Velocity Ratios			
Systolic Velocity		*Diastolic Velocity*	
% Stenosis	*Ratio*	*% Stenosis*	*Ratio*
Normal	____	Normal	____
50%–79%	____	50%–79%	____
> 80%	____	> 80%	____

29. Transcranial Doppler is performed by using a ______________ pulsed Doppler.

30. As many as ______________% to ______________% of patients may have temporal bones too thick to allow adequate ultrasound penetration for transcranial Doppler.

APPENDIX

A

Quality Assurance

Quality assurance in the vascular laboratory is an essential component of the routine activities of that department, and implies a constant attempt to ensure that testing, reporting, and equipment meet the standards necessary for maintaining the best possible results. To reach and maintain that standard, equipment and personnel must be brought up to a level of acceptable performance.

Previously, we discussed the value of statistics when evaluating the performance of testing procedures and vascular specialists. High levels of accuracy require that noninvasive testing correlate well with the "gold standard." It is also important, however, to ensure that information from the ultrasound, Doppler, or plethysmographic equipment is valid, that is, produced by equipment that is functioning properly. It is like the guitar player who tunes the guitar before playing it. By adjusting the tones of certain strings to match the gold standard of a tuning fork, the player can be assured that the chords played are clear and melodious. In addition, the player will be in harmony with other players in the band.

When we measure an aorta or a peak velocity Doppler signal of an internal carotid artery, we depend on the ultrasound system to display accurate measurements. A peak systolic velocity that suggests severe internal carotid artery disease had better be correct! Otherwise, a patient may receive an unnecessary arteriogram. Measuring an aortic diameter accurately is also critical. The stability or progression of an aneurysm is very important information to the vascular surgeon.

Ultrasound systems and Dopplers, therefore must be checked periodically to ensure that measurements obtained are precise when compared with a gold standard. Like the tones and notes of a musical instrument, the engineer adjusts the image quality, settings, and calculations of the vascular testing equipment. The primary areas of instrument performance that must be evaluated are

1. image quality
2. Doppler quality

IMAGE QUALITY

The primary method for evaluating ultrasound imaging performance is the American Institute for Ultrasound in Medicine (AIUM) test phantom (Fig. A-1). The test phantom is a device that looks like a small fish tank filled with a material that matches the acoustic impedance of soft tissue. Within this material is a series of pins and tubes placed at precise depths and distances away from each other. The ultrasound system is then used to detect these objects, and the measurements of either depth, diameter, or distance are compared with the known measurements of the phantom. In addition, the system's axial and special resolution can be evaluated by noting the system's ability to detect two separate pins placed very close to each other in an axial and lateral plane. Other testing parameters are also available with the AIUM test phantom.

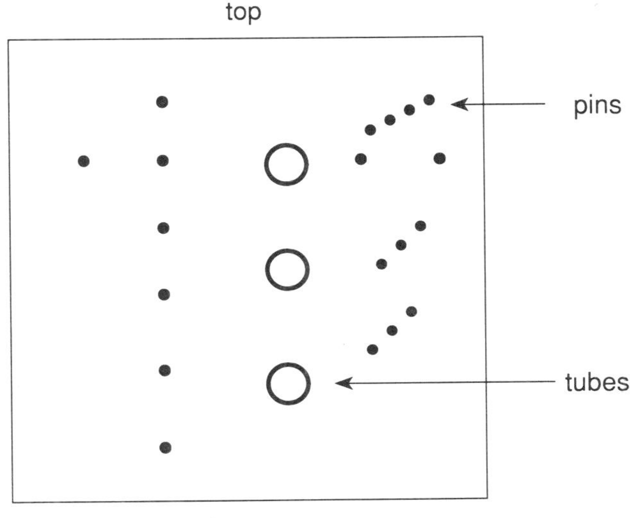

Fig. A-1. The AIUM test phantom. The phantom contains various pins and tubes at specific depths and distances from each other. Measurements of the test phantom, which is considered the gold standard, are compared with the ultrasound system to ensure accuracy of measurements.

DOPPLER QUALITY

Doppler velocity accuracy is evaluated with a string phantom. A string phantom looks like a small fish tank filled with water with a string running through a series of pulleys (Fig. A-2). The string is moved through the pulleys by an electric motor at a precise speed, which is controlled by a small computer chip. The Doppler transducer is placed in a clamp and aimed at the moving string. Velocity measurements are obtained on the system and compared with the known velocity of the moving string. Any variance of that velocity is corrected by a qualified engineer.

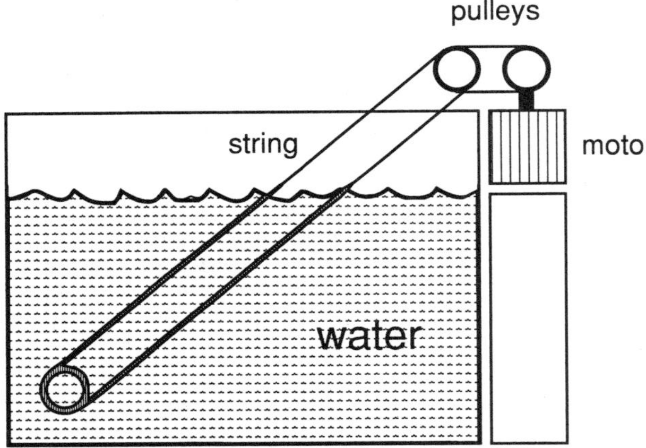

Fig. A-2. The string phantom is used to measure Doppler frequency/velocity accuracy. The transducer head is placed in the water at various angles and measures the speed of the moving string at various depths. Doppler measurements are then compared with the string phantom, which is considered the gold standard.

PREVENTATIVE MAINTENANCE

Your vascular testing equipment is a major financial investment, and like any investment, it is essential to care for your equipment by maintaining the system in good running condition. When you tune up your car and change the oil, your car doesn't necessarily run better or faster immediately after. You will notice after time has passed, however, that with consistent and regular maintenance, the car will have fewer breakdowns and retain its value.

Vascular testing equipment will also have less "down time" if the equipment receives regular preventative maintenance. Because most equipment manufacturers provide regularly scheduled maintenance visits, it's not necessary for the vascular specialist to perform these sophisticated tests. There are a few steps that may be taken on a regular basis, however, to protect your vascular testing equipment.

1. Regular inspection and cleaning of transducers, cuffs, and equipment
2. Proper storage of transducers, cuffs, cables, and gel
3. Routine cleaning of equipment air filters
4. Proper warm-up of the system before testing

ULTRASOUND SAFETY

Diagnostic ultrasound and vascular testing is termed *noninvasive*, which means safe and painless. This does *not* imply, however, that all ultrasound is completely safe. Some therapeutic ultrasound is so powerful that it dissolves kidney stones. Other therapeutic ultrasound is used to actually destroy tissue, such as tumors. Nevertheless, diagnostic ultrasound is, in general, safe. In fact, the AIUM has made the following statement:

> No confirmed biological effects on patients or instrument operators caused by exposure at intensities typical of present diagnostic ultrasound instruments have ever been reported.

The key to this statement is the phrase, "intensities typical of diagnostic ultrasound." In fact, the Food and Drug Administration sets specific limits on the amount of power and the intensities that can be used for specific diagnostic procedures. As long as the vascular specialist uses the preset levels that are most often programmed in the system, adverse biological effects can be avoided. Excessive ultrasound intensities may cause biological effects in the form of heating. In severe cases, they may even cause cavitation, which means to form a hollow space. This does not normally occur with diagnostic frequencies, however.

EXPRESSIONS OF INTENSITY

There are several different expressions of intensity used. The most common form is spacial peak time average (SPTA). SPTA measures the amount of ultrasound intensity at a specific site over a period of time. The acceptable level of SPTA measurements is dependent on

1. whether the probe is focused or unfocused
2. the specific application for which the probe will be used

In other words, focused ultrasound will produce higher levels of intensities than will unfocused probes, and intensities considered safe for the abdomen may not be safe for the eye. This rule of thumb for ultrasound safety is to

1. not exceed the reccmmended limits of ultrasound intensity
2. limit the amount of time a patient is exposed to ultrasound

Section Review

1. Quality assurance of image quality and measurements is best obtained on a ______________________.

2. Quality assurance of accurate Doppler velocity measurements is best obtained on a ______________________.

3. List four preventative maintenances that may be performed by the vascular specialist on noninvasive vascular testing equipment.

   a. ______________________

   b. ______________________

   c. ______________________

   d. ______________________

4. The most common expression used to express levels of ultrasound intensity is ______________________.

5. Unusually high levels of ultrasound intensities may cause

   a. ______________________

   b. ______________________

6. The two rules of thumb used in preventing biological hazards with ultrasound are

   a. ______________________

   b. ______________________

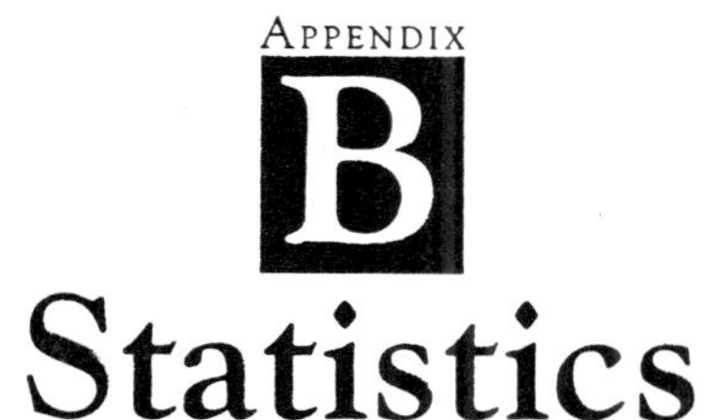

Statistics

Statistics concerns the gathering of facts. Facts are usually accumulated as numbers and presented to show certain information. For example, it is not scientific to simply say you have a "busy" laboratory or department unless you can back that up with the number of studies and how many vascular specialists are available to perform them. It is also not scientific to say that your laboratory or department has a "high rate of accuracy" unless that can be backed up with facts. How many cerebrovascular studies that your lab performed were proved right or wrong? How do you determine whether your studies were correct? What system is available to you to help determine the accuracy of your lab?

RELIABILITY

Reliability is the consistency of obtaining similar results in similar circumstances. A laboratory or ultrasound department is considered reliable when the results of tests produced are consistently correct when compared with the "gold standard." The current gold standard for vascular testing remains the arteriogram or venogram. However, surgical pathology may be the most accurate.

CHI SQUARE

The Chi square (pronounced "Kye," as in sky) is a statistical test that, in sum, compares the difference between what you expect and what you observe. For example, what you expect might be duplex finding of 50% to 79% stenosis of an internal carotid artery. What is observed would be an arteriogram that either agrees or disagrees with your findings.

The more tests you perform that agree with the gold standard, in this case the arteriogram, or the narrower the differences between the expected and the observed, the greater your accuracy. On the other hand, the more your studies disagree with the gold standard, the greater the difference between the expected and observed, and the poorer your accuracy.

The Chi square is designed as a box containing four letters (A through D) (Fig. B-1). Each letter represents results of the expected and of the observed findings. In this example, we will define "your test" as the noninvasive test, or what is expected. The "arteriogram" stands for the gold standard, or what is observed. There are four possible results that the vascular specialist can report:

Gold Standard (Arteriogram)

Your Tests (Duplex)		+	–
	+	**A**	**B**
	–	**C**	**D**

Fig. B-1. The Chi square.

1. **True Positive (A):** Both the noninvasive test and the arteriogram agree that the test was positive.
2. **False Positive (B):** The noninvasive test indicated the study was positive, but the arteriogram indicated it was negative.
3. **False Negative (C):** The noninvasive study showed the study was negative, but the arteriogram showed it was positive.
4. **True Negative (D):** Both the noninvasive study and the arteriogram agree that the study was negative.

ACCURACY

Accuracy is defined as the ability to give the right answer; that is, accuracy in finding disease when disease is present and not finding disease when there is no disease present (by the gold standard).

Accuracy is derived from the Chi square by the following formula:

$$\frac{\text{True Positives} + \text{True Negatives}}{\text{Total Number of Tests}} = \frac{A + D}{A + B + C + D}$$

SENSITIVITY

The ability to find disease when disease is present is called *sensitivity*. Sensitivity is derived from the Chi square by the following formula:

$$\frac{\text{True Positives}}{\text{True Positives} + \text{False Negatives}} = \frac{A}{A + C}$$

SPECIFICITY

Accuracy is also the ability to document a normal study when there is no disease found by arteriogram. This is called *specificity*. Specificity is derived from the Chi square by the following formula:

$$\frac{\text{True Negatives}}{\text{True Negatives} + \text{False Positives}} = \frac{D}{D + B}$$

POSITIVE PREDICTIVE VALUE

The Chi square also helps determine whether a test has the ability to predict that a population will likely have a positive study. The positive predictive value (PPV) is derived from the number of positive noninvasive tests found to be negative by the arteriogram. In other words, the more accurate the noninvasive study in finding disease when disease is present, the higher the PPV. The PPV is derived from the Chi square by the following formula:

$$\frac{\text{True Positives}}{\text{True Positives} + \text{False Positives}} = \frac{A}{A + B}$$

NEGATIVE PREDICTIVE VALUE

Conversely, the negative predictive value (NPV) is derived from the number of negative noninvasive tests that were found positive by the gold standard. The more accurate your tests in finding no disease when no disease is present by arteriogram, the higher your NPV. The NPV is derived from the Chi square by the following formula:

$$\frac{\text{True Negatives}}{\text{True Negatives} + \text{False Positives}} = \frac{D}{D + C}$$

Section Review

You want to document your lab's *accuracy* for detecting DVT. You have performed *100 duplex ultrasounds*; *venograms* have also been performed on these patients.

From your collected data, you said that of those 100 patients examined, 75 had a positive DVT study and 25 had a negative DVT study. However, the venogram report states that of the 75 patients you said had a positive study, 70 were positive and 5 were negative. Of the 25 patients you said did not have a DVT, 20 had a negative study and 5 had a positive study.

From this data, determine your

1. Accuracy ____________________
2. Sensitivity ____________________
3. Specificity ____________________
4. Positive predictive value ____________________
5. Negative predictive value ____________________

Index